Deafness and Mental Health

Deafness and Mental Health

Edited by

Laszlo K. Stein, Ph.D.
Director
David T. Siegel Institute for Communicative Disorders
Michael Reese Medical Center
Chicago, Illinois

Eugene D. Mindel, M.D.
Psychiatrist
David T. Siegel Institute for Communicative Disorders
Michael Reese Medical Center
Chicago, Illinois

Theresa Jabaley, M.A.
Assistant Director and Clinical Audiologist
David T. Siegel Institute for Communicative Disorders
Michael Reese Medical Center
Chicago, Illinois

Grune & Stratton
A Subsidiary of Harcourt Brace Jovanovich, Publishers
New York   London   Toronto   Sydney   San Francisco

Library of Congress Cataloging in Publication Data
Main entry under title:

Deafness and mental health.

Includes expanded and updated papers from the
First National Symposium on Mental Health Needs of
Deaf Adults and Children, held in Chicago in June
1975 and sponsored by the David T. Siegel Institute
of Michael Reese Hospital.
Includes bibliographies and index.
Contents: The deaf child: Studies of behavior
problems of deaf children / Kathryn P. Meadow.
Early identification and parent couseling / Laszlo
K. Stein, Theresa Jabaley. The parent-pro-
fessional / Jacqueline Z. Mendelsohn. Psychological
evaluation of the deaf and hard of hearing / [etc.]
1. Deaf—Mental health—Congresses. 2. Children,
Deaf—Mental health—Congresses. I. Stein,
Laszlo K. II. Mindel, Eugene D. III. Jabaley,
Theresa. IV. National Symposium on Mental Health
Needs of Deaf Adults and Children (1st: 1975:
Chicago, Ill.) [DNLM: 1. Deafness. 2. Mental
health. 3. Mental health services. WV 270 D277]
RC451.4D4D42   362.4'2   81-2853
ISBN 0-8089-1347-6   AACR2

Grune & Stratton, Inc.
111 Fifth Avenue
New York, New York 10003

Distributed in the United Kingdom by
Academic Press Inc. (London) Ltd.
24/28 Oval Road, London NW 1

Library of Congress Catalog Number 81-2853
International Standard Book Number 0-8089-1347-6

Printed in the United States of America

Contents

v

Preface

In the early 1950s the first systematic research aimed specifically at understanding the personal and intrafamily patterns of adjustment to deafness was initiated. These efforts, conducted by researchers and therapists in psychiatry, psychology, social work, sociology, and linguistics, sought to extend to deaf people mental health services heretofore denied them because of ignorance or neglect.

The research and clinical programs advanced in 1955 at the New York State Psychiatric Institute and Rockland Psychiatric Center were followed over the next decade by the formation of investigative teams and clinical services at the Psychosomatic and Psychiatric Institute, Michael Reese Hospital in Chicago, the St. Elizabeth's Hospital in Washington, D.C., and the Langley-Porter Neuropsychiatric Institute in San Francisco.

By 1974, a number of us who work in the area of deafness and mental health felt sufficient interest, knowledge, and clinical experience had been developed to warrant a formal exchange of information through a symposium, an edited book, or both. As a result, in June 1975, the David T. Siegel Institute of Michael Reese Hospital sponsored the First National Symposium on the Mental Health Needs of Deaf Adults and Children. Nearly 250 mental health workers, teachers, rehabilitation specialists, and advocates for deaf people met for three days in Chicago to listen and respond to presentations covering a wide range of treatment, language, and societal issues.

Our original intent was to publish the proceedings of the symposium in their entirety, but this proved impractical. Instead, we developed a publication concentrating on those topic areas and papers that generated the greatest interest among the symposium's faculty and participants. Whenever possible, we invited symposium faculty to be contributors, but, again, this did not always prove possible. In final form, this book combines expanded and updated versions of several papers presented at the symposium, along with papers covering subjects we felt would be of particular relevance both to experienced clinicians and to people recently attracted to the field.

The book is divided into three parts. Part I is devoted to the deaf child. In Chapter I, Meadow presents information that is of critical importance to anyone involved in planning, justifying, or implementing services for deaf children with emotional/behavioral problems. Next, because the future social, emotional, and educational growth of the deaf child is so intimately dependent on the nature of the early parent–child relationship, two chapters on this subject are included. One, by Stein and Jabaley, addresses the issue from a programmatic viewpoint; the other, by Mendelsohn, provides a more personal view by a counselor who also happens to be a parent of a deaf child. In Chapter 4, Vernon and Ottinger provide a guide for psychologists and teachers on the special nature of testing and evaluating the abilities of the deaf child or adult. In Chapters 5, 6, and 7, the issue of treatment is approached from three different perspectives by Litoff and Feldman, Mindel, and Lennan. These chapters serve to emphasize that vastly differing treatment plans may be needed to meet the unique needs of the deaf child—an obvious but often ignored point.

In Part II, four chapters are devoted to therapy approaches with the deaf adult. In Chapter 8, Altshuler and Abdullah concentrate on the deaf inpatient unit and the relationship between psychopharmacologic and interpersonal therapies. This topic is particularly timely in view of the growing concern over the wisdom of the extreme view against hospitalization that has prevailed over the past decade. Levin, in Chapter 9, brings a frankly psychoanalytic viewpoint to his work with deaf patients. This should not discourage those who may have limited background in traditional analytic theory. Many of Levin's points on patient–therapist relationships apply regardless of the psychotherapy employed. Many deaf adults enter into counseling through initial contact around vocational issues. In Chapter 10, Stewart combines academic and clinical experience with unique personal insights (due to his own deafness) in presenting a very personal account of the counseling process. That many people outside the professional mental health community perform important supportive functions is demonstrated in Chapter 11 by Walsh's observations as a minister working with the deaf.

Four chapters on what we chose to refer to as societal issues form the third and final section of the book. The issue of communication with the deaf patient—specifically the use of sign language by therapists—created lively and, at times, impassioned debate at the symposium. Stokoe and Battison, in Chapter 12, approach the question of the interrelatedness of deafness and mental health with language, particularly sign language, from the perspectives of an anthropologist and a linguist. Their view that a deaf person is not a hearing person with something lacking, but rather a person who has had to learn and develop different ways of functioning, is to them a crucial difference that hearing therapists should understand.

Noble moral intentions are often not enough to secure individual rights for the deaf. Legal recourse may be necessary before equal and appropriate social, educational, and psychiatric services can be provided. In Chapter 13, DuBow and Goldberg, attorneys who have advocated the legal rights of deaf people, provide examples of how the law can be used to help in instances where the needs of deaf people have been ignored.

Vernon and Harris, both psychologists, have distinguished themselves in advocating the rights and self-determination of deaf people. The significance of work for deaf people and the need for job training opportunities, vocational rehabilitation, and career guidance as they relate to mental well-being, are convincingly described by Vernon in Chapter 14. Harris, in Chapter 15, advocates that the deaf community must assume a stronger activist role in determining its future. Harris, like Stewart, is deaf. His perspectives for the 1980s may well serve as the scale by which we measure how well all of us, both deaf and hearing, achieve our goals in providing mental health services for deaf people.

Our attempt has been to bring together a series of papers that include information we feel is basic to anyone who has or plans to have any extended contact with deaf people—be that in the role of therapist, rehabilitation counselor, teacher, or friend. We have included papers that are original and innovative but that always maintain a practical clinical orientation.

Laszlo K. Stein, Ph.D.
Senior Editor

Contributors

Syed Abdullah, M.D.
Chief, In-Patient Unit
Rockland Psychiatric Center
New York State Department of Mental Hygiene
New York, New York

Kenneth Altshuler, M.D.
Chairman, Department of Psychiatry
University of Texas Health Science Center
Dallas, Texas

Robbin M. Battison, Ph.D.
Associate Research Scientist
American Institute for Research
Washington, D.C.

Sy DuBow, J.D.
Legal Director
National Center for Law and the Deaf
Washington, D.C.

Valerie J. Feldman, M.Ed.
Child Development Specialist
David T. Siegel Institute for Communicative Disorders
Michael Reese Medical Center
Chicago, Illinois

Larry J. Goldberg, J.D.
Clinical Lawyer Supervisor
National Center for Law and the Deaf
Washington, D.C.

Robert I. Harris, Ph.D.
Senior Clinical Psychologist
Director of Research and Training
Mental Health and Hearing-Impaired Program
St. Paul-Ramsey Medical Center
Assistant Professor of Psychiatry
University of Minnesota
St. Paul, Minnesota

Theresa Jabaley, M.A.
Assistant Director and Clinical Audiologist
David T. Siegel Institute for Communicative Disorders
Michael Reese Medical Center
Chicago, Illinois

Robert K. Lennan, Ed.D.
Assistant Superintendent, California School for the Deaf
Riverside, California

Fred M. Levin, M.D.
Psychiatrist, David T. Siegel Institute for Communicative Disorders
Michael Reese Medical Center
Chicago, Illinois

Susan Goldstein Litoff, M.A.
Psychotherapist, Coordinator of Child and Adolescent Services, MENDAC
David T. Siegel Institute for Communicative Disorders
Michael Reese Medical Center
Chicago, Illinois

Kathryn P. Meadow, Ph.D.
Director, Child Development Research Unit
Educational Research Laboratory
Gallaudet College Research Institute
Washington, D.C.

Jacqueline Z. Mendelsohn
Executive Director
International Association of Parents of the Deaf, Inc.
Silver Spring, Maryland

Eugene D. Mindel, M.D.
Psychiatrist
David T. Siegel Institute for Communicative Disorders
Michael Reese Medical Center
Chicago, Illinois

Paula Ottinger, M.A.
Assistant Coordinator
Teacher Training Program
Education of the Deaf
Western Maryland College
Westminster, Maryland

Laszlo K. Stein, Ph.D.
Director
David T. Siegel Institute for Communicative Disorders
Michael Reese Medical Center
Chicago, Illinois

Larry G. Stewart, Ed.D
Clinical Director and Psychologist
Community Mental Health Services for the Deaf
Santa Ana, California

William C. Stokoe, Ph.D.
Department of Linguistics
Gallaudet College
Washington, D.C.

McCay Vernon, Ph.D.
Professor of Psychology
Western Maryland College
Westminster, Maryland

David Walsh, C.Ss.R.
Chancery Office
Corpus Christi, Texas

PART I

The Deaf Child

Kathryn P. Meadow, Ph.D.

1

Studies of Behavior Problems of Deaf Children*

This chapter reviews existing studies on the prevalence and type of behavioral problems in deaf children. There are many definitional complexities inherent in any effort to estimate or to specify the extent to which any population group is subject to emotional or behavioral disturbances. Thus, before reviewing the studies that have been attempted with groups of deaf children, it is important to discuss some of the relevant issues.

The diagnosis, the description, the label, or the definition applied to a behavioral problem is influenced greatly by the particular professional discipline of the ascribing person. For example, a child may be called ''mentally ill'' by a psychiatrist, ''emotionally disturbed'' by a psychologist, or ''behavior disordered'' by a special educator (Hobbs, 1975, p. 57). That same child may be seen by a sociologist to be stigmatized and handicapped further by the labels used by helping professionals. Each diagnostic term implies an asumption about the cause of the problem, the kind of treatment to be employed, and the prognosis for improvement. For example, ''mental illness'' is a term more likely to be applied by medical professionals, who are also more likely to prescribe drugs for the treatment of the difficulty.

The process of identifying, classifying, or labeling the aberrant behavior of both children and adults has long been recognized as having important implications for future treatment and potential cure. The American Psychiatric Association has published successive revisions of its *Diagnostic and Statistical Manual* in a con-

*This chapter appeared in a different form in *Deafness and Child Development*, published by the University of California Press, 1980, and was prepared while the author was affiliated with the University of California, San Francisco, with partial support from Maternal and Child Health (Grant No. MC-R-060160) and from the Office of Education (Grant No. OEG-0-1441).

tinuing effort to evolve a system that is acceptable and useful to its members. The World Health Organization and the Group for Advancement of Psychiatry both have appointed committees to develop classifications. A useful review of the existing classification systems of emotional disorders in children has been written by Prugh, Engel, and Morse (1975). A study of the definitions and rates of prevalence for a wide variety of handicapping conditions was undertaken and recently published as a two-volume study. Classification of the various conditions was considered to be so important that the set was entitled *The Futures of Children* (Hobbs, 1975). Table 1-1 which was extracted from that study, illustrates some of the handicapping conditions of children, gives approximate numbers of children with each condition, and considers the importance of definition in the development of the estimates. Table 1-1 shows that there are 1,400,000 children in the United States who are in need of psychiatric care, according to the figures of the Joint Commission on Mental Health. Of these children, 100,000 are receiving treatment in residential centers; over 500,000 are receiving special education because of their emotional or behavioral problems. Hobbs (1975, p. 58) points out that emotional disturbance is most difficult to diagnose in its mild and moderate forms. While professionals and lay persons alike may agree on the identification of a seriously disturbed child, there will still be a considerable difference of opinion on what the condition should be called.

DANGERS OF CLASSIFICATION

Diagnostic labeling is most often the target for criticism by those concerned with the rights of children (and of adults, too, for that matter). Even though there is much diagreement among professionals about the specific meaning of particular diagnostic categories, once a diagnosis has been assigned, it usually remains in the files or records that follow a child from one school or treatment center to another. Thus, there are dangers in attaching diagnostic labels to children.

These dangers are greater when the problems are mild or moderate because the behavior may represent short-term responses to current stresses. If the child's situation at home or at school improves, the problematic behavior may also improve. However, if a label has been assigned, the label itself can influence the reactions of others to the child, thus reinforcing unacceptable behavior.

Another danger inherent in classifying aberrant behavior is that it encourages a static view that actually may be more related to differential rates of development or maturity. The traditional approach to the classification of childhood mental disorders was derived from and is tied to the classification of adult disorders. This means that professionals may be tempted to view the child as a miniature adult, thereby ignoring developmental patterns that reflect maturational lags. Labeling may also encourage the idea that disturbance in childhood leads inevitably to disturbance in adulthood, although this is not the case (Phillips, Draguns, & Bartlett, 1975, p. 40).

Table 1-1

Prevalence of Handicapping Conditions Among Children in United States

Condition	Definition	Source	Number
Mental retardation	Significantly subaverage intellectual functioning (below 70 IQ) Ages 0–19	Bureau for the Education of the Handicapped	1,700,000
	Served in special school programs		875,000
Emotional disturbance	Need psychiatric care Ages 0–18	Joint Commission on Mental Health	1,400,000
	In residential mental health treatment centers	Joint Commission on Mental Health	100,000
	Special educational provisions	U.S. Office of Education	556,000
Economic disadvantage	Lacking money for minimum basic needs up to $4275/yr nonfarm family of four up to $5044/yr nonfarm family of five	Joint Commission on Mental Health	10,500,000
Visual impairments	Visually impaired or partially seeing	Bureau for the Education of the Handicapped	70,000
	Served in special education programs	Bureau for the Education of the Handicapped	24,000
Hearing impairments	Deaf Hard-of-hearing Served in special programs	Bureau for the Education of the Handicapped	52,000 350,000 80,000
Speech and language disorders	Speech-impaired Special programs	Bureau for the Education of the Handicapped	2,440,000 1,360,000

Information extracted from Hobbs, 1975.

THE NEED FOR CLASSIFICATION OF CHILDREN

While there are inherent dangers for children in labeling and/or classifying their behavior as problematic, handicapped, abnormal, deviant, or exceptional, there are some positive reasons for classifying. If services are to be provided to children who need them, it is necessary to know who and how many children need services, what kinds of problems they have, and what kinds of special treatment are needed. Teachers and school administrators, who have the most direct contact with the children and are most familiar with their special problems, can knowledgeably inform legislators and administrators of state and federal agencies about the kinds of attention needed by these special children.

The people who are most often concerned with the classification of aberrant behavior in children are those whose motivation is grounded in an ideology of help and service rather than of punishment (Rains et al., 1975, p. 90). This is in contrast to other classifications of persons who are seen as deviant; for example, the vagrant or the drug addict. In both instances, however, it is often the interests of the persons who do the classifying that are served by inflating estimates of exceptional children needing services or of deviant adults requiring punishment. A system of checks and balances is needed to insure that judgment of the diagnosticians is not swayed by self-interest in the eventual provision of services or correctional systems.

One frequent criticism of classifying or labeling those who are ''different'' is that attaching the label can be the first step in confining an individual to an institution. Once officially designated by a label that implies unmanageability in the community, a person is channeled to a setting where behavior *can* be managed; for the criminal, the jail; for the mentally ill, a state mental hospital. A proper and humane concern for the rights of individuals, therefore, can center on the eventual, perhaps unintended, result of the overly facile application of a label.

EXCLUSION AS A RESULT OF LABELING

A possible and unintended consequence of assigning a label to an individual is the reduction in the numbers of alternatives for special services. This can happen to a young child—and especially to a young deaf child—who is diagnosed as ''emotionally disturbed.'' The application of this label may become the rationale for exclusion from school, the most significant institution outside of the family. Once a deaf child has been labeled emotionally disturbed and thus excluded from school, the burden for future care becomes the exclusive concern of the family. The deaf emotionally disturbed child becomes so special, so deviant, so exceptional that he or she fits into no existing program. There are very few alternatives for this child. Parents often are forced to spend extra time begging administrators for educational opportunities that should have been guaranteed. All exceptional children with special needs have a difficult time getting equal opportunity. Sadly, most new programs for handicapped children develop as a result of pressure exerted by parents rather than from actions by professionals, administrators, or legislators. Deaf children with emotional problems fall somewhere between, rather than into, most established educational programs. They are excluded from programs for deaf children because of their aberrant behavior. They are excluded from programs for emotionally disturbed children because of their deafness. The rationale for their exclusion from both kinds of programs may stem from a complex mixture of objective and subjective, rational and irrational, factors. Specialists in the education of the deaf may be frightened of bizarre behavior, and unable to accept a child who is different. Specialists in the education of emotionally disturbed children (or in mental health treatment, for that matter) simply may be frightened of deafness. A major tool in the treatment of emotional disturbance is effective communication.

A child who is unable to communicate because of a handicap represents a dual threat to a professional whose skills depend on language. Also, it is unreasonable to expect a teacher to absorb a child with special needs into a group that already makes unusual demands on energy and skill.

The paradox in labeling is that if a child is not defined as "extra special," he or she has no chance to receive the extra special services needed. However, if the child *is* defined as "extra special," some existing resources may be removed. Often, the only viable answer to this double bind evolves from the creative application of definitions by administrators who combine expertise with compassion.

CLASSIFICATION OF CHILDREN BY TEACHERS AND PARENTS

Teachers are more likely to label the child who is active, impulsive, and aggressive as emotionally disturbed than the child who is shy, withdrawn, and uncommunicative. Our culture values and encourages children who are quiet, polite, and easy to manage. If a child says nothing and bothers no one, he or she may be considered to have model behavior. Noisy exuberance, more prevalent in boys than in girls, may result in more boys being diagnosed as disturbed.

The kinds of behavior labeled as disturbed may also be related to the specific preferences of individual teachers. Teachers' preferences for students are related to temperament to some extent, in the same way that mothers' temperaments influence their abilities to relate to their infants. An active, responsive infant may fulfill the expectations of one mother, while another mother could find the same infant unmanageable. Although such factors must be considered in discussing behavioral classifications of children, the fact remains that both teachers and parents make judgments of children's behavior that agree with those made by mental health professionals (Berlin, 1967; Bower, 1958).

Children's behavioral disorders are more likely to be defined in terms of social relationships rather than in terms of intrapsychic pathology. Thus, the perception of the "deviant child" almost always occurs in a context of adult expectations for acceptable patterns of behavior. These expectations may be idiosyncratic to a particular adult, and may reflect a judgmental evaluation of a child's behavior that might not be considered justified by everyone (Phillips, Draguns, & Bartlett, 1975, p. 41).

STUDIES OF THE PREVALENCE OF BEHAVIOR PROBLEMS IN DEAF CHILDREN

In reviewing prevalence studies of behavior problems in deaf children, it is essential to know both the definitions of problematic behavior that are used, and the identities of those making the assessments. No attempt has been made to ascertain the numbers of hearing-impaired children who are institutionalized because of mental illness, nor even to count those deaf children who are assigned to special educational classes because of serious emotional or behavioral problems. The absence of these data reflects the relative lack of interest in, knowledge about, and provisions for deaf emotionally disturbed children. It is generally agreed that there are many children who could legitimately be classified in this way (Schein, 1975). Most of the cited studies have been conducted on children who are enrolled in schools for the deaf. Thus, those children who have been excluded from schools precisely because they are emotionally disturbed would not be included in the studies. In fact, Schein (1975, p. 96) reported that in one suburban county, his group found that nearly 10 percent of school-age deaf children were not enrolled in educational programs because they had emotional or behavioral problems too severe to be managed in existing classrooms. Vernon (1969, p. 71) reported that 9 percent of students enrolled in the school that he studied were later excluded because of severe emotional problems. These two sources would indicate that the prevalence studies to be discussed probably show rates that are below the true prevalence rate of behavioral problems in deaf children.

Table 1-2 summarizes five sources of data yielding estimates of the prevalence of behavioral problems in deaf children. These studies indicate rates of behavioral disturbance ranging from about 9 percent to more than 22 percent. A review of the individual studies illustrates a number of problems related to (1) the base population surveyed; (2) definitions and methods of assessing problematic behavior, and (3) the identity of the person who makes the determination about any particular child.

Annual Survey of Hearing-Impaired Children and Youth

Each year since 1968–1969, the Office of Demographic Studies at Gallaudet College has conducted a survey of all schools and some classes in the United States offering special educational programs for deaf students. Each year, survey forms have been mailed to participating programs, with requests for information about each of the enrolled children. These survey forms have included items for listing handicaps in addition to deafness; emotional and/or behavioral problems are additional categories that have appeared each year. In 1968–1969, 12.4 percent of deaf students surveyed were considered to have emotional and/or behavioral problems. In 1969–1970, this rate was 12.9 percent; in 1970–1971, the rate was 9.6 percent; and in 1971–1972 it was 9.2 percent (Gentile & McCarthy, 1973).

It will be noted from Table 1-2 that the numbers of children on which these rates are based vary from slightly more than 21,000 in the first survey year to almost 34,800 in the 1970–1971 school year. Thus, we are immediately confronted with a major difficulty in estimating the prevalence of any condition in a particular subgroup of a population: contacting all members of that population on which to base the ''count'' of those with a specific characteristic.

The Bureau for the Education of the Handicapped has estimated that in the United States there are 52,000 deaf children and 350,000 hearing-impaired children

Table 1-2
Summary of Prevalence Studies: Emotional and Behavioral Problems of Deaf Children

Source	Population	Definition	Identity of Rater/ Diagnostician	Prevalence Rate (%)
Gentile & McCarthy, 1973	Hearing-impaired children in school programs (annual survey) 1968–1969 (N = 21,130) 1969–1970 (N = 29,131) 1970–1971 N = 34,795) 1971–1972 (N = 33,711)	Emotional and behavioral problems Emotional or behavioral problems	Doctors, psychologists, teachers, others	12.4 12.9 9.6 9.2
Schlesinger & Meadow, 1972	Children enrolled in one state residential school for the deaf (N = 516)	Severely emotionally disturbed Requires disproportionate share of time	Teachers and dormitory counselors	11.6 19.6
Vernon, 1969	Children enrolled in one state residential school for the deaf with known etiology for hearing loss (N = 358)	Poor emotional adjustment on 5-point rating scale	Teachers	20.7
Graham & Rutter, 1968	All deaf children ages 10–11 living on Isle of Wight (N = 13)	Psychiatric disorders. Battery of ratings, tests, interviews, and observations	Parents, teachers psychiatrists	15.4
Freeman, Malkin, & Hastings, 1975	All deaf children living in Greater Vancouver, British Columbia (N = 120)	Moderate or severe psychiatric disorder. Global ratings	Parents and teachers	22.6

up to 19-years-old, of whom 80,000 are being served in special educational programs (Hobbs, 1975). Thus, the prevalence rates for behavioral problems are based on a population considerably smaller than the universe of deaf school children. This situation is not unusual for large-scale surveys. When the numbers involved are as large as these, it is possible that a considerable increase in the population base (that is, in the *denominator* of the fraction reflected as "prevalence rate") will result in a change of only a few tenths of a percent. If the children who are excluded from the survey do not differ in those characteristics that are of particular interest here, the rate may not be changed significantly. However, in the case of deaf children with emotional or behavioral problems, it is clear that those who have the most severe problems are precisely those who are not included in the survey, for the simple reason that they are excluded from school programs.

Participation in the survey is voluntary. As it has become more well established, administrators are probably becoming more convinced of the value of the reports that are based on the data and are therefore more willing to participate. Procedures for contacting and processing the data are becoming more highly organized. Differences in the procedure for collecting information on emotional and behavioral problems are reflected in the prevalence rates reported for the years 1968–1969 and 1969–1970, and those reported for the years 1970–1971 and 1971–1972. The rates for the first 2 years are 12.4 percent and 12.9 percent, respectively, while the rates drop for the last 2 years to 9.6 percent and 9.2 percent (Gentile & McCarthy, 1973).

During the first 2 years of the survey, emotional problems and behavioral problems were entered on the report form as separate categories. Some children were classified under both headings and thus were included twice in the combined rate computed for those years. Schein (1975, p. 93) reported that when duplication in the two similar categories was eliminated, the rate of emotional and/or behavioral disturbances among all hearing-impaired students reported in the survey was 10.6 percent. The Office of Demographic Studies combined the categories on the report form beginning in 1970–1971. This is probably the reason for the apparent decline in the rate of emotional/behavioral problems (Gentile & McCarthy, 1973, p. 4).

Included in the survey form are spaces for specifying the person making the diagnosis of additional handicaps. In 1971–1972, the children with emotional and behavioral problems were identified by medical doctors (17.3 percent), by psychologists (31.4 percent), by teachers (36.0 percent), or by others (15.4 percent). Medical doctors and psychologists classified about 20 percent of the children as severely handicapped by their behavioral problems. Teachers placed about 13 percent of the children in the severe category. There is no way of knowing whether these discrepancies were a function of differences in the children assigned to the various professional groups for classification, or whether they reflect differences in definitions of problem behavior.

Studies Conducted at State Residential
Schools for Deaf Students

Two of the studies of deaf children from which prevalence rates for behavioral problems can be computed were conducted at state residential schools for the deaf (Vernon, 1969; Schlesinger & Meadow, 1972). Vernon's study focused on the relationship between causes of deafness and prevalence of additional handicaps as related to measures of the functional abilities of deaf children. The study reported by Schlesinger and Meadow (1972) was designed specifically to provide an estimate of the prevalence of behavioral disorders in students at a particular residential school, for the purpose of identifying mental health needs.

Both of these studies are subject to the advantages and the limitations imposed by the selective nature of the population of deaf children enrolled in state residential schools. One advantage is that there is a fairly large population base on which prevalence rates can be computed. Vernon used school records pertaining to all children who were admitted or who were given preadmission evaluations by school personnel from 1953 to 1964 ($N = 1468$). This enabled him to select the 358 children whose deafness was caused by one of the following conditions: maternal rubella, meningitis, prematurity, complications from Rh factor, or heredity. The school enrollment in the Schlesinger and Meadow study was 516.

Some characteristics of residential schools may lead to overestimates of the prevalence of behavioral problems in deaf students, while others may lead to underestimates. The fact that these schools are public schools means that they are less selective in their enrollment criteria than are most private schools. In spite of the mandate to provide educational services for all, public schools still exclude children whose physical or emotional problems are extreme or whose intellectual potential makes the educational program inappropriate for them. The state residential schools, compared to the day schools and classes, may serve a disproportionate number of children from rural areas. Residential schools probably have more deaf children whose parents are deaf than do other kinds of schools; they may also have a disproportionate number of children from unstable families or broken homes. (This is because residential school placement may be viewed more positively by single parents who have the entire financial and emotional responsibility of caring for a handicapped child in addition to the entire financial and emotional responsibility of caring for a family.) All of these factors might influence the prevalence rate for behavioral problems. The point to be made here is that any time rates are reported based on a single school population, or on a population with a known selective bias, the data must be interpreted with caution.

The two studies conducted in residential schools used teachers as evaluators of students' behavior. The Schlesinger and Meadow study utilized dormitory counselors in addition to teachers. Vernon used school records in addition to teachers' ratings of students' behavior, and also administered psychological tests.

THE SCHLESINGER AND MEADOW SURVEY

The Schlesinger and Meadow survey was designed specifically for the purpose of identifying those children at a state residential school who were considered by their teachers or dormitory counselors to be severely emotionally disturbed and in need of psychiatric treatment. This particular definition was selected because the survey was to be used as one basis for defining the extent of the need for mental health services and a justification for a request for funding these services. The survey form that was utilized gave school personnel two choices: either they could identify problem children as severely disturbed and in need of psychiatric help, or they could identify children as not severely disturbed, but needing a disproportionate share of the teacher's time or requiring other special attention. There were two reasons for this choice: (1) they believed that by giving an option for identifying less severely disturbed children, they could place more confidence in the more severely disturbed ratings; and (2) this same format had been used previously in a mental health survey conducted in Los Angeles county and therefore provided a comparative base for the survey at the school for deaf children. Teachers and counselors were not asked to attach specific behaviors to individual children. However, the survey forms included some suggestions about the kinds of behaviors that might lead school personnel to identify a child as needing treatment or disproportionate care: withdrawal from peers; overdependency; hyperactivity; nervous habits such as tics; truancy; accident-proneness; chronic illnesses without identifiable physical causes; and marked aggressive behavior.

Of the 516 students in the school, 11.6 percent were considered to be severely disturbed and in need of psychiatric treatment. An additional 19.6 percent were considered to have behavioral problems leading to disproportionate demands on teachers' and counselors' time. Compared to these figures, 2.4 percent of students in Los Angeles county were identified as severely disturbed and an additional 7.3 percent were identified as needing disproportionate time from teachers in the classroom. Thus, the survey at the school for the deaf showed a prevalence of behavioral problems 3–5 times greater than the rate for children in the Los Angeles county school system.

THE VERNON STUDY

Vernon studied the relationship between etiology of deafness and the nature of secondary disabilities in children who attended or who received evaluations by a state residential school for the deaf from 1953 to 1964. Since this study included assessments of the psychological adjustment of some of the children, it is possible to utilize Vernon's findings in our effort to survey prevalence of behavioral problems. Most of Vernon's data are based on children for whom there was firm evidence that their deafness resulted from one of the following causes: heredity, Rh factor, prematurity, meningitis, or maternal rubella. Thus, he eliminated all children whose deafness was caused by other factors (32 percent of the total school population of 1468) or by unknown factors (30 percent of the total). The large numbers of the total school population not covered in Vernon's measures of psychological adjustment make his study less useful for present purposes than it would be if the total population had been assessed. However, it can be noted here that when Meadow and Schlesinger tabulated cause of deafness and prevalence of behavioral problems, those children with ''unknown'' etiologies were significantly more likely to be rated as emotionally disturbed (Schlesinger & Meadow, 1972, p. 161). This suggests that Vernon's figures may reflect minimum rather than maximum estimates of behavioral problems.

Vernon used three basic approaches to measure the psychological adjustment of the children in his study: (1) Teachers were asked to rate the child's adjustment as superior, above average, average, below average, or poor; (2) school records were tabulated in order to determine the numbers of children who were dismissed from school because of emotional disturbance; and (3) psychological evaluations performed at the time pupils were admitted to school were categorized as reflecting "normal adjustment" or "severe problems which profoundly jeopardize . . . ability to function adequately in the school setting." The proportion of children considered by teachers to demonstrate poor psychological adjustment (20.7 percent) was very close to the proportion of students whose psychological test evaluations indicated that they were emotionally disturbed (22.5 percent). There was considerable variation in the proportion of the various etiologic groups rated as disturbed. According to the teachers' ratings, these proportions range from a low of 10 percent for the group with hereditary deafness to a high of 31 percent for children whose deafness resulted from maternal rubella (Vernon, 1961, p. 70). Nine percent of the children whose records were evaluated had been dismissed from school because of severe emotional disturbance (p. 71). This figure is very close to the one reported by Schein (1975), whose staff found that 10 percent of the deaf children in one county were not attending school because of the severity of their behavioral problems.

British and Canadian Studies

The last two studies to be discussed in detail were both conducted outside of the United States: one was done as part of a larger study of the education, health, and behavior of school-age children living on the Isle of Wight; the other was concerned specifically with deaf children living in the Greater Vancouver area, British Columbia.

DEAF CHILDREN ON THE ISLE OF WIGHT

The Isle of Wight, an island located 4 miles off the coast of England, was selected for a comprehensive study of handicapping conditions of all children living there (Rutter, Tizard, & Whitmore, 1970). This is an extremely important study for those interested in any aspect of physical, intellectual, or emotional deficiencies in children because of the completeness of the survey, and because of the care with which the research was conducted. A series of surveys was carried out in 1964 and 1965, examining the relationship between various kinds of handicapping conditions, with elaborate case-finding and testing techniques developed to investigate each of several questions. Since this chapter concerns the prevalence of behavioral or psychiatric disorders in deaf children, consideration will be limited to a paper reporting the findings on organic brain dysfunction and child psychiatric disorders (Graham & Rutter, 1968). For this study, subgroups were selected from within the total population of 11,685 children, ages 5–14. These subgroups included (1) children with brain disorders, that is, those with epilepsy, cerebral palsy, and other disorders indicating "lesions above the brain stem"; (2) children with physical disorders not involving the brain; and (3) a random sample of the general population of 10- and 11-year-olds without any physical handicaps. These groups of children were carefully screened and examined by medical teams to determine their physical condition.

The psychiatric status of the children was studied by means of (1) a behavioral questionnaire completed by teachers; (2) similar questionnaires completed by parents; (3) interviews with parents about the children's behavior, relationships, and emotions; and (4) a psychiatric examination of the children. Based on these data, a determination was made of the presence or absence of psychiatric disorder in each child.

The rate of psychiatric disorder in the Isle of Wight children ranged from 6.6 percent for the general population of nonhandicapped children, to a high of 58.3 percent for children who had signs of brain disorder that included fits. Deaf children showed a rate of 15.4 percent, more than twice as high as that shown by the nonhandicapped children (Graham & Rutter, 1968, p. 696). It should be noted, however, that this rate is based on only 13 deaf children. This is a drawback of this particular study for those who are specifically interested in the relationship of sensory disability and psychiatric disorder. Large general populations will include only a few deaf or blind children because of the low incidence of these handicaps. The approach used by the Vancouver group, discussed below, is more useful for our purposes because the study subjects were all deaf children.

THE VANCOUVER STUDY

One of the most important studies for assessing the prevalence of behavioral problems in deaf children is the one conducted by Freeman, Malkin, and Hastings (1975) of all deaf children living in the Greater Vancouver area. The results of this study have special credence for the following reasons:

1. *All* deaf children between the ages of 5 and 15 were included as subjects. This means that a number of different schools were represented. The authors believe that only a few cases were not included. This means that the danger of bias from elimination of cases with behavioral problems is less severe.
2. The number of children ($N = 120$) is large enough for the figures to have good reliability—at least as compared to the Isle of Wight study.
3. The investigators are specialists in problems of deafness, and therefore sophisticated about the information that is critical, and about the methodological pitfalls to be avoided.
4. Identification of children with behavioral problems was done by combining the judgments of parents, of teachers, and of medical records. Thus, the danger of idiosyncratic bias in the identification of individual children was avoided.
5. A control group of children with normal hearing, matched with the deaf children for age, sex and neighborhood was included.

A behavioral rating scale completed by parents and teachers was used as a major source for the global ratings reported as psychiatric disorders. This scale was a slightly modified version of the one used by Rutter et al. in the Isle of Wight study described in the preceding section. Some of the items included on this scale were frequency of temper tantrums, toileting accidents, truancy, stealing, eating problems, restlessness, fighting, disobedience, excessive fearfulness, and bullying (Rutter et al. 1970, pp. 419–421).

On the global ratings that incorporated scales completed by parents and teachers, 22.6 percent of the Vancouver deaf children were judged to have a psychiatric disorder of moderate or severe degree. Severe referred to those with a major impairment (6.1 percent) such as "no social relations; bizarre behavior; extremely anxious; persistent major delinquency" (Freeman et al., 1975, p. 396).

COMPARISONS OF PREVALENCE RATES FOR
DEAF AND HEARING CHILDREN

The five sources of data on behavioral problems of deaf children that were summarized in Table 1-1 have been reviewed in the preceding pages. The rates of psychiatric disturbance or emotional/behavioral problems shown in the various studies range from about 9 percent to about 22 percent. How does this compare to the prevalence of behavioral problems among children in the general population?

The Joint Commission on Mental Health of Children (1970) estimated that 2 percent of young people under 25 "are severely disturbed and need immediate psychiatric care. Another 8 to 10 percent are in need of help from mental health workers." The study of all school children in Los Angeles County (State, of California, 1960) on which Schlesinger and Meadow based their survey form, identified 2.4 percent of the students as severely disturbed, and an additional 7.3 percent as having behavioral problems. Schlesinger and Meadow's prevalence rates are 3–5 times higher than those reported in the Los Angeles study. Freeman et al. give no specific comparative rates of psychiatric disturbance for the deaf and hearing children who participated in their study. However, their results do not contradict the results of other studies they have reviewed, including the Schlesinger and Meadow survey. They also report that deaf children were significantly more likely than hearing children to be described by their mothers as disobedient, restless, possessive, too dependent, too fussy, having bad habits, and having stolen things.

The only source that shows rates somewhat lower than the others are the surveys conducted annually by the Office of Demographic Studies (ODS). Altshuler (1975) had the opportunity to check the reporting that was done by one school to the Office of Demographic Studies. As psychiatric consultant, he had been asked to evaluate 40 children from the school during the course of 9 months. He found that slightly more than one third had been designated as emotionally/behaviorally disturbed in the report that the school had sent to the ODS. This led Altshuler to believe that the 8-percent estimate is a significant underrepresentation (Altshuler, 1975). This discrepancy may indicate that teachers and school administrators are less reluctant to label a child when they believe that this procedure may lead to some actual help in the classroom than they are when they assume that the labeling is solely for research purposes.

This point of view differs from that taken by Furth (1973) in his discussion of the high rates of behavioral disorders reported by Schlesinger and Meadow. Furth believes that teachers in schools for the deaf tend to exaggerate the severity of the behavioral problems of their pupils and that the high prevalence rates reflect the opinions of the adults rather than the personalities of the child (Furth, 1973).

There probably is no definitive way of resolving this discrepancy in viewpoints. However, from the evidence available in the surveys and studies conducted to date, it seems that ample evidence exists to conclude that the rate of behavioral problems in deaf children is significantly higher than in the general population of school-age children.

TYPES OF BEHAVIOR PROBLEMS
OBSERVED IN DEAF CHILDREN

It is common for deaf children and deaf adults to be described as lacking in social and emotional maturity. Levine (1956) includes the following traits in deaf adolescent girls: egocentricity, easy irritability, impulsiveness, and suggestibility. Hess (1960) found similar traits in a group of 8–10-year-old children. Myklebust (1960) found deaf persons immature in caring for others. Altshuler (1974) and Rainer et al (1969) characterized deaf patients as demonstrating "egocentricity, a lack of empathy, dependency." Lewis (1968) summarized current opinions and findings on the personality traits of deaf children by noting that they are often described as egocentric, immature in self-awareness, lacking in self-confidence and initiative, and having a tendency to be rigid rather than flexible. Some of these descriptions resulted from clinicians' experiences with deaf patients. A number of research studies have utilized the Vineland Social Maturity Scale* (Doll, 1965) to measure this particular complex of variables. Streng and Kirk (1938), Avery (1948), Burchard and Myklebust (1942), and Schlesinger and Meadow (1972) all found that deaf children scored lower than hearing children of comparable ages in scales that equate maturity with self-help skills.

Another approach to the description of behavioral problems in deaf children is through the use of behavioral symptom check lists that parents and teachers are asked to complete. These kinds of ratings were the basis for most of the prevalence studies cited in previous sections of this chapter. Reivich and Rothrock (1972) analyzed one set of behavior ratings completed by teachers in a state residential school for the deaf in an effort to summarize the kinds of behavior most often checked by teachers to describe their deaf students. By using a computer they were able to complete a minute analysis of the traits that were considered to be present in at least 10 percent of the 327 students who were rated. Three groupings of traits seemed to account for most of the disturbed behavior. These groupings were traits (1) related to unacceptable conduct usually seen as a hyperactive lack of control;

---

*This scale is based on mothers' or other observers' reports of children's abilities to perform in the areas of self-direction, locomotion, occupation, communication, social relations, and self-help. A score or "social quotient" is derived that takes account of the child's chronological age and the kinds of activities he or she might be expected to do at different ages.

(2) related to personality and labeled as ''anxious inhibition''; or (3) related to immaturity and labeled as ''preoccupation.'' Hyperactive lack of control was further described as behavior that was impulsive, unreflective, and uninhibited.

A different method evaluating personality is by means of psychological tests. This was the basis for Levine's (1956) description of deaf adolescents. In this early work, she utilized the Rorschach test with a group of deaf girls. More recently, she and Wagner (1974) utilized the Hand Test in an effort to describe personality patterns in a group of deaf persons.

Examples of the behavioral disorders that are reflected in psychiatric diagnoses are available from two illustrative sources. Both of these are from special populations. One is Williams' (1970) classification of 51 children who were either students in or applying for admission to a school for emotionally disturbed deaf children in England. He points out that those children who are referred for admission were more likely to be those ''whose maladjustment is disturbing to their environment'' (Williams, 1970, p. 3). The category with the largest proportion of children (43 percent) was that of an antisocial disorder. About 20 percent of the group was diagnosed as psychotic, with lesser proportions in several other diagnostic classifications.

The second special group of deaf children for whom psychiatric diagnoses are available is made up of 65 rubella children, subjects of a study conducted at the New York University Medical Center (Chess, Korn, & Fernandez, 1971). Four of these children had a hearing loss of unspecified severity, three of whom had a psychiatric disorder; 14 had a moderate hearing loss, seven of whom had a psychiatric disorder; 47 had a severe hearing loss, 16 (34 percent) of whom had a psychiatric disorder. The largest single group of children in this study was that diagnosed as having a reactive behavior disorder. Some degree of mental retardation was found in 12 of these children, and 5 were found to be autistic (p. 50). The authors comment on the fact that children with multiple physical handicaps are more likely to receive a psychiatric diagnosis as well. They also point out the high rate of mental retardation and autism relative to the general population.

THE GENESIS OF BEHAVIOR PROBLEMS
IN DEAF CHILDREN

Ideas about the bases of behavioral problems and of mental illness depend to some extent on the training, experience, and general orientation of the individuals performing the diagnosis. Theories range from almost complete reliance on physiologic or biochemical explanations to almost complete reliance on psychological or experiential explanations. However, most professionals would agree that some combination or interaction of physical, biologic, social, and psychological factors is usually necessary in arriving at an understanding of abnormal behavior. The question of etiology is particularly confusing when deafness is a part of the picture, because some of the diseases or conditions that cause deafness may also cause other problems that result in behavioral disorders. For example, there are genetic syndromes where deafness is part of a complex of difficulties; high fevers that accompany diseases such as meningitis may cause both deafness and brain damage—the same is true for deafness resulting from incompatibility of blood types in parents, and for deafness resulting from maternal rubella (Vernon, 1969; Mindel & Vernon, 1971). However, the interaction of physiologic and psychological factors in the creation of conditions often described as neurologic impairment, minimal brain dysfunction, or hyperkinesis is not fully understood. A few years ago, these terms became overused. They grew to be convenient catch phrases disguised as diagnoses, and were used to describe impairments in language, motor or sensory functioning, and intellectual abilities, all of which were supposed to be related to the inadequacy of or damage to the central nervous system. Hobbs (1975, p. 75) noted that the concept of brain damage or neurologic impairment is virtually useless when trying to establish a specific syndrome.

Several of the authors of the prevalence studies described above make it clear that they exercised extreme caution in ascribing the label or diagnosis of brain damage to children included in their study groups (Freeman, Malkin, & Hastings, 1975; Chess, Korn & Fernandez, 1971; Graham & Rutter, 1968). One danger of defining a child's behavioral problems as the result of brain damage is the possibility that parents and professionals will cease their efforts to effect situational changes that might help to alter the unacceptable behavior. This possibility relates to our earlier discussion on the dangers of labeling. Altshuler points out (1974, p. 372) that symptoms such as hyperactivity, irritability, withdrawal, aggression, and sleeping and eating problems can result from a variety of causes.

The tensions to which deaf children and their families are subjected are numerous. They are related to the general stress experienced by families with handicapped children, and to the specific stress that accompanies the reduced ability to communicate (Meadow, 1968; Mindel & Vernon, 1971).

Schlesinger and Meadow (1972) have analyzed the development of deaf children from the perspective of Erik Erikson's eight stages of man, pinpointing the areas where communication and response to diagnosis are most likely to have an influence. The least is known about the deaf child's development in the earliest stage—infancy—when basic trust and attachment to the maternal figure are being established. Because the diagnosis of deafness is very often delayed until after the first year of life has passed, we know very little about what happens to the deaf child during infancy or whether the deaf child responds differently than the hearing child to persons and objects in the environment.

Williams (1970, pp. 12–13) collected retrospective developmental data from parents of the deaf children he examined upon their application to a school for emotionally disturbed deaf children. Ten of the 51 children receiving the examination were diagnosed as psychotic. He had data on 8 of these. Half were said to have slept excessively during their first year of life, and to have shown failure to anticipate being picked up and negativism. Six of the 8 were described as excessively placid and indifferent. Six showed gaze avoidance. Data were available for 22 of the nonpsychotic children. In these children, parents' complaints were of excessive wakefulness (6 cases), excessive crying (7 cases), feeding difficulties (5 cases), and irritability (4 cases). Five of these children showed gaze avoidance as well.

Erikson suggests that, during the period from 1½ to 3 years of age, the basic developmental task is the establishment of autonomy: the sense of existence as a separate human being with control over one's own body and environment. The period from 3–6 years is seen as especially important for the development of initiative: a feeling of the purposefulness of life and self. The child with hearing has increasing command of linguistic symbols during these two periods encompassing the years from 1½ to 6 years. The deaf child not only fails to understand the restrictions placed upon him or her while searching for autonomy and initiative, but he or she also cannot communicate.

The behavioral problems identified by parents, teachers, and mental health professionals alike are tied to the kinds of developmental expectations that caretakers have for children at differing ages. Thus, in the study of rubella children ages 2½–4, the following areas of behavioral deviation were defined: sleep problems, 46 percent; feeding and eating problems, 53 percent; elimination problems, 37 percent; mood difficulties (separation anxiety, withdrawn behavior, temper tantrums), 72 percent; discipline problems, 64 percent; deviant motor activity (hyperactivity), 55 percent; peculiar habits and rituals, 67 percent (Chess, Korn, & Fernandez, 1971).

Freedman, Cannady, and Robinson (1971) followed the development of five congenitally deaf girls, all rubella babies. They said that "It is characteristic of all these little girls that they tend to translate their wishes into action more readily than might be anticipated from the observation of children of similar age with normal hearing." Their description of one of these five children reflects the kinds of experiences related to language deficiencies that many deaf children have. This particular child was left at 38 months of age in the care of her grandparents when her father was hospitalized. The mother made no preparations for the separation and disappeared for several days. Following this event, the child regressed and became quite disturbed.

Parents of deaf children often feel they do not have the command of communication necessary to explain complicated events. Thus, we have known children whose worlds changed drastically from one day to the next, with no explanation for the disappearance of a parent or grandparent, for a move from one house to another or from one city to another, for a trip to the hospital with frightening and painful procedures performed.

Lesser and Easser (1972, p. 462) have suggested that the impulsiveness of deaf children is closely connected with the lack of adequate communicative channels for expressing needs and feelings. They believe that such impulsiveness is "directly related to the organization of emotions for the self and the understanding . . . of the emotions by the self. Once an affect can be named, it can come under the sway of ego control . . . This delay in organizing the 'emotional self' is clearly related to the deaf child's difficulty with empathic responses."

Social skills that enable children to get along with others are developed through language. Heider's (1948) study of pairs of deaf and hearing children reflected this. She found that the hearing children were more able than the deaf children to gain control of a social situation without arousing either aggression or withdrawal in another child. The social relationships of the deaf children appeared to be more diffuse, less structured, and less sharply oriented than the social relationships of the hearing children.

A study completed by Herren and Colin (1972) illustrates the greater difficulty deaf children had in progressing from competition to cooperation when confronted with a task requiring cooperation. They state that "the delayed progression from competition to cooperation shown by the deaf is bound to an intellectual handicap secondary to language deprivation."

Since parent–child communication is by definition a two-way process, differences in parental definition of the child's handicap and capabilities influence performance dramatically. This is illustrated in a striking way in the study of rubella children. There was a marked discrepancy between the children's ability to perform self-help activities, and their actual performance of them. Among the children for whom information was available, half were capable of performing 80 percent of the activities necessary for dressing themselves. Fewer than half actually performed even 25 percent of these activities (Chess et al., 1971, p. 94).

Thus, there are many ways in which physical, psychological, familial, experiential, and linguistic factors interact to contribute to the creation, treatment, and outcome of behavioral problems of deaf children.

CONCLUSIONS

Recognition of the high levels of behavioral disturbance in deaf children is a first step in the provision of mental health services to treat the problems. Provision of services is a first step in the prevention of future problems. Both parents and children can be helped by mental health professionals and by sensitive teachers to communicate in more effective ways and to give and to accept additional responsibility for performance of developmental tasks. Although there are too few programs, centers, and professionals trained and equipped to work in the important areas of prevention and remediation of the behavioral problems of deaf children, those that have been engaged in this work have demonstrated that they can be effective. The size of the problem is great, but theoretical knowledge and practical experience for dealing with the behavioral problems of deaf children are expanding.

REFERENCES

Altshuler, K.Z. The social and psychological development of the deaf child: Problems, their treatment and prevention. *American Annals of the Deaf*, 1974, *119*, 365–376.
Altshuler, K.Z. Identifying and programming for the emotionally handicapped deaf child.

In D.W. Naiman (Ed.), *Needs of emotionally disturbed hearing impaired children*. New York: Deafness Research and Training Center, New York University Press, 1975.

Avery, C. The social competence of pre-school acoustically handicapped children. *Journal of Exceptional Children*, 1948, *15*, 71–73.

Berlin, I.N. Preventive aspects of mental health consultation to schools. *Mental Hygiene*, 1967, *51*, 34–40.

Bower, E.M. A process for early identification of emotionally disturbed children. *Bulletin of the California State Department of Education*, 1958, *27*.

Burchard, E.M.L., & Myklebust, H.R. A comparison of congenital and adventitious deafness with respect to its effect on intelligence, personality, and social maturity. *American Annals of the Deaf*, 1942, *87*, 140–154, 241–251, 342–360.

Doll, E.A. *Vineland social maturity scale: condensed manual of directions*. Circle Pines, Minn.: American Guidance Service, 1965.

Chess, S., Korn, S.J., & Fernandez, P.B. *Psychiatric disorders of children with congenital rubella*. New York: Brunner/Mazel, 1971.

Freedman, D.A., Cannady, C., & Robinson, J.A. Speech and psychic structure: A reconsideration of their relation. *Journal of the American Psychoanalytic Association*, 1971, *19*, 765–779.

Freeman, R.F., Malkin, S.F., & Hastings, J.O. Psychosocial problems of deaf children and their families: A comparative study. *American Annals of the Deaf*, 1975, *120*, 391–405.

Furth, H.G. *Deafness and learning: a psychosocial approach*. Belmont, Calif.: Wadsworth Publishing Company, 1973.

Gentile, A., & McCarthy, B. *Additional handicapping conditions among hearing impaired students, United States: 1971–72* (Report No. 14, Series D). Washington, D.C.: Gallaudet College, Office of Demographic Studies, 1973.

Graham, P., & Rutter, M. Organic brain dysfunction and child psychiatric disorder. *British Medical Journal*, 1968, *3*, 695–700.

Heider, G.M. Adjustment problems of the deaf child. *Nervous Child*, 1948, *1*, 38–44.

Herren, H., & Colin, D. Implicit language and cooperation in children: Comparative study of deaf and hearing children. *Enfance*, 1972, *5*, 325–337 *Psychological Abstracts*, 1973, *50*, 9192).

Hess, W. *Personality adjustment in deaf children*. Unpublished Ph.D. dissertation, University of Rochester, 1960.

Hobbs, N. *The futures of children: categories, labels, and their consequences*. San Francisco, Calif.: Jossey-Bass, 1975.

Joint Commission on Mental Health of Children. *Crisis in child mental health: Challenge for the 1970's*. New York: Harper & Row, 1970.

Lesser, S.R., & Easser, B.R. Personality differences in the perceptually handicapped. *Journal of the American Academy of Child Psychiatry*, 1972, *11*, 458–466.

Levine, E.S. *Youth in a soundless world: A search for personality*. New York: New York University Press, 1956.

Levine, E.S. Psychological contributions. *Volta Review*, 1976, *78*, 23–33.

Levine, E.S., & Wagner, E.E. Personality patterns of deaf persons: An interpretation based on research with the Hand Test. *Perceptual and Motor Skills*, 1974, *39*, 1167–1236.

Lewis, M.M. *Language and personality in deaf children*. Slough, England: National Foundation for Educational Research. Occasional Publication Series No. 20, 1968.

Meadow, K.P. Parental responses to the medical ambiguities of deafness. *Journal of Health and Social Behavior*, 1968, *9*, 299–309.

Mindel, E.D., & Vernon, M. *They grow in silence—The deaf child and his family*. Silver Spring, Md.: National Association of the Deaf, 1971.

Myklebust, H.R. *The psychology of deafness, sensory deprivation, learning and adjustment*. New York: Grune & Stratton, 1960.

Phillips, L., Draguns, J.G., & Bartlett, D.P. Classification of behavior disorders. In N. Hobbs (Ed.), *Issues in the classification of children* (Vol. 1). San Francisco, Calif.: Jossey-Bass, 1975.

Prugh, D.G., Engel, M., & Morse, W.C. Emotional disturbance in children. In N. Hobbs (Ed.), *Issues in the classification of children* (Vol. 1). San Francisco, Calif.: Jossey-Bass, 1975.

Rainer, J.D., Altshuler, K.Z., & Kallmann; F.J. (Eds.). *Family and mental health problems in a deaf population* (2nd ed.). Springfield, Illinois: Charles C Thomas, 1969.

Rains, P., Kitsuse, J.I., Duster, T., et al. The labeling approach to deviance. In N. Hobbs (Ed.), *Issues in the classification of children* (Vol. 1). San Francisco, Calif.: Jossey-Bass, 1975.

Reivich, R.S., & Rothrock, I.A. Behavior problems of deaf children and adolescents: A factor-analytic study. *Journal of Speech and Hearing Research*, 1972, *15*, 84–92.

Rutter, M., Tizard, J., & Whitmore, K. (Eds.). *Education, health and behaviour. Psychological and medical study of childhood development*. New York: Wiley, 1970.

Schein, J.D. Deaf students with other disabilities. *American Annals of the Deaf*, 1975, *120*, 92–99.

Schlesinger, H.S., & Meadow, K.P. *Sound and sign: Childhood deafness and mental health*. Berkeley, Calif.: University of California Press, 1972.

State of California. *Mental health survey of Los Angeles County*. Sacramento: Department of Mental Hygiene, 1960.

Streng, A., & Kirk, S.A. The social competence of deaf and hard of hearing children in a public day school. *American Annals of the Deaf*, 1938, *83*, 244–254.

Vernon, M. *Multiply handicapped deaf children: Medical, educational, and psychological considerations* (CEC Research Monograph). Washington, D.C.: Council for Exceptional Children, 1969.

Williams, C.E. Some psychiatric observations on a group of maladjusted deaf children. *Journal of Child Psychology and Psychiatry*, 1970, *11*, 1–18.

Laszlo K. Stein, Ph.D.
Theresa Jabaley, M.A.

2

Early Identification and Parent Counseling

The two most common factors in the environment of deaf children that can account for their emotional or behavioral differences are (1) the lag in language development and its effect on family communication and socialization, and (2) the psychological response of parents to the diagnosis of a hearing handicap. Rainer et al. (1963) and Grinker (1969) emphasized the significance of parental response when they noted that many of the mental health problems of the deaf adult can be traced to deficiencies in early parent–child relationships, unrealistic expectations by parents, and the inability of parents to cope in a healthy manner with the fact that their growing child is different from other children and to a certain extent will always be different. Additional evidence for the importance of the parent–child relationship in the life of a deaf child is found in Mindel and Vernon (1971) and Schlesinger and Meadow (1972). From these studies, and our own clinical experience (Stein, Merrill, & Dahlberg, 1974), we conclude that the most common forms of emotional and behavioral difficulties that beset the adult deaf person are to a very large extent attributable to inadequacies in the parent–child bond.

Educators of the deaf have traditionally stressed the need for parent involvement. In the educational model, parent involvement is typically viewed as focusing on educational issues. The parent, principally the mother, is seen by the teacher as an adjunctive teacher who will reinforce, through drills at home and other activities outside the classroom, the language and educational programs prescribed by the teacher. As important as this form of parent participation is, it is only one aspect of the parent–child relationship. Lacking (perhaps unintentionally because of ignorance or deliberately because of philosophical bias) is concern for the psychological trauma the parent may be experiencing over having a handicapped child.

Parent counseling limited to educational issues assumes that the parent, again

23

principally the mother, is capable of listening to and accepting the advice offered. She is expected to follow the instructions of the teacher and as "a good mother" devote herself completely to the education of her hearing-impaired child. Rarely, if ever, is the issue openly faced of whether the mother, father, and other members of the immediate family are capable of coping with the deep personal feelings the hearing-impaired child may have generated within each of them. Nor is it considered that well-intentioned counseling attempts by physicians, audiologists, and educators of the deaf may fail because the parents of a hearing-impaired child may not be able to act upon the advice given due to the psychological trauma they have suffered.

It is our contention that parental acceptance and a healthy parent–child relationship can significantly influence the later well-being and achievement of a deaf child. Early intervention, emphasizing parental acceptance, parent–child interaction, and an effective program of language development, is seen as the best preventive mental health measure for reducing the high prevalence of emotional/ behavioral problems among deaf children and adults. Although we believe that the ideal early intervention model must incorporate the elements of early diagnosis, comprehensive medical service, a sound strategy for language development, and techniques fostering a healthy parent–child bond, we will limit ourselves to the psychological responses and needs of parents.

BACKGROUND

In an earlier publication, aimed primarily toward physicians and audiologists, we described a psychotherapeutic model for counseling parents of hearing-impaired children (Stein 1979). Our interest in this area began in 1966 and was prompted by two related developments. The first was our concern for the unusually large number of hearing-impaired infants being referred to our institute (The David T. Siegel Institute for Communicative Disorders) as a result of the rubella epidemic of the mid-1960s. Because many of the children were born with cataracts and cardiac problems that were among features of the rubella syndrome, the deafness was also detected as early as age 1½–2 years. Thus, we had a large number of younger deaf children with a range of other disabilities and prognoses. It soon was apparent to our staff that the deaf babies would require special attention if they were to have any chance to develop language and socialization skills during the critical first 3 years of life. At the time, most preschool programs were geared only for 3–5-year-old children; this was commonly the age of definitive diagnosis. Those few programs that did accept infants were often quite limited in their approach and scope. The second concern involved awareness of psychiatric studies showing that many of the emotional/behavioral problems of deaf adults were in large part attributable to, or at the very least exacerbated by, inadequacies of early parent–child relationships (Grinker, 1969). These concerns about the prevailing educational approach with deaf infants, particularly in the areas of language development and the nature of early parent–infant relationships prompted our formation of an innovative nursery program for deaf infants and their parents in 1967. Fundamental to that program was the use of sign language in conjunction with aural/oral training, the fostering of the parent–infant bond through interactive language-learning activities, and individual and group counseling sessions conducted by staff child psychiatrists, clinical psychologists, and psychiatric social workers. Other staff members, including audiologists, otologists, and physicians, became aware of the feelings of parents in the crisis of diagnosis and also became sensitive to the emotional aspects of parent–child and parent–professional relationships.

In the following sections, we discuss impressions from 15 years in counseling parents of deaf children. This experience was not only with parents from a broad metropolitan population area—inner city, middle-income city, and upper-middle-income suburban—but also with parents from rural and smaller urban communities attending workshops and institutes conducted in other parts of the state. The experiences and responses of parents from wide geographic, socioeconomic, and ethnic backgrounds are thus represented. It is our hope that mental health professionals and educators of the deaf will obtain a sense of what the birth of a deaf child means to parents and what psychotherapeutically oriented counseling requires of both parent and therapist.

DIAGNOSIS

Until relatively recently, the diagnosis of deafness in an infant or a child under 3 years of age was uncertain and in a real sense, a medical dilemma (Meadow, 1968). Unless the infant was an obvious risk for hearing impairment—with a history of hereditary deafness or maternal rubella during the first trimester of pregnancy—the possibility of congenital hearing loss was largely ignored. Pediatricians, rightly or wrongly, were often accused of dismissing the possibility of hearing loss or the concerns of the parents. In truth, the failure to identify hearing loss during infancy can be blamed on two factors: (1) the frequently cited lack of awareness or knowledge among pediatricians about hearing disorders, which unfortunately was true in too many instances; and (2) the equally important but sometimes overlooked fact that no one definitive test to rule out deafness in an infant existed.

Unlike adults, infants and young children under 3 or 4 years of age cannot tell an examiner whether they can hear a test signal or not. Only through a lengthy series of observations of an infant's reflexive response or lack of response to sound could hearing impairment be detected. Physical examinations, including x-rays, are of limited value in the detection of hearing loss due to inner ear damage. Although a number of major hospital centers specializing in hearing loss in childhood were capable of diagnosing the presence of deafness quite early using behavioral or subjective methods, the relative low incidence of congenital hearing loss, estimated to be 2 in 1000 births, limited the number of such facilities and the public support required for the needed additional resources.

Public attention generated as a result of the rubella epidemic in the mid-1960s, passage of mandatory special education laws at both the state and federal level, growing demands by handicapped citizens for equal rights and opportunities, and increasing interest in early childhood development are some of the major reasons for improvement in efforts to diagnose hearing loss at an earlier age. Yet, despite the best efforts of professional and parent organizations toward advancing the concept of neonatal screening programs and registry of infants at high risk for hearing impairment, the actual diagnostic testing of infant hearing was still based on behavioral methods. The success and accuracy of these methods depended on the skill and experience of the audiologist to discern a true response to sound in a young child and to differentiate it from a visual or a situational response, lack of response, or chance. Needed was a more objective and definitive test, one not dependent on the cooperation of the child and the subjective skill of the examiner.

In the early 1970s, published reports appeared on what is now rapidly being accepted as the method of choice in diagnosing hearing loss in infants (Hecox & Galambos, 1974; Jewett & Williston, 1971; Schulman-Galambos & Galambos, 1975; Sohmer & Feinmeser, 1967; Stein, 1975, 1976). Auditory Brainstem Response (ABR), or Brainstem Evoked Response (BSER or BER), is an electrophysiologic test that records the changes in the electrical activity of the human brain in response to sound. Somewhat similar to the brain wave test or electroencephalogram (EEG), neural activity of the auditory (VIIIth) nerve and the auditory pathways in the brainstem is recorded through electrodes pasted to the head and analyzed by means of a small average response computer. The only requirement of the infant or child is to lie quietly, preferably asleep. A mild sedative, chloral hydrate for example, may be prescribed to help the more active or fussy infant sleep for the hour or so needed to complete the test. With newborns, testing is frequently done after feeding during natural sleep. Although ABR in its present form does not provide a complete picture of hearing for all frequencies, it does reveal whether or not the infant has a hearing loss and the degree of that loss in the 2000–4000 Hz range. Hearing in this frequency range is critical for the understanding and subsequent development of speech. A loss of hearing for the mid-high and high frequencies as measured by the ABR technique does indicate whether the infant is educationally hearing-impaired.

At the present time, ABR can identify hearing loss in newborns and infants. This, as anyone who has experienced or witnessed the anxiety of parents around the uncertainties of diagnosis knows, is a remarkable advance. Although a relatively simple procedure for use with infants, the complexity of the electronic equipment needed and the technical skill required of the examiners restricts current use to hospital centers. ABR will not replace the audiologist and the requirement for conventional audiologic testing with hearing-impaired children. What ABR does promise is a means for identification of hearing loss in newborns and infants, who, once identified, can be referred for any indicated medical, audiologic, or habilitative follow-up. Whether all newborns or newborns judged at high risk for hearing impairment—with low birthweight, history of familial hearing loss, prenatal or natal difficulties, etc.—eventually will be screened by ABR or some other physiologic test, such as the Crib-o-gram (Simons, 1980), is not certain at this time. But what does seem definite is that the increasing availability and utilization of electrophysiologic or physiologic testing in hospital centers will substantially reduce the uncertainty and delay that previously existed around the early diagnosis of hearing loss in infants.

It remains to be seen if we can take advantage of the technical advances that have been made in the early identification of hearing loss and provide appropriate language stimulation and parent–infant services. Such states as California and Utah have already legislated mandatory hearing screening or registry of the newborn at risk for hearing loss. Other states are either comtemplating or drafting similar legislation. With few exceptions, notably Utah (Clark & Watkins, 1978), little consideration has been given to development of comprehensive parent–infant programs once hearing loss has been identified. This is particularly true for large urban metropolitan areas, where the availability and quality of special education services vary widely because of the jurisdictional, bureaucratic, and fiscal problems of the school systems and social agencies involved. Add to this the socioeconomic and ethnic diversity of the population to be served, and the magnitude of the task becomes apparent. In our own program we are attempting to at least partially address some of these issues through a Model-Demonstration Program Grant from Bureau of the Education of the Handicapped (BEH), which incorporates the various medical, academic, and psychological elements into a unified parent–infant program for hearing impaired infants 0–3 years of age.

We chose for this paper to give a rather full explanation of the problems associated with the early diagnosis of hearing loss and the tremendous potential that recent developments in medical technology have given us in testing infant hearing as background to the role of the parent. The principal advantage of diagnosis during the newborn period is that language stimulation activities can be started sooner and, theoretically, full advantage can be taken of the critical language-learning period. This means very little, however, without the early and adequate development of a healthy parent–infant relationship. Parental response is still crucial, whether the hearing impairment is diagnosed at birth or at 3 years of age. It is a critical time that can have far-reaching effects on the future of the child and the emotional well-being of the parent. Poorly handled, the impact on the parent may be so disruptive and pervasive, and their ability to accept and cope with the situation may be so limited, that subsequent attempts to initiate effective therapy and education are neutralized. Despite the importance attributed to the time of diagnosis, many parents will not have proper support, and the mental health worker may have to retrace and help overcome parental feelings that stem from circumstances surrounding the initial diagnosis.

PARENTAL RESPONSES

First-Stage Responses

Almost invariably, parental reaction to the diagnosis of deafness includes expressions of anger at professionals. Typically, these are first directed toward the physicians whom the parent feels failed to inform them of the consequences of the mother's pregnancy or failed to provide proper medical care. In most circumstances, this initial anger is replaced by expressions of anger toward those professionals the parents associate with the diagnosis. It is not uncommon to hear a parent complain about how little time the doctor spent with them. Nor is it uncommon to hear anger expressed at professionals who, either through ignorance or through well-intentioned but mistaken attempts to spare feelings, gave false reassurances.

Although a certain amount of parental anger at professionals is a way of denying guilt by projecting blame on outside factors, it is important for the therapist to separate what may be actual from what is imagined. It should be remembered that during the diagnostic stage, many parents may not display acceptance and understanding despite the best efforts of audiologists and otologists. As we pointed out earlier, this initial stage is defined by shock, anger, and denial. Most of the information imparted to parents during the diagnostic process, regardless of how skillfully done, may not be heard because at this stage parents really do not want to know these things. This, in part, may explain some of the frustrations experienced by professionals who spend hours talking with parents and then hear them later say "But I was never told!" It is also a period when parents are searching for other opinions and "miracle" cures. Often this results in what has been termed *shopping behavior*. Parents may visit the same professional or a number of different professionals or clinics with the hope of finding either clearer or more acceptable explanations for their child's problem. Professionals often show irritation at the shopping parent; however, Buscaglia (1975), after reviewing several studies on shopping behavior, suggests that many parents seeking additional opinions may not be necessarily rejecting recommendations and information but simply requesting services different from those they have received. Despite mixed opinions on whether shopping behavior should be discouraged (either at the time of initial diagnosis or later when the parent may be seeking alternative educational programs), it seems clear that several factors contribute to the satisfaction that parents express toward any contact with a professional.

The time spent with parents and what is said is obviously important; however, the attitude shown by the otologist, audiologist, teacher, or therapist is an obvious yet sometimes overlooked factor. Objectivity does not mean feeling must be absent. Unpleasant or painful information may be rejected by the parent when that information comes from the professional who displays a seemingly uninterested or unfeeling attitude (Beck, 1959). Much of what actually transpires during a counseling session can be significantly facilitated if the professional is able to recognize and identify with the feelings, emotions, and torments that the parent is experiencing. An empathic response on the part of the professional implies the understanding of the other person's thoughts, feelings, and actions in an intellectual sense. Empathy does not mean commiseration in the sense of superficial solace. Rather, it is an ability to understand one's own feelings as well as the feelings of those you are trying to help. As Ross (1964) points out, the professional engaged in counseling parents must possess not only the professional attributes of objectivity, knowledge, and the technical skill of interviewing, but also the human qualities of acceptance, understanding, warmth, and honesty.

These are important factors for the mental health worker or counselor to remember if placed in the position of counseling parents at the time of diagnosis or, possibly, having to help parents later retrace and overcome negative feelings surrounding the initial diagnosis. If possible, it is desirable for both parents to attend any initial interview or conference to avoid later misunderstanding due to failure or unwillingness to communicate about issues that are obviously difficult for both of them. It may be necessary to spend considerable time on medical or educational issues before more direct exploration of feelings is attempted. In certain situations, it may be more effective for several professionals to be involved in these informational sessions, although the therefore more formal counseling sessions may inhibit an easy exchange of information. The most important thing for the mental health worker or counselor to remember is that during this initial stage, parents in all likelihood are still wondering if their child can hear (denial), and that they have a need to displace their anger and sorrow toward someone else.

Second-Stage Responses

When parents find it increasingly difficult to deny the existence of a hearing loss, expressions of anger at their child often surface. This again may be a manifestation of anger displayed outwardly at someone else, but also may signify feelings of confusion and concern about how to raise a deaf child. This is often reflected around the issue of discipline. Even parents who have successfully raised hearing children express distrust of their own instincts about showing displeasure, as well as love. At this point, many parents appear very willing to accept the advice of professionals, even if such advice goes against their own instincts. Doubts and insecurities, feelings of helplessness and inadequacy, lead many parents to look toward others rather than to themselves for answers to their problems.

These expressions of anger by parents frequently lead to expressions of the sadness they feel in relating to their deaf child. This sadness is often expressed as a "lost" feeling because they have no idea of how their deaf child perceives the world and of what lies ahead. This grief may be handled in several ways. The fear of possible isolation from the child is sometimes expressed in discussions of their own isolation as a parent of a hearing-handicapped child. Others, including well-meaning grandparents and extended family members, do not understand or appreciate their struggles. Feelings of being alone as a parent exacerbate feelings of isolation from their child. Concerns over the effect of deafness on the deaf child's thinking and feeling and the fear that the child will gravitate away from the parent into the deaf community may be openly expressed by some parents but totally repressed by others. As a means of compensating for these emerging feelings of sadness and isolation, some parents busy themselves in extra outside activities; others may overindulge their children with gifts; and still others attempt to maintain a stiff-upper-lip position because "If you can't do anything about it, why cry?"

Expressions of anger and sadness often may be suppressed by a return to discussions of concrete issues: medical cures, validity of hearing tests, benefits of hearing aids, oralism versus total communication, etc. Later in this stage, discussions of solutions tend to wane and be replaced by a "hard-work ethic." This is reflected by comments such as "If we work hard, things will be all right; teachers will not be mad at us and blame us; and we have to prepare our children so they will work hard to learn." It is not uncommon to find seemingly dedicated parents who, in reality, may have displaced all expressions of feelings with an exaggerated work ethic. This may be followed by expressions of wanting to get out from it all. The parents may feel caught in the dilemma between giving an overwhelming kind of caretaking to their child and abandoning him or her—in a sense giving over total care to the school.

Third-Stage Responses

An emerging theme centering on the acceptance of hearing-impaired children by their parents and the outside world marks the transition from sadness and anger to the development of adaptation and coping behavior. The parents might introduce the notion of their own acceptance by first discussing acceptance of their child by other children, teachers, and members of the extended family. Examples of how painful it is not to be accepted and how hard people try to win friends are often given. Parents who might be quite strict with their child explain, "My child has to be hardened because it will be a difficult world for a hearing-impaired child." They feel they must prepare their hearing-handicapped child for all kinds of ugly eventualities because the handicapped are rejected and ridiculed. Typical are stories such as the mother in the neighborhood who would not let her daughter play with the deaf child or the godmother who could not feel close to the child after learning she was deaf. By talking about acceptance of their child by others, the parents may actually be grappling with their own sense of acceptance. Parents in this stage may show indications of understanding that the sadness they feel and the issue of their own acceptance must be handled. Some may approach this in a rather direct fashion, but others may discuss it more indirectly through other people, such as a friend whose husband died sometime ago but who still feels sad because she never really mourned his death.

If there is one ideal goal to be reached, it is that parents handle the sadness they feel through the natural process of mourning or normal grief. The natural mourning process implies that the individual has been able to deal with feelings of loss—in the case of a hearing-impaired child, the loss of the expected "perfect" child—in contrast to inward manifestations of self-accusation and feelings of guilt. It is a period when the parent can openly express feelings of personal responsibility, guilt, shame, and wishing the problem away. The parents may openly ask, "Why me?" The mourning process that the parent experiences with a handicapped child has been compared to that experienced at the death of a loved one. In a sense, this may be true when compared to the loss of the expected perfect child. Unfortunately, with the deaf child, it cannot be resolved in the same way. As the child grows, new problems of adjustment will appear for both the child and the parent. There will be constant reminders that the hearing impairment imposes certain limitations requiring reevaluation of previously held aspirations. Nevertheless, the parent who achieves insight into feelings that such problems create has a far better chance to summon the resources and means to adapt and cope with each new problem.

We have attempted to highlight the sequence of reactions and concerns that a parent of a hearing-impaired child may experience. Obviously, there can be no absolute prediction as to how an individual parent will respond. Some will be able to tap inner resources through previous experience with crisis situations or through the support provided by family, and with relative ease achieve satisfactory adaptation to the birth of a hearing-impaired child. Others may never be able to successfully cope with their feelings and will remain in a state of sorrow long after their child has reached adulthood.

COUNSELING STRATEGIES

In our experience, the optimal time for involving parents in either individual or group psychotherapy is as soon as possible after the diagnosis is conclusive. This is the time when feelings of shock, anger, and guilt are most accessible. Ideally, there should be a smooth transition from diagnosis to enrollment in a parent–infant program. The availability of a mental health worker can help the parents make this transition. It has been our impression that parents who have been exposed to a period of educational guidance may be diverted from dealing with their true feelings, because they have been offered, at least feel they have been offered, solutions that promise great hope. The mother may involve herself completely in educational activities and the father withdraw into the provider role, thus forming a defense against potentially painful confrontations with their feelings through channels accepted by society.

The role of the father is very important, but unfortunately he is almost entirely excluded from the very beginning. From the time of diagnosis on, the father usually receives most of the information about his child secondhand from the mother. Unless extraordinary efforts are made on the part of both the parents, the father often gradually retreats to a secondary role because he either feels or is made to feel, less expert than his wife, and therefore fears he might not do the right thing with his child. The father in this situation may find himself with strongly conflicting feelings. On the one hand, he may interpret the male role as one of strength; on the other, he may want to give way to deep feelings of sorrow and failure. The burden of having produced an imperfect child can stimulate intense feelings in both parents, but in his role as provider the father can withdraw, whereas the mother is forced to assume the immediate responsibility for the day-to-day care of the child. Under these circumstances, the presence of a hearing-impaired child can have a disruptive effect on marital relations.

The gradual emotional and physical withdrawal of the father may result in the mother becoming angry and resentful. The responsibility of the deaf child added to the already demanding requirements of motherhood often presents an overwhelming burden. Compounding all of this is the changing role of women in contemporary society. Other than role of wife, mother, or mother of a deaf child, more women are seeking to reaffirm individual identity through outside activities. The dependency of the deaf child on the mother and the restrictions on her activities imposed by such dependency can seriously affect the healthy development of mother–child and mother–family relationships. Inability to share the hurt can result in both parents becoming remote from each other. The father finding his own life disrupted and his needs unmet may not show his resentment toward his child, because, in our society, this is unacceptable. He may, however, show it toward his wife who now becomes the object of his anger. An already strained marriage may not be able to survive the burden of a handicapped child, and individual or marital therapy may be indicated.

The preceding section addressed the potential impact of a handicapped child on traditional husband–wife families. Changes in American life style, however, made families maintained by female householders with no husband present the fastest growing type of family in the country during the 1970s, according to Census Bureau figures released in late 1980 (Rawlings, 1980). Among factors contributing to this shift are (1) childbearing outside marriage; (2) the dissolution of traditional families through separation, divorce or widowhood; (3) the inclination and ability of women to establish or maintain independent families rather than residing with parents or other relatives as they might have done at one time; and (4) the disproportionate population increase in the young adult ages. According to this same Census Bureau study, in 1979 12 percent of all white families were maintained by female householders, while 20 percent of Hispanic and 41 percent of black families were maintained by women.

This growing trend of single-parent (mother–child) families or families maintained by female householders, opens an entirely new dimension to parental involvement with the handicapped child. Added to the question of personal feelings generated by the birth of a hearing impaired child is how can the mother assume the increased demands for the day-to-day care of the child and still maintain a provider and head of household role. The female householder with a deaf child is becoming an increasingly important area of concern—one that mental health workers and teachers cannot ignore.

The proliferation of parent groups for hearing-impaired children at both the local and national level attests to the fact that parents want to meet other parents. If nothing else, such largely social groups serve to reduce parental feelings of being alone. These groups can also provide a convenient way for parents to obtain information on schools and the availability of special services. More active parent groups can serve a very important advocacy role. Rarely, however, do these groups deal with parental feelings and emotions in a direct and planned manner. Attempts at incorporating a form of psychotherapeutic counseling within the framework of an established parent group invariably meets resistance because of the parental wish to avoid painful feelings. The mental health worker interested in organizing and conducting a psychotherapeutically oriented parent group will probably find it best to keep such a group separate from the school- or community-sponsored parent group or association.

The increasing ability to diagnose hearing impairment at or very soon after birth may have a significant effect on parental acceptance. One common and bitter complaint of parents has been the delay between the time they first suspected that something was wrong and the time their child was finally enrolled in a parent–infant or educational program. The time period beginning with the pediatrician who mistakenly allayed the parent's fears, to the uncertainty of sometimes conflicting diagnostic impressions, to enrollment of the child in an appropriate educational program may have been months, or possibly a year or more. Rawlings (1971) reported that a 1969–1970 survey indicated that only 11.2 percent of 26,888 hearing-impaired students started education prior to 3 years of age, 53.1 percent started between 3 and 5 years of age, and fully 29.8 percent had no education prior to age 6. Our own experience shows that over the 5-year period ending in 1979, the mean age at time of enrollment in our program was 2.2 years. In contrast, the mean age at time of enrollment in our program at the present time is 11 months. Age at time of enrollment may be even further reduced by increased use of electrophysiologic or physiologic testing with newborns at risk for hearing impairment. Even in instances where the child is not at risk for hearing impairment and is otherwise developing normally, the time from when the parent first suspects something might be wrong to the time of enrollment in a parent–infant program is being substantially reduced. An example is provided by a recent case where the mother had casually asked the pediatrician if she should begin toilet training her 2-year-old, who had not yet begun to talk. The pediatrician immediately arranged an appointment with an otolaryngologist who, in turn, referred the child to us for ABR testing. The elapsed time from the mother's first inquiry to the diagnosis of profound deafness was 24 hours. By the following week, the child had been enrolled in a local parent–infant program and arrangements were being made to fit him with wearable amplification. Interestingly, the response of both the mother and father to the diagnosis of deafness was very similar to the sequence of stages of response we described earlier; however, with support, both appeared to negotiate these stages in an accelerated and seemingly healthy fashion. The diagnosis immediately following ABR testing involved both parents and thus did not require the mother alone to remember and interpret the information later to other family members. The shock and grief of both parents was intense and surfaced immediately. This was soon followed by statements of denial and disbelief such as "Look at him— he's healthy and bright—he can't be *deaf*—are you telling us he hears *nothing?*" By the end of the session, the parents were discussing the dreaded impact on the grandparents and the hopefulness of the parent–infant program. There were many new surges of hopefulness as the parents moved through the various stages asso- ciated with diagnosis of a handicap, and each time the hope was relinquished, the pain was revived. The feelings of these parents were explored carefully, and throughout the counseling, support of other parents and professionals remained available to them. For this particular family, we can only speculate as to whether the sensitivity of the pediatrician, the immediate availability of the diagnosis, and supportive counseling made the difference or whether these parents would have responded favorably under any circumstances. At this time, we anticipate that early diagnosis may reduce some of the problems parents of hearing-impaired children have experienced in the past, but may also introduce an entirely new set of emo- tional responses.

CONCLUSIONS

In our view, the ideal early intervention program must include early diagnosis, comprehensive medical services, a productive strategy for language development, and enhancement of the parent–infant bond. Such a program provides direct inter- vention with the child and a psychotherapeutic counseling experience for the parents to help them achieve a satisfactory emotional adjustment to the birth of a hearing- handicapped child. As a preventive measure, work with parents is seen as the best hope of reducing the high prevalence of emotional and behavioral problems among deaf children and adults.

REFERENCES

Beck, H. Counseling parents of retarded children. *Children,* 1959, *6,* 225–230.
Buscaglia, L. *The disabled and their parents, a counseling challenge.* New Jersey: Charles B. Slack, 1975.
Clark, T., & Watkins, S. *The SKI*HI model* (3rd ed.). Champaign-Urbana, Illinois: Edu- cational Resources Information Center, 1978.
Grinker, R.R. *Psychiatric diagnosis, therapy and research on the psychotic deaf.* Wash- ington, D.C.: U.S. Department of Health, Education and Welfare Social and Rehabil- itation Service, 1969.
Hecox, K., & Galambos, R. Brainstem auditory evoked responses in human infants and adults. *Archives of Otolaryngology,* 1974, *99,* 30–33.
Jewett, D., & Williston, J. Auditory-evoked far-fields averages from the scalp of humans. *Brain,* 1971, *94,* 681–696.

Meadow, K. Parental response to the medical ambiguities of congenital deafness. *Journal of Health and Social Behavior,* 1968, *9,* 299–309.

Mindel, E., & Vernon, M. *They grow in silence—The deaf child and his family.* Silver Spring, Md.: National Association of the Deaf, 1971.

Rainer, J.D., Altshuler, K.Z., Kallman, F.J., et al. (Eds.). *Family and mental health problems in a deaf population* (2nd ed.). Springfield, Ill.: Charles C Thomas, 1963.

Rawlings, B. *Summary of selected characteristics of hearing impaired students.* Washington, D.C.: Office of Demographic Studies, Gallaudet College, 1971.

Rawlings, S. Families Maintained by Female Householders 1970–79. Current Population Reports, Special Studies, Series P-23, No. 107. Bureau of the Census, U.S. Department of Commerce, Washington, D.C., 1980.

Ross, A.O. *The exceptional child in the family.* New York: Grune & Stratton, 1964.

Schlesinger, H., & Meadow, K. Emotional support to parents: How, when and by whom. In D. Lillie (Ed.), *Parent programs in child development centers: First chance for children,* (Vol. 1). Chapel Hill, N.C.: University of North Carolina Press, 1972.

Schulman-Galambos, C., & Galambos, R. Brainstem auditory evoked responses in premature infants. *Journal of Speech and Hearing Research,* 1975, *18,* 456–465.

Simmons, B. Patterns of deafness in newborns. *Laryngoscope,* 1980, *90,* 448–453.

Sohmer, H., & Feinmesser, M. Cochlear action potentials recorded from the external ear in man. *Annals of Otolaryngology* 1967, *76,* 427–435.

Stein, L. *Clinical study of brainstem evoked response (BER) with untestable and high risk children.* Paper presented at the American Speech and Hearing Association, Washington, D.C., 1975.

Stein, L. Electrophysiological test of infant hearing. *American Annals of the Deaf,* 1976, *121,* 322–326.

Stein, L. Counseling parents of hearing impaired children. In L. Bradford & W. Hardy (Eds.), *Hearing and hearing impairment.* New York: Grune & Stratton, 1979.

Stein, L., Merrill, N., & Dahlberg, P. *Counseling parents of hearing-impaired children—a psychotherapeutic model.* Paper presented at the American Speech and Hearing Association, Las Vegas, Nev., 1974.

Jacqueline Z. Mendelsohn

3

The Parent–Professional:
A Personal View

I am the mother of a deaf child. Before assuming my present position in the International Association of Parents of the Deaf, I was also a counseling psychologist in a school program for deaf students. My husband is a psychiatrist who has worked with deaf children and adults. As parents and mental health professionals, we have been thrust into experiencing deafness both personally and professionally.

My personal involvement has been the impetus for seeking solutions to questions that are more apt to arise in the parent–child relationship than in the classroom or the psychotherapist's playroom. My professional viewpoint may be colored by personal bias, thereby affecting both my objectivity and my objectives; however, I hope such shortcomings are overcome by perspective gained through continuing experiences and observations made at home, in association with other parents and professionals, and in the classroom. It seems appropriate to begin where it began for us—with Joshua.

Our son, Joshua, was diagnosed profoundly deaf 1 month before his third birthday. It is difficult to remember when we first became aware that Joshua was different from other infants. We never noticed that he did not turn his head when we entered the room; we were vaguely aware of his lack of babbling but were not particularly bothered. He showed no signs of a physical handicap. My only memory of these early times was when Joshua was 11-months-old. I called a friend who was a psychiatrist and asked for an appointment. I was seeking help because I thought I was not coping well as a mother. I had done well with our older child, Aaron, but when Joshua was an infant I experienced undefined anxiety. Something was not right, but I could not define the problem. As Joshua grew older, his behavior became difficult. He did not listen when we said no. He did not respond when we called his name. In general, he ignored us except for a great deal of pulling and pushing when he wanted something from us. Periodically we would

37

drop pots on the linoleum floor as he sat in his highchair, slam the door when he wasn't looking, or slap our hands behind his head. He responded to all these "sounds." Whenever we approached our pediatrician with questions about his hearing he comforted us, saying, "don't worry, he'll outgrow it."

At the time of Joshua's birth, my husband had graduated from medical school and was doing his internship in pediatrics. During his entire period in training he received only brief review of the anatomical and physiologic basis of deafness. No practical application of the material was offered. As a result, he never learned to appreciate the different behaviors or responses of deaf children until he had to understand them in his own son. It is not terribly surprising that our pediatrician and several other professionals with whom we dealt had minimal knowledge of deafness, cursory understanding of the deaf child, and little or no information of the needs of parents. Thus, the appropriate referral to the knowledgeable professionals was too long in coming.

Joshua's behavior became more physical. He slammed drawers and doors; he flipped light switches on and off; he climbed out of his crib to find us in the night. I remember visiting my mother and tying shut all the doors and drawers in her kitchen to keep Joshua from banging them during our visit.

When Joshua was 2-years-old, we asked a friend who was an audiologist to test his hearing. The diagnosis was that he could hear. Our search for answers continued. The strain between my husband and myself grew because of our individual anxieties. I kept my worries to myself, since I was afraid to appear foolish or hysterical. As the tension grew worse, I blamed myself for being a bad mother, wondering what I was doing that was so wrong. When I became tired of self-blame, I blamed my husband. I was looking for a rescuer and could not find one.

Between the ages of two and three, Joshua had sleeping problems. We could not know that a deaf child in a dark room is completely isolated except for touch and is understandably too anxious to sleep. Consequently, and without full understanding, we stayed in his room until he slept and then crawled out on our bellies so our shadows would not wake him. We took Joshua to another pediatrician who assured us that there was nothing to worry about, then to a neurologist who diagnosed Joshua (with a tuning fork) as "hearing but asphasic," and then to a psychiatrist who diagnosed him as having an "overanxious reaction to childhood." We all went into therapy; I went individually; my husband went individually; we went together. Aaron and Joshua went. For almost 9 months my days were spent driving back and forth to the psychiatrist looking for explanations about our difficult child and the stresses surrounding him.

Over a period of time, communication between my husband and myself increased and improved. We were beginning to voice our worries and hopes to each other again. Joshua's behavior had quieted down, but he was still neither talking nor responding to our voices. On the recommendation of our psychiatrist, we again took Joshua in for a hearing test. This time we did not go to someone who was as personally involved as our friend had been.

I was told by this audiologist that Joshua had a "hearing problem." I was told to put an ''auditory trainer'' on him and ''he would learn to recognize sounds.'' I accepted all this information. Barry, however, felt that the information was not clear and went back to the audiologist. The audiologist told Barry that Joshua was profoundly deaf and that the hearing aid might help him hear some very loud sounds. It was Barry who came home and gave me the diagnosis of Joshua's deafness. As I wept I realized that I had been grieving for a long time and my tears were a ''letting go.'' We had been searching for so long that after the initial shock we were relieved to have a diagnosis.

Within a week we were involved with the Mental Health Services for the Deaf Program, at the University of California, San Francisco, learning sign language and participating in a parent group. Talking with parents who were at different stages in their understanding of deafness gave us the strength we needed for this vulnerable time in our lives. We now had tangible tasks to guide us rather than vague fears to continuously unsettle our lives. The problems we faced could be met by formulating the right questions and seeking answers from inside ourselves or from appropriate mentors from the outside world.

The intensity of those experiences during the early years and the energy needed to resolve and understand each crisis undoubtedly fueled my interest in becoming professionally involved with deafness and in directing my curiosity toward an understanding of the psychodynamics of family members at various stages in their lives. As I look at my past and current experiences with Joshua and consider the stories shared with me by many parents and siblings of deaf children, I recognize key periods in a family's development relative to the growth of their deaf child. These are periods during which families are more vulnerable, more in need of open channels for communication as well as intrafamilial and external supports. I call these periods the ''prediagnostic phase'' and the ''diagnostic phase.'' Quite obviously, any significant change may temporarily shake a family's stability—birth, separation, loss, moves, job changes, etc. Here, however, the underlying issue is the introduction of a disabled child into a family.

PREDIAGNOSTIC PHASE

The birth of a child is in itself a potential crisis for a husband and wife. It is a time that demands a redefinition of roles, a transformation from husband and wife to father and mother. In order to adjust to these changed roles, the parents must learn to clarify their expectations of parenthood and each other through clear, direct modes of communication. When the birth and development of a child is accompanied by anxiety due to a feeling that the child may have a handicap, strain is common. Many parents have reported that the prediagnostic period is often much more difficult to live through than the period after the diagnosis is established.

Anxiety often leads to self-doubt and/or blame embodied in such questions as ''Why can't *I* be a more effective parent?'' and ''Why aren't *you* a better parent?'' Husbands and wives become hostile toward each other and withdraw. Sharing, bonding, and nurturing mechanisms are disturbed in a family with an undiagnosed deaf child. At a time when support between partners is important, the prediagnostic period becomes more often a time of isolation. As the stressed parent tries to cope with the changing relationship, he or she may put a lid on strong feelings that need to be shared. This tendency to repress feelings may promote a denial of the child's symptoms. Anxiety may be handled by a variety of ego defenses, some more disabling to the parent than others. For example, one parent may respond by showing physical symptoms requiring more attention from the spouse and draining energy from the primary focus, the handicapped child. Another may sublimate the anxiety by turning toward outside interests.

A major factor contributing to anxiety is the lack of parental gratification. Deafness is an invisible handicap where unease remains ill-defined because the real handicap of the deaf child is unclear. The child may not turn and smile on hearing the parent's voice. Such behavior may be seen as negative rather than based on a physical deficit. Parents need to feel love from their children and a child who gives little response often leaves the parent feeling empty. I have experienced, as have many of the parents I have worked with, the feeling of being a ''bad'' parent or of being a little ''crazy'' for not being able to define what was wrong with my child and with my parenting. I was caught in the isolation of an undefined stress.

DIAGNOSTIC PHASE

When parents are given the diagnosis that they have a handicapped child, they experience feelings of shock, helplessness, confusion, and anger. Even if deafness had been anticipated because of rubella or familial deafness, the confrontation with the handicap as a reality is overwhelming. The fantasies of presenting a ''perfect gift'' to one's spouse, or presenting the world with a potentially great person may be crushed with diagnosis.* A child is seen as the extension of self, a fulfillment of the parents' dreams themselves.

A disabled child does not fit into the family ''plan.'' In our family, I imagined that I would be the ideal mother, raising a family of intelligent, college-bound children. With Joshua's diagnosis came the questions, ''Can we have a normal life with a deaf child in the family?'' ''What about schools?'' ''What about the future?'' ''Will I have to support him the rest of his life?''

At the time of diagnosis, there is a failure of traditional defenses and a massive attack on self-esteem with resulting depression, feelings of helplessness, free-floating anxiety, and other symptoms. Each parent needs large amounts of ego bolstering, attentive and empathic listening, and constructive planning. The spouse may be able to provide some support as may the extended family. Professionals in the field of health, mental health, education, and vocational planning become very important resources during the diagnostic period.

---

*With little or no personal knowledge of deafness, parental expectations of their child often fall short of the true abilities of an individual who is deaf.

Regardless of the degree of external supports, all parents experience some mourning symptoms upon the diagnosis of their child's deafness. They are grieving the "death of hearing," the death of their dreams of a perfect gift, a perfect child.

Denial

Mourning is a complicated process and may be seen as having several stages. The first stage of the mourning process is denial. During this period, parents resist and ignore the idea that there may be a handicap. Denial is a protection from the anxiety that pervades the family. Accompanying denial is the tendency to shop for cures, seek miracles, or search for doctors to change the diagnosis or prognosis. Denial impedes the communication between parents and professionals who need to put the family on track by focusing on the reality of the disability, the current knowledge on deafness, and the first steps toward family adjustment.

Anger

Often accompanying denial is the next mourning stage, anger. Anger goes in many directions: toward those professionals who work with our children, toward ourselves for producing a handicapped child, and toward the child just for existing. The anger that focuses on the child may be expressed in many ways. Parents may subtly or overtly reject their deaf child. Others may overprotect the child. Both rejection and overprotection show an overidentification with the handicap rather than with the child. Parents who stay locked in either of these positions tend to have more difficulty in concluding their grieving. Many teachers with whom I have worked observe anger when they have an interaction with the parents, seeing the parents as attacking any suggestions they make toward resolving school problems. Should the teacher then become defensive, cooperation becomes impossible.

Parents need strong emotional support during this phase. They need a listening ear, a person (or persons) to whom they can talk and with whom they can share the emotional crisis of having a handicapped child. Ideally, the spouse can offer the most support.

The extended family can be another source of strength. Unfortunately this source of support may not be available because a spouse, a grandparent, or an extended family member may also have difficulty accepting the handicapped child. Professionals also can provide support. Unhappily, it has been my observation that by the time parents have reached the diagnostic stage, their feeling toward professionals are often negative. There have been too many experiences of improper diagnosis, or unrealistic suggestions by professionals.

Reactions to Professionals

Parents tend to be suspicious of any new professionals entering their lives. It is a time when parents are often overwhelmed by advice from well-meaning professionals involved in various aspects of the diagnostic or educational process. The person who informs the parents of the diagnosis may present the handicap in such a bleak and threatening way that the parents see no hope for themselves or their child. Other professionals may be reluctant to speak directly about the handicap and will minimize the problem. They may emphasize the normality of the situation. Most of all, many professionals do not have the skill nor the time to really listen to the parents. Some may tend to be overly directive; others, too vague, superficial, or uninvolved. Parents need honest, clear, direct statements from professionals who are at the same time ready to explore questions and be sensitive to the parents' feelings.

As a parent struggles with raising a handicapped child, he or she not only seeks answers to a variety of questions, but also seeks constancy and reassurance. The professional who can be empathic, positive, and supportive while helping the parent understand and accept the responsibilities of a handicapped child can significantly aid the parent in working through the grief and denial.

Resolution

Some degree of resolution of the grieving process follows the denial and anger stages, particularly if outside intervention is early enough and appropriate in its focus. At this point, parents come to grips with having a deaf child. Resolution simply means the acceptance of having a disabled child in the family. This acceptance allows the family to work with the handicapping condition and be less overwhelmed. It is at this stage when parents can best accept advice, information, and education from professionals. The parents make the commitment to deal effectively with the deafness by learning sign language, speech cues, taking part in school programs, and developing relationships with the child that are qualitatively similar to the hearing sibling. The parents make a commitment to educate themselves about deafness in order to choose appropriate ways for meeting the child's educational, emotional, and physical needs. At this stage, parents are able to admit that they need help and that it does not lessen them to seek an outside source with reliable information on techniques for raising healthy deaf children.

It is well accepted that early parent involvement is of primary importance for the optimal development of the deaf child. I have found that parents who do not resolve their mourning to a significant extent in the initial diagnostic stages rarely, if ever, become fully involved. Those who do not learn an effective communication system with the child during the early years will never really catch up, missing out on many key experiences as well as depriving themselves of the richness of their child's inner life and deeper feelings.

Parents often need help in sorting out the child from the handicap. As a parent–professional, I have the advantage of living with a deaf child. This gives me the ability, on a personal level, to help parents learn to separate which behaviors of their child may be due to the child's personality and which may be due to the handicap. Too often parents make excuses for their child's lack of social development by saying that the child is deaf and therefore doesn't understand. Professionals can help the parents put the child in a proper perspective rather than have the deafness become all-consuming. The following personal anecdote will illustrate this phenomenon.

We went to a psychiatrist to better understand Joshua's behaviors. After we described in rich detail his disruptive behaviors, the psychiatrist asked, "How old is Joshua?" We replied, "Two years old." He then asked, "How tall is he?" We measured from the floor the size of a 2-year-old. Raising his eyebrows, the psychiatrist responded. "I thought from your description of Joshua and his behaviors that he was ten-feet-tall and had arms and legs that encompassed the house." This statement put our child back in perspective for us. We were the adults, Joshua was the child, young in age, small in size. I share this experience with parents I work with in order to help them also bring their child and deafness into proper perspective. Parents accept my opinions and advice because they know I live with the same difficulties they do. I am careful not to judge a parent, but rather I empathize with them while clarifying normal development and maturation. I give parents permission to accept the fact that their lives are more complicated by a deaf child. It is important that parents have feelings of frustration, anger, and grief without thinking that they are bad parents. I have seen that parents who admit to the frustrations of having a deaf child develop stronger, more positive relationships with their child than parents who pretend that nothing in their lives has changed.

METHODS OF HELPING PARENTS

As a professional, I have worked with parents in two general formats: My husband and I have given workshops for parent groups in a particular community, and I have provided educational and therapeutic services to parents whose children have attended the Alaska State Program for the Deaf. The families I see range from those who are just beginning to experience having a deaf child in their lives to those who have lived with a deaf child for years. As we have talked in group or individual sessions, personal statements highlight the nature of present adjustments and the degree to which people have resolved their personal mourning. One mother states, "My son is just like me, he keeps it all inside." Another mother describes her family life before the diagnosis of their child, "My husband was gone a lot. I had most of the responsibility. He didn't want to take my boy anywhere. I hated being alone." This particular couple had a great deal of difficulty sharing their feelings about the problems they were having with their child. At another time this mother added, "My fantasy is to have a more understanding husband who would care more. Neither of us show feelings. I would like to see him cry."

During counseling sessions, I watch particularly for styles of interaction between the parents and with me. In our sessions I often see that for the first time partners are sharing their feelings about their emotional stress. One husband related,

"I'm not as brittle as my wife is about feeling. She thinks things don't bother me but they do. I just don't talk about them."

The stress experienced by parents at the time of the initial session is due not only to the stress of the diagnostic phase but also to the experience of registering their child in a school program for the deaf. It becomes a time of confrontation. The child is handicapped. The child needs special programs. The invisible handicap suddenly becomes visible. The families who have had time between diagnosis and entrance into school often experience the same stress; they see concrete evidence that their child does have special needs. One mother related, "My husband gives me a lot of confidence at times. When the teacher says something is wrong, he shares this with me. Otherwise, I don't think anyone can understand what it's really like to have a deaf child." When I tell parents that I have a deaf child, there appears to be a relaxation on their part. One parent exclaimed, "You really know what I am talking about."

Group involvement has been a particularly useful way of having parents share their feelings about their deaf children. When groups and workshops are held, I have observed that mothers attend more consistently and that parents of younger children predominate. As previously stated, I have found that it is crucial to intervene early and to encourage both parents to be involved in order to minimize the avoidance and divisiveness that can easily develop in families. The groups initially focus on immediate issues, such as communication skills, eating and sleeping patterns, attitudes of siblings or extended family members, and community involvement. I use a reality approach, avoiding jargon, reaching and teaching, sharing mutual experiences. I seek to bring out emotions and provide a forum for the feelings of inadequacy so often repressed by parents when dealing with their day-to-day struggles.

I have found that being a "parent–professional" has given me a valuable "ticket of admission" to the group, allowing me to use my counseling skills without seeming threatening as professionals can sometimes seem. The group approach appears to be particularly successful for reaching parents who are resentful towards professionals; i.e., those who "diagnose" or "inform in an impersonal manner." Many parents speak of experiences of traveling from professional to professional with their children while they look for the correct diagnosis. Often parents find it hard to speak candidly to experts who they fear might minimize their subjective experiences. Parents do express these feelings to each other, often gaining support for their ways of raising a deaf child. In this way, mutual learning occurs without the ambivalence that may be aroused in parents by professionals.

As parents become more trusting of and comfortable with others in the group they find it easier to express deep feelings. They find they are able to begin to say such things as, "I can't cope. I'm in pain. My life is in disarray. There are times when I hate deafness." Then they learn that they need not be overwhelmed by their child's handicap, that they need not reject their child. Deafness can become a part of a family's life. Many have already experienced the satisfaction of a deaf child well-integrated into the family.

The ultimate goal, which parents and professionals have alike for the deaf child, is that the child may reach his or her whole potential. Positive expectations aid the child in building feelings of positive self-esteem. In working with families, I have found that parents who receive positive support and information in turn convey to their children positive expectations and feelings.

CONCLUSIONS

This paper would not be complete without a statement or two about some of the difficulties of being both a parent and a professional. Wearing two hats can be an exhausting experience. A major source of difficulty for me has been in finding a balance between my professional training and my emotional involvement as a parent of a deaf child. On one hand, I find myself closely in tune with parents, enabling them to be able to talk to me as they have not been able to talk to other professionals. I can identify with families, often to their benefit, as long as I do not overidentify and project my own experiences. I feel a certain intuitive sense in working with children and parents and in relating to other professionals in the community. Perhaps the fact that I can more easily emphathize with families having deaf children makes me a more available and therapeutic resource. I am, after all, one of them.

On the other hand, I find myself overidentifying with parents seeking my assistance, thus becoming less effective as an objective resource. Sometimes I'm overly directive showing personal successes that may not fit their family model at all. What works for me does not necessarily work for them. Parents have projected anger onto me because of the success of my son. Thus, what could possibly be an area of sharing becomes enmeshed in the dangers of comparing the abilities of different children. I have noticed a tendency in myself to parent deaf children in the therapy groups I have held. This crossing of roles may cause the children to pull back or take stands similar to the ones they would take with their own mothers or fathers, thus diminishing my effectiveness as an adult who cares and is different from the parent.

Finally, I often struggle with the reality of being a parent–professional in a program where organizational needs are not always compatible with parental ones. I sometimes find myself straddling the fence, prepared to leap to the aid of one side or the other, only to feel in the end a sense of isolation and diffused identity. Being a member of both camps does not necessarily make one a good mediator.

I am confident that the role of parent–professional is a noble, unique, and relevant one, and that the fellow professional and fellow parent will view the parent–professional as a valued colleague and objective therapist. Bringing both experiences into one person can add a new dimension to the provision of services for deaf children and their families. It is my hope that the parent–professional may help to simplify the process of proper intervention at the proper time.

REFERENCES

Altshuler, K. Psychological development of the deaf child—Problems, their treatment and prevention. *American Annals of the Deaf,* 1974, *119,* 365–375.

Anthony, E.J. & Koupernik, C. *The child in his family* (Yearbook of the International Association for the Child Psychiatry and Allied Professions; Vol. 2). New York: John Wiley and Sons, 1973.

Barsch, R.H. *The parent of the handicapped child. The study of child rearing practices.* Springfield, Ill.: Charles C Thomas, 1968.

Bennington, K.F. Counseling the family of the deafened adult. *Journal of Applied Rehabilitation Counseling,* 1972, *3,* 178–187.

Bernhards, K.S. Parent education and mental health. *Bulletin of Institute of Child Study,* 1954, *16,* 3–15.

Brill, R. *Total communication as a basis of educating prelingually deaf children.* Frederick, Md.: Presented at the Communication Symposium, 1970.

Curtis, M. Counseling in schools for the deaf. *American Annals of the Deaf,* 1976, *121,* 386–388.

Gregory, S. *The deaf child and his family.* New York: Halsted Press, 1976.

Hampton, P.J. Group psychotherapy with parents. *American Journal of Othopsychiatry,* 1962, *32,* 918.

Hefferman, A. A psychiatric study of fifty children referred to hospitals for suspected deafness. In G. Caplan (Ed.), *Emotional problems of childhood.* New York: Basic Books, 1955.

Heisler, V. *A handicapped child in the family. A guide for parents.* New York: Grune & Stratton, 1972.

Mathis, S. *The organization and administration of parent education at the Carver School for the Deaf.* Paper presented at the Convention of American Instructors of the Deaf, Little Rock, Arkansas, June, 1971.

Meadow, K. Schlesinger, H. & DeVos, W. *Mental health services for the deaf.* Hearing and Speech News Reprint No. 38-2-14. Washington, D.C.: National Association of Hearing and Speech Agencies.

Mindel, E.D. A child psychiatrist looks at deafness. *Deaf American,* 1968, *20,* 15–19.

Mindel, E.D. *Program development for young deaf children: Issues and Rationale.* In Craig, W.N. & Barkaloo, H.W. (Eds.). *Psychologist to deaf children: A developing perspective.* Pittsburgh, Penn.: School of Education, The University of Pittsburgh, 1968.

Mindel, E.D., & Vernon, M. *They grow in silence.* Silver Spring, Md.: National Association of the Deaf, 1971.

Mindel, E.D., & Vernon, M. Out of the shadows and the silence. *Journal of the American Medical Association,* 1972, *220,* 1127–1128.

Rainer, J., Altshuler, K., & Fellman, F. *Family and mental health problems in a deaf population.* Springfield, Ill.: Charles C Thomas, 1963.

Rotter, P. Working with parents of young deaf children. In R. Hardy & J. Cull (Eds.), *Educational and psychosocial aspects of deafness.* Springfield, Ill.: Charles C Thomas, 1974.

Sanderson, R. A personal theory of counseling. *Journal of Rehabilitation of the Deaf,* 1974, *7,* 22–28.

Schlesinger, H. Beyond the range of sound. The non-otological aspects of deafness. *California Medicine,* 1969, *110,* 213–217.

Schlesinger, H. & Meadow, K. *Sound and sign. Childhood deafness and mental health.* Berkeley: University of California Press, 1972.

Shapiro, R.J., & Harris, R. Family therapy in treatment of the deaf: A case report. *Family Process,* 1976, *15,* 83–97.

Smith, A. *Parent counseling.* Report of the Proceedings of the Deaf, Washington, D.C., 1960.

Susman, A. *Attitudes towards deafness: Psychology's role: Past, present and potential.* Keynote address to the Commission of Psychology, VII World Congress of the Deaf, Washington D.C., 1975.

Vernon, M. Pschodynamics surrounding the diagnosis of a child's deafness. *Rehabilitation Psychology,* 1972, *19,* 127–134.

McCay Vernon, Ph.D.
Paula Ottinger, M.A.

4

Psychological Evaluation of the Deaf and Hard of Hearing

The increasing demand for services for deaf people brings a parallel need for improvements in the quality and availability of psychological evaluation for these individuals. Psychologists, rehabilitation counselors, school personnel, and other professionals involved with deaf children and adults are often hampered in their efforts to provide effective services because they are unable to obtain a psychological evaluation that provides adequate, accurate information about the client. Such evaluation requires familiarity not only with the various psychometric instruments and procedures, but also with the psychological, educational, communicational, and vocational ramifications of deafness as well. There are, unfortunately, few psychologists who have the necessary training and experience.

The purpose of this paper is to review testing instruments and techniques that have been evaluated by the authors through use with deaf persons. By describing and briefly evaluating the basic psychometric instruments and procedures, it is hoped that a useful reference will be provided for professionals who refer deaf people for psychological evaluation, as well as for psychologists and others having the responsibility of testing deaf persons and/or interpreting such test results. In this way, the probability of obtaining accurate evaluations on deaf adults and youngsters will be increased, thus better serving their needs.

GENERAL CONSIDERATIONS

It is helpful first to establish certain general principles for evaluating deaf clients, and to define what is meant by the term deafness. Within this paper, deafness means lack of sufficient hearing to understand conversational speech, since birth, or loss of hearing before having learned language (before approximately

49

3 years of age). Many of the principles discussed here will also apply, though sometimes to lesser degrees, to the adventitiously deafened and to the hard of hearing, with their varying levels of hearing loss and varying language and communication competencies.

Below are listed some concepts that are fundamental to all types of psychological evaluations of deaf clients. These concepts underlie the discussion on the various facets of evaluation that comprise the balance of the chapter.

1. Of crucial importance is the fact that psychological tests involving verbal language to measure intelligence, personality, and aptitude are not generally valid with a hearing-impaired client. Such tests measure the language deficiencies imposed by a hearing loss; they do not measure intelligence, emotional stability, or other capabilities.
2. Evaluations administered by persons not experienced in testing deaf and hard-of-hearing clients may have appreciably greater error than when administered by one so practiced.
3. Group testing of the deaf and hard-of-hearing is a highly dubious procedure and should at best be regarded as only a screening technique (Hiskey, 1955; Lane & Schneider, 1941; Levine, 1960, p. 221; Myklebust, 1962; Vernon & Mindel, 1978).
4. Often, the congenitally hard-of-hearing client is, from a psychodiagnostic point of view, much more like a congenitally deaf client than speech and responses to sound would suggest. It is therefore vital that tests be given that are suitable for use with a person having a profound hearing loss, in addition to tests ordinarily used with hearing people. Where large differences occur between these two sets of test responses, they often show that the client performed better on the non-language tests. The latter findings should be judged as the more valid in such circumstances.

TYPES OF TESTING

Following are suggestions on the choice of evaluation instruments and their use with deaf adults and children. A review of testing instruments is provided in Tables 4-1 and 4-2. These tables are intended to serve as a concise, easy reference. They are based on our personal experience and the scanty relevant literature available. The tests described are in wide use by psychologists working in schools and agencies for the hearing-impaired (Brill, 1962; Levine, 1960, pp. 222–224; Levine, 1971; Myklebust, 1954, pp. 298–302; Myklebust, 1960, pp. 69–76, 161–177; Myklebust, 1962; Sullivan & Vernon, 1979; Vernon, 1967; Vernon & Brown, 1964).

Intelligence Testing

A clear understanding of the following factors should precede any effort to administer or to interpret the results of intelligence tests with deaf clients.

Table 4-1

Evaluation of Some Intelligence Tests Most Commonly Used with Deaf and Hard-of-Hearing Children and Adults

Test	Age Range Covered	Evaluation
Wechsler Performance Scale for Children—Revised (WISC-R)	9–16 years	This is at present the best test for deaf children ages 9–16. It yields a relatively valid IQ score, and offers opportunities for qualitative interpretation of factors such as brain injury or emotional disturbance (Wechsler, 1955, pp. 80–81). It has good interest appeal and is relatively easy to administer and reasonable in cost.
Wechsler Performance Scale for Adults (1955)	16–70 years	This is at present the best test for deaf adults. It yields IQ scores and offers opportunities for qualitative interpretation of factors such as brain injury or emotional disturbance (Wechsler, 1955, pp. 80–81). It has good interest appeal, is relatively easy to administer, and is reasonable in cost. The rating is the same as the rating on the Wechsler Performance Scale for Children.
Leiter International Performance Scale (1948 Revision)	4–12 years (also suitable for older mentally retarded deaf subjects)	This test has good interest appeal. It can be used to evaluate relatively disturbed deaf clients who could not otherwise be tested. This test is expensive and lacking somewhat in validation. In general, however, it is an excellent test for young deaf children. Timing is a minor factor in this test. One disadvantage is in the interpretation of the IQ scores because the mean of the test is 95 and the standard deviation is 20. This means that the absolute normal score on this test is 95 instead of 100 as on other intelligence tests. Scores of, for example, 60, therefore, do not indicate mental deficiency but correspond more

(continued)

51

Table 4-1
Evaluation of Some Intelligence Tests Most Commonly Used with Deaf and Hard-of-Hearing Children and Adults (*continued*)

Test	Age Range Covered	Evaluation
Progressive Matrices (Raven, 1948)	9 years–adulthood	to about a 70 on a test such as the Wechsler or Binet. Great care must be taken in interpreting Leiter IQ scores for these reasons. Raven's Progressive Matrices are good as a second test to substantiate another more comprehensive intelligence test. The advantage of the Matrices is that it is extremely easy to administer and score, taking relatively little of the examiner's time, and is very inexpensive. It yields invalid test scores for impulsive deaf subjects, who tend to respond randomly rather than with accuracy and care. For this reason, the examiner should observe the client carefully to assure that she or he is really trying.
The Revised Beta (Levine, 1960, pp. 203, 206, 269)	Adults	The Revised Beta is a non-language test involving mazes, spatial relations, matching, and similar performance type items. It provides an adequate measure of the intelligence of deaf adults.
Ontario School Ability Examination (Amoss, 1949)	4–10 years	This is a reasonably good test for deaf children within these age ranges.
Nebraska Test of Learning Aptitude (Heider, 1940; Hiskey, 1955)	4–12 years	This test is comparable in value to the Ontario, and is standardized for both hearing and deaf children.
Chicago Non-Verbal Examination (Brown, Stein, & Rohrer, 1947)	7–12 years	This test rates fair if given as an individual test and very poor if given as a group test. The scoring is tedious, and reliability is rather low.

Grace Arthur Performance Scale (Arthur, 1947)	4.5–15.5 years	This is a test that is poor to fair due to the fact that timing is heavily emphasized, norms are not adequate, and directions are somewhat unsatisfactory. This test is especially unsatisfactory for emotionally disturbed children who are also deaf. With this type subject, this test will sometimes yield a score indicating extreme retardation when the difficulty is actually one of maladjustment. It is also poor for young deaf children who are of below average intelligence because they often respond randomly instead of rationally.
Merrill-Palmer Scale of Mental Tests (Sutsman, 1931)	2–4 years	The Merrill-Palmer is a fair test for young deaf children, but it must be adapted in order to be used and requires a skilled examiner with a thorough knowledge of deaf children.
Goodenough Draw-A-Man Test (1926)	8.5–11 years	Directions are very difficult to give young children in a standardized manner. Scoring is less objective than would be desired, so this test is relatively unreliable. It does, however, have some projective value in terms of personality assessment.
Randalls Island Performance Test (1932)	2–5 years	This is one of the few nonverbal instruments available for measuring preschool children. It consists of a wide range of performance and manipulative tasks, which, used by a competent examiner, provide diagnostic and insightful information. This test is relatively expensive, but valuable.

53

Table 4-2
Personality Tests Used with Deaf and Hard-of-Hearing Children and Adults

Test	Age Range Covered	Evaluation
Draw-A-Person (Machover, 1949)	9 years–adulthood	This is a good screening device for detecting very severe emotional problems. It is relatively nonverbal and is probably the most practical projective personality test for deaf subjects. Its interpretation is very subjective, and in the hands of a poor psychologist it can result in rather extreme diagnostic statements about deaf clients.
Thematic Apperception Test (TAT) or Children's Apperception Test (CAT) (Stein, 1955)	Can be used with deaf subjects of school age through adulthood who can communicate well manually or can communicate very well in written language.	This is a test of great potential, if the psychologist giving it and the deaf subject taking it can both communicate with fluency in manual communication. It is of very limited value otherwise unless the deaf subject has an exceptional command of the English language. This test could be given through an interpreter by an exceptionally perceptive psychologist, although it is more desirable if the psychologist can do his or her own communicating.
Rorschach Ink Blot Test (Rorschach, 1942)	Can be given to deaf subjects as soon as they are able to communicate fluently manually or if they can communicate with exceptional skill orally.	In order for the Rorschach to be used, it is almost absolutely necessary that the psychologist giving it and the deaf subject taking it be fluent in manual communication. Even under these circumstances, it is debatable if it yields much of value unless the subject is of above-average intelligence. It would be possible with a very bright deaf subject who had a remarkable proficiency in English to administer a Rorschach through writing, but this would be a dubious procedure.
The House Tree Test (Buck, 1949)	School age through adulthood	This is a procedure similar to the Draw-A-Person test. It requires little verbal communication and affords the competent clinician some valuable insight into basic personality dynamics of the subject.
Bender-Gestalt (Bender, 1938)	Best for ages 12 years–adulthood	A useful projective test for personality and also for the detection of brain damage. Because of the rather high prevalence of brain damage among deaf people, it is often valuable to administer a Bender-Gestalt to clients who have severe learning problems or who give evidence of bizarre behavior.

First and foremost, it is necessary to re-emphasize the importance of using nonverbal tests in assessing the IQs of deaf persons. Many authors have written on the incorrectness of using verbal tests because such tests yield results that are a measure of language impairment due to hearing loss, rather than a measure of intelligence (Brill, 1962; Burchard & Myklebust, 1942; Heider, 1940; Levine, 1960, pp. 217–221; Lloyd, 1976, pp. 195–224; Myklebust, 1954, pp. 25, 237; Myklebust, 1962; Sullivan & Vernon, 1979). To validly measure intelligence, test instruments for a hearing-impaired population must be the nonverbal, performance type. Tragic consequences have resulted when verbal tests have been given to deaf people. Some people have been misdiagnosed as mentally deficient on the basis of verbal measures. Some have been committed to institutions for the retarded. Only years later have they been found to be of average or above average intelligence when re-evaluated using correct procedures (Lloyd, 1976, pp. 195–224). There have also been many cases of deaf people being denied proper vocational rehabilitation and education because improper tests were employed.

It is possible, however, to obtain valid intelligence test scores for deaf clients using nonverbal performance tests. The discrepancy between verbal and nonverbal tests is illustrated by the fact that it is possible for a deaf person to score at the genius level on a performance IQ test and at the retarded level on a verbal IQ test, or even on the verbal scale of the same tests.

It should be noted that not all nonverbal tests are suitable for use with deaf persons. A major consideration is that, while many have non-language items, they may nevertheless require verbal direction (Heider, 1940; Lane & Schneider, 1941; Lloyd, 1976, pp. 195–224; Myklebust, 1960, p. 62; Wechsler, 1955, pp. 159–161; Zeckel, 1942; Zeckel & Kalb, 1937). Results obtained in testing a client who does not clearly understand the task at hand are obviously open to criticism.

Hard-of-hearing clients may give the impression of being able to understand verbal tests, but this is often an artifact (Levine, 1971; Myklebust, 1962; Lloyd, 1976, pp. 195–224). In testing such persons, it is essential to begin with a performance measure, and then, if desired, to try a verbal instrument. When the score yielded by the former is appreciably higher, the probability is that this is the more valid score, with the lower score on the language-dependent test being due to the subject's hearing impairment rather than being a true measure of intelligence. There are rare occasions when a verbal test may be used with a deaf or hearing-impaired adult who has exceptional language achievement; this, however, is not the rule. Generally, the inclusion of verbal IQ scores in a report is indicative of a poor psychological evaluation of a deaf client, especially if these results are not carefully qualified.

The performance part of many conventional intelligence tests constitutes only half or less of the total test procedure. Therefore, to approach the validity expected of a full IQ test, it is necessary to give at least two performance scales.

Special Considerations in Intelligence Testing
With Children

In addition to the principles discussed above, the following factors are relevant to testing deaf children.

Even more than with hearing subjects, scores on preschool and early-school deaf and hard-of-hearing children tend to be unreliable (Heider, 1940; Hiskey, 1950; Lloyd, 1976, pp. 195–212). For this reason, low scores in particular should be viewed as questionable in the absence of other supporting data.

There is far more danger that a low IQ score is inaccurate than a high one (Vernon & Brown, 1964). This is due to the many factors (fatigue, tension, etc.) that can lead to a child's not performing to capacity; whereas, in contrast, there are almost no conditions that can lead to an artificial performance above capacity.

Intelligence tests for young deaf or hard-of-hearing children (age 12 or below) that base the score on completion within a standardized predetermined time are not as valid in most cases as are other tests that do not stress time (Vernon & Brown, 1964). This is because these children often react to the timing by either working in great haste and ignoring accuracy or else disregarding the time factor completely. In either instance, the result is not necessarily a reflection of intelligence.

As mentioned above, tests administered to any deaf client by psychologists without prior experience in working with the deaf or hard-of-hearing are much more subject to error than are those administered by a psychologist familiar with the subtleties of deafness. This is especially true for hearing-impaired youngsters. One of the reasons for this is felt to be the seemingly atypical attentive set that these children display in testing situations, which has been frequently cited in the professional literature (Levine, 1971; Lloyd, 1976, pp. 195–212; Zeckel, 1942). For example, deaf children will often answer randomly rather than ask for an explanation of directions they do not understand. Or they may exhibit visual attention patterns that seem "atypical" to those psychologists unused to working with deaf children. Examples include such behaviors as highly concentrated visual attention on the examiner (in an attempt to decipher what is being said or required of them), or seeming to be very visually distractable (substitution of vision for the role of audition in maintaining awareness of their environment).

Personality Evaluation

As in the case of intelligence testing, it is important to take into account certain basic factors prior to evaluating specific personality tests.

Personality evaluation of deaf individuals is a far more complex task than IQ testing. For this reason, test findings should be carefully interpreted in the light of case history data and personal experiences with the client. In fact, it is often wise for professionals with knowledge and experience in the field of deafness to view with skepticism results reported by examiners who are unfamiliar with deafness when these findings sharply contradict their own impressions of a deaf person with whom they are familiar.

Due to the communication problems inherent in severe hearing loss, personality tests are more difficult to use with deaf subjects than with the general population (Graham & Kendall, 1960; Levine, 1971; Lloyd, 1976, pp. 195–212; Myklebust, 1954, p. 313; Myklebust, 1960, pp. 121–122; Zeckel, 1942; Zeckel & Kalb, 1937). Not only do these tests depend on extensive verbal interchange or reading skills, but they also presuppose a confidence in the testing procedure on the part of the subject that is difficult to achieve when the person examined does not fully understand what is being said or written. Paper and pencil personality measures are perhaps suitable for hearing-impaired persons with well-developed expressive and receptive language ability; however, such individuals are the exception, and even here the problems of test administration and interpretation make the meaningfulness of results doubtful (Graham & Kendall, 1960; Levine, 1960, pp. 225–226; Levine, 1971; Myklebust, 1954, pp. 121–122; Myklebust, 1962; Vernon & Brown, 1964). If projective measures like the Rorschach or Thematic Apperception Test are used, fluency in manual communication (the language of signs) by the examiner is essential.

There is some question as to whether the norms for the personality structure of hearing people can be appropriately applied to deaf and hard-of-hearing subjects (Lloyd, 1976, pp. 195–212; Zeckel, 1942; Zeckel & Kalb, 1937). Conceivably, deafness alters the perceived environment enough to cause a different organization of personality, in which normality then differs from what it is for a person with normal hearing (Bender, 1938; Hathaway & McKinley, 1951, p. 256; Lloyd, 1976, pp. 195–212; Myklebust, 1954, pp. 115–118; Zeckel, 1942). Although this is presently an unresolved issue, it is one that is frequently raised by scholars in the field of deafness and should be considered in any discussion on the personality of those with severe hearing losses.

The use of interpreters to translate the psychologist's directions into finger spelling and sign language is a questionable procedure because the interpreter must not only be fluent in manual communication, but sophisticated about psychology and testing (Vernon, 1967; Zeckel & Kalb, 1937). Obviously, such an individual would be doing the examining, not interpreting it for another. Therefore, reported results involving an interpreter are not likely to be valid.

In personality evaluations, it is important to note that the seeming confusion and disassociation reflected in the writing of deaf clients with low-level verbal skills rarely indicates equally deranged thought processes. It is usually only the result of language deficiency. Psychologists unaware of this have been known to equate the written language of semiliterate deaf persons with that of schizophrenics. Misdiagnoses have occurred based in large part upon this confusion.

Few personality tests have had wide and successful application with deaf or hard-of-hearing persons because of the difficulties listed above. Those more commonly and effectively used with children and adults are evaluated in Tables 4-1 and 4-2.

Screening Tests for Psychoneurologic Dysfunction

Because of the high incidence of brain dysfunction among deaf children, especially those who a teacher is likely to refer for psychlogical evaluation, discussion of some tests used to diagnose and measure this condition is included here (Vernon, 1961; Vernon & Mindel, 1978). A thorough assessment of neurologic impairment would generally include one or more of these psychological instruments plus neurologic and audiologic techniques of diagnosis (Vernon, 1961; Vernon & Mindel, 1978). A brief discussion of some tests and items from tests that are useful for detecting brain injury follows.

Bender-Gestalt (Bender, 1938).   This is probably the most widely used screening instrument for the detection of gross neurologic impairment. Standardization of norms continues; interpretation requires extensive training and experience. However, the Bender-Gestalt is a valuable part of a test battery for deaf subjects (Vernon & Mindel, 1978).

Wechsler Performance Scale (Wechsler, 1949; Wechsler, 1955).   Quantitative pattern analysis of these scales is of debatable validity as a diagnostic tool for neurologic dysfunction. There is fairly general agreement, however, that in the hands of a capable clinical psychologist, a partial qualitative type of diagnosis is possible (Levine, 1960, pp. 228–229; Myklebust, 1954, p. 301; Vernon & Mindel, 1978).

Memory-For-Designs Test (Graham & Kendall, 1960).   This test is similar in principle to the Bender-Gestalt and has considerable value. Its precise scoring technique controls for variation in age, intelligence, and vocabulary level.

Ellis Visual Designs Test (Strauss & Kephart, 1955, pp. 149, 219).   This test has potential but lacks validation (Vernon & Mindel, 1978).

Strauss-Werner Marble Board Test (Strauss & Kephart, 1955, pp. 152, 215).   This test is potentially excellent but is very difficult to obtain. Scoring instructions are inadequate (Levine, 1960, p. 229; Levine, 1971).

Hiskey Blocks (Heider, 1940).   This test requires a great deal of visualization and abstract ability and is of value for this reason (Heider, 1940; Myklebust, 1954, p. 300; Vernon & Mindel, 1978).

Rorschach (1942).   The use of this test requires not only competency in administration, but also fluency in the use of manual communication. Results reported where these conditions are not met are highly questionable.

Kohs Blocks (Kohs, 1923).   These are similar to the block design subtest of the Wechsler Scales, but have more designs. A qualitative diagnosis is possible, but norms are lacking for organic involvement.

The Diamond Drawing from the Stanford Binet (Terman & Merrill, 1937, p. 230). This test has good validity, is generally available, and can be easily administered.

Various measures of motor ability and development. Among these would be the rail-walking test, tests of laterality, and certain items on the Vineland Social Maturity Scale that pertain to motor development.

CASE HISTORY DATA

The past is still the best predictor of the future. For this reason complete background information on a client, especially if he or she is deaf and may not be accurately evaluated with regular psychological procedures, is of extreme importance. The best psychiatric and psychological evaluations are often based 75 percent upon background information.

With deaf children, it is often possible to obtain complete and insightful information by contacting their school(s). Integrated educational programs, i.e., facilities where the deaf and hearing attend together, may offer valuable data if they have teachers or counselors who are qualified to work with deaf youth.

With a deaf child, all of the information normally included in a case history should be taken. Additional information relevant to the disability is helpful. This would involve the parents' description of the nature of the problem; its etiology and onset; history of the diagnosis and of previous and present professional services relative to the hearing impairment (including schools); medical/developmental history (including vision); familial history of deafness; communication in the home; and family attitudes and coping behaviors toward the hearing loss.

In a case history of an adult, some factors to consider are the client's performance on jobs, whether or not she or he has habitually demonstrated any particular problems or assets, what kind of circumstances have led to success or failure, and what specific educational and vocational skills he or she has mastered.

COMMUNICATION SKILLS

It is in the realm of communication that deafness presents its major handicap. For this reason, it is important that an evaluation include an assessment of communication skills.

There are numerous aspects of communication that should be appraised in the deaf client. Ability with written language (reading and writing) is the first of these. The importance of this skill has been shown by research demonstrating that this is the communication method most widely used by deaf persons at work (Boatner, 1964, pp. 62–69; Lunde & Bigman, 1959). It is vital to determine the client's degree of skill in written language, since this will have important ramifications in determining the type and level of occupational skills open to him or her.

Another area of evaluation having considerable relevance to the deaf adult in the world of work is that of oral communication skills—speech and speech reading.

To be able to speak intelligibly is especially important and helpful. Speech-reading ability is an asset, but even the most skilled deaf lip reader generally finds this an inadequate way to obtain important information and will usually prefer writing. When one remembers that many English words look alike when spoken, it is understandable that the confusion of speech-reading would lead a deaf person to prefer written communication.

Finally, it is helpful to evaluate the deaf client's ability to communicate via manual communication (finger spelling and the language of signs) since this is the means of communication most frequently employed by deaf adults among themselves. Such an evaluation, however, requires that the evaluator have sufficient expertise in these modes to draw legitimate conclusions.

Communication evaluation for deaf children often combines the efforts of the psychologist, audiologist, and speech and language specialist, as well as involving parental input. The child's ability, both expressive and receptive, in written, oral/aural, and manual modes of communication should be specifically evaluated. This information will be relevant to interpretation of the child's performance in other areas of evaluation, as well as to decisions about current functioning and programming/treatment needs.

One final point must be remembered when evaluating communication skills. Many extremely bright and capable deaf persons lack the ability to speak and lip-read. It is of critical importance that the rehabilitation counselor or psychologist not confuse difficulty in communication in any mode, with lack of intelligence. For example, though any individual deaf client may or may not be fluent in manual communication, the majority of deaf individuals will be. Since (like other languages) American Sign Language has its own grammar—not that of English—it may easily happen that a congenitally deaf individual may have a very high IQ and be quite fluent in American Sign Language, yet have written English language that is not developed grammatically. The rehabilitation counselor and the psychologist must be keenly aware of these factors if they are to be fair and helpful to a deaf client.

EDUCATIONAL ACHIEVEMENT

When an estimate of educational achievement is desired, school records should be consulted as the most likely source for such information. There are numerous achievement tests available for all content and skill areas. One of the most widely used within schools for the deaf is the Stanford Achievement Test series, which has been revised for use with deaf students by the Office of Demographic Studies at Gallaudet College.

Rehabilitation counselors and others working with adult deaf clients will also, in many cases, want a measure of the client's level of educational achievement. The most appropriate tests for obtaining this information are the Metropolitan Achievement Tests. This series has norms for deaf and hearing subjects and is easy to administer, but the examiner must make certain that the client understands and successfully completes the sample items for each subtest. Another critical point in using this or any achievement tests is to choose a battery that is at a level appropriate to the person being tested.

In interpreting results of achievement tests with deaf persons, it is important to keep in mind that only about 5 percent of graduates from day and residential schools for the deaf attain a 10th-grade level in educational achievement; 41 percent, 7th or 8th grade; 27 percent, 5th or 6th grade; and approximately 30 percent are 4th grade or below. Most in the last category are termed functionally illiterate by present governmental standards (McClure, 1966).

These figures are given so that a rehabilitation counselor will understand some of the educational problems of deafness and have some baseline data about the norms to be used in judging the educational achievement of a particular client.

APTITUDE AND INTEREST TESTING

In working with deaf adults and older teenagers, a basic part of a complete rehabilitation evaluation is aptitude testing, i.e., finding out the particular abilities that a client may have. As there are hundreds of aptitude tests on the market, it is not feasible to list or discuss them individually. Levine (1960) has discussed this topic thoroughly and well; however, certain information about the following three areas is often of great value because these kinds of aptitudes are directly related to the types of work most deaf people do: (1) manual dexterity; (2) mechanical aptitudes; and (3) spatial relations.

It is important in selecting from the many measures of aptitude available to choose tests that are not primarily dependent on language for either their directions or administration.

Interest tests are almost without exception highly verbal and, therefore, can generally not be used effectively with a deaf person. There are pictorial tests designed for use with clients who are deaf, but they are narrow in scope and offer limited data for a psychological evaluation.

We would be remiss to discuss tests in a rehabilitation framework without mention of the General Aptitude Test Battery (GATB). The standard version of this test discriminates against a deaf client. With the exception of certain parts, it yields more misinformation than help. Fortunately, an adaptation of the GATB for use with deaf clients is now available through the auspices of the Vocational Rehabilitation Administration.

RECOMMENDED TEST BATTERIES

Suggested Test Batteries for Deaf and
Hard-of-Hearing School-Age Children

Because an adequate psychological assessment should properly be based on a series of tests rather than a single instrument, the following test batteries are suggested for the various age groups of a school population.

Preschool. Measurement of intelligence should be based on at least two of the following IQ tests: the Leiter International Performance Scale, the Merrill-Palmer Scale of Mental Tests, or the Randalls Island Performance Tests.

There are no suitable personality tests or tests for neurologic dysfunction for deaf preschool children. Clinical judgment and medical, audiologic, and case history data must be exclusively depended upon for evaluation in these areas.

Early school through age 9. IQ tests should include at least two of the following: the Leiter International Performance Scale, WISC-R Performance Scale, Nebraska Test of Learning Aptitude, Ontario Test of School Ability, Goodenough Draw-A-Man Test, or Progressive Matrices. Human figure drawing interpretation and Bender-Gestalt responses should be used to screen for personality deviations and organic brain dysfunction.

Ages 9 through 15. The most appropriate measure of intelligence for this age range is the WISC-R Performance Scale. It can best be supplemented with Progressive Matrices, the Chicago Non-Verbal Test, or the Leiter International Performance Scale. Human figure drawings and the Bender-Gestalt become increasingly valid measures in this age range and are the best screening techniques for personality disturbance and brain damage.

Age 16 through graduation. The WAIS Performance Scale stands out as the superior measure of intelligence for this age range. The second measure for intelligence found most valid is the Progressive Matrices. The Memory-For-Designs Test can be added to the Bender-Gestalt and Draw-A-Person Test as a screening measure for organic brain dysfunction. Vocational tests should be added at this time. Their selection is a highly individual matter depending on the subject and available vocational educational facilities.

Recommended Evaluation for Deaf
and Hard-of-Hearing Adults

An evaluation workup for adult deaf clients is most often done for rehabilitation purposes. For such an evaluation to be complete, the following kinds of information should be included: (1) a measure of intelligence; (2) an evaluation of personality structure; (3) an appraisal of communication skills; (4) aptitude and interest testing; (5) case history data.

Details on choice of tests and procedural guidelines for each of these areas have been provided above, and in the tables that follow. In addition, school records (or other sources) may provide much valuable information.

REFERENCES

Amoss, H. *Ontario School Ability Examination*. Toronto, Canada: Ryerson Press, 1949.

Arthur, G. *A point scale of performance tests* (Rev. Form II). New York: Psychological Corp., 1947.

Bender, L. *A visual motor Gestalt test and its clinical use*. New York: American Orthopsychiatric Association, 1938.

Boatner, B. New England Survey of the young adult deaf. In J. T. Ott (Ed.), *Proceedings of a national workshop on improved opportunities for the deaf*. Knoxville, Tennessee: Sponsored by the Vocational Rehabilitation Administration, 1964.

Brill, T. The relation of Wechsler IQs to academic achievement among deaf students. *Exceptional Children*, 1962, *28*, 315.

Brown, A., Stein, S., & Rohrer, R. *Chicago non-verbal examination*. New York: Psychological Corp., 1947.

Buck, J. The H.T.P. technique, a qualitative and quantitative scoring manual. *Journal of Clinical Psychology*, 1948–1949, 4–5.

Burchard, E. M., & Myklebust, H. R. A comparison of congenital and adventitious deafness with respect to its effect on intelligence, personality, and social maturity (Part II social maturity). *American Annals of the Deaf*, 1942, *87*, 241–250.

Goodenough, F. *Measurement of Intelligence by Drawings*. Chicago: World Book, 1926.

Graham, F. K., & Kendall, B. S. *Memory-For-Designs Test: Revised general manual*. Perceptual Motor Skills Monograph Supplement 2-VII, 1960.

Hathaway, S., & McKinley, J. *Minnesota multiphasic personality inventory manual* (Rev. ed.). New York: Psychological Corp., 1951.

Heider, G. M. The thinking of the deaf child. *Volta Review*, 1940, *42*, 774–776, 804–808.

Hiskey, M. S. Determining the mental competence levels of children with impaired hearing. *Volta Review*, 1950, *52*, 406–408, 430–432.

Hiskey, M. S. *Nebraska Test of Learning Aptitude for young deaf children*. Lincoln: University of Nebraska Press, 1955.

Kohs, S. *The Block Designs Test*. Chicago: Stoelting, 1923.

Lane, H. S., & Schneider, J. L. A performance test for school age deaf children. *American Annals of the Deaf*, 1941, *86*, 441.

Levine, E. S. *The psychology of deafness*. New York: Columbia University Press, 1960.

Levine, E. S. Mental assessment of the deaf child. *Volta Review*, 1971, *73*, 80–96.

Leiter, R. *The Leiter International Performance Scale*. Chicago: Stoelting, 1948.

Lloyd, L. L. *Communication, assessment and intervention strategies*. Baltimore: University Park Press, 1976.

Lunde, A. S., & Bigman, S. K. *Occupational conditions among the deaf*. Washington, D.C.: Gallaudet College, 1959.

Machover, K. *Personality projection in the drawing of the human figure*. Springfield, Ill.: Charles C Thomas, 1949.

McClure, W. J. Current problems and trends in the education of the deaf. *The Deaf American,* 1966, *18,* 8–14.

Myklebust, H. *Auditory disorders in children.* New York: Grune & Stratton, 1954.

Myklebust, H. Guidance and counseling for the deaf. *American Annals of the Deaf,* 1962, 370–415. Vol. 107.

Myklebust, H. *The psychology of deafness.* New York: Grune & Stratton, 1960.

The Randalls Island Performance Series (Manual). Chicago: Stoelting, 1932.

Raven, J. *Progressive matrices.* New York: Psychological Corp., 1948.

Rorschach, H. *Psychodiagnostics.* Berne, Switzerland: Hans Huber, 1942.

Stein, M. I. *The Thematic Apperception Test.* Cambridge: Addison-Wesley, 1955.

Strauss, A., & Kephart, N. *Psychopathology and education of the brain-injured child.* New York: Grune & Stratton, 1955.

Sullivan, P., & Vernon, M. Psychological assessment of hearing impaired children. *School Psychology Digest,* 1979, *8,* 271–299.

Sutsman, R. *Mental measurement of pre-school children.* Yonkers-on-Hudson, New York: World Book, 1931.

Terman, L. M., & Merrill, M. A. *Measuring intelligence.* New York: Houghton-Mifflin, 1937.

Vernon, M. The brain injured (neurologically impaired) deaf child: A discussion of the significance of the problem, its symptoms and causes in deaf children. *American Annals of the Deaf,* 1961, *106,* 239–250.

Vernon, M. A guide to the psychological evaluation of deaf and severely hard of hearing adults. *Deaf American,* 1967, *19,* 15–18.

Vernon, M., & Brown, D. W. A guide to psychological tests and testing procedures in the evaluation of deaf and hard of hearing children. *Journal of Speech and Hearing Disorders,* 1964, *29,* 4–14, 422.

Vernon, M., & Mindel, E. Psychological and psychiatric evaluation. In D. Rose (Ed.), *Audiologic Assessment* (2nd ed.) Englewood Cliffs, N.J.: Prentice Hall, 1978, pp. 125–145.

Wechsler, D. *Wechsler Intelligence Scale for Children.* New York: Psychological Corp., 1949.

Wechsler, D. *Wechsler Adult Intelligence Scale.* New York: Psychological Corp., 1955.

Zeckel, A. Research possibilities with the deaf. *American Annals of the Deaf,* 1942, *87,* 173–191.

Zeckel, A., & Kalb, J. A. A comparative test of groups of children born deaf and of good hearing by means of the Porteus Maze Test., *American Annals of the Deaf,* 1937, *84,* 114–123.

Susan Goldstein Litoff, M.A.
Valerie J. Feldman, M.Ed.

5

Treatment Issues with Deaf Children: An Eriksonian Perspective*

According to Erikson (1963, 1968), it is in the first 3 years of life that a child develops ego controls and advances toward developing autonomy. During this time, the foundations are laid for becoming a healthy, independent adult. Our clinical experiences with emotionally disturbed deaf children suggest that their maladaptive behavior is clearly linked to unresolved psychological issues of early childhood. Paraphrasing Erikson, these children have not successfully resolved the crisis associated with the second stage of early development, the stage of "autonomy versus shame and doubt."

Most of the children we have seen for treatment exhibit two kinds of problems: first, lack of control of impulses, and, second, lack of control of environment. In the first instance, the child cannot effectively modulate internal tensions and therefore creates conflict in the environment in order to reduce anxiety. In the second instance, the child assumes a passive stance because of feeling unable to change the environment.

We have seen deaf adults manifest similar difficulties. Why are these adults responding to environmental stresses in the same way as toddlers? Have there been neither refinements nor modifications of coping behavior? Why is a 26-year-old deaf man asked to leave his workshop program for kicking and punching a peer without provocation and a 9-year-old boy excluded from the public elementary school system for exactly the same reasons? Such behavior in a 2-year-old can be expected. At the age of 9, however, there will be social repercussions that affect

---

*The use of the masculine gender throughout this chapter has been maintained for several reasons. First, it is felt that attempting to neutralize the large number of gender-specific referents would serve only to make the material more cumbersome to read and less personalized. Secondly, it reflects the much higher incidence of emotional and behavioral disturbances in deaf boys as compared to deaf girls.

both child and family. For a 26-year-old the repercussions go beyond the immediate family into the community. What stands in the way of the development of more acceptable social skills? To answer these questions, we will look at Erikson's developmental theory and its applicability to the development of appropriate social behavior.

THE THEORETICAL FRAMEWORK

Erikson posits eight stages of psychosocial development. They are (1) basic trust versus mistrust; (2) autonomy versus shame and doubt; (3) initiative versus guilt; (4) industry versus inferiority; (5) identity versus role confusion; (6) intimacy versus isolation; (7) generativity versus stagnation; and (8) integrity versus despair. Rudiments of each stage are present at birth, and each stage lays the groundwork for the next. Vestiges of each stage remain throughout the entire life cycle, reintegrated and reassimilated again and again. The stages are universal; the duration and the intensity of each may differ according to cultural and societal expectations and needs. The interested reader is referred to *Childhood and Society* for a more complete discussion of Erikson's work (Erikson, 1963).

In the earliest months of life, the infant experiences and responds to the world. Nourishment, nurturance, and comfort for the infant are provided by the primary caretaker, usually the mother. It is through the mother's quality of caretaking and through the quality of the ongoing mother/infant relationship that the infant ultimately develops a sense of basic trust or mistrust about the world. For purposes of this discussion let us assume that the children we speak of have successfully established a sense of basic trust.

The second of the eight stages, autonomy versus shame and doubt, generally occurs between the ages of 18 months and 3 years. During this time the infant begins to be able to stand, and can now explore an environment of expanded boundaries. Having established trust in a primary caretaker and knowing that basic needs will be fulfilled, the infant begins to physically and psychologically separate from the mother. The infant becomes the "toddler" and starts to gain greater control over his body *and* bodily functions. Toilet training becomes a major issue, and the child can now decide when to hold on and when to let go. With the polarization of choices occurring during this stage, it is no wonder that the intrapsychic and psychosocial transactions become the foundation for so many neurotic conflicts of later life.

During the second stage of psychosocial development, a sense of self-control emerges. In order to establish controls, the child needs to receive, and to feel he has received, firm, reassuring, and well-guided controls from parents. Autonomy and pride gradually develop from the child's knowing that he has the ability to make a choice—a choice perceived as good. Sometimes parents are unable to provide the firm outer controls and consistent limits when the child most needs them. They may be unable to say "no" when the child throws food all over the floor; they may spend evenings at home, rather than going out, afraid that the child will overwhelm the babysitter with tantrums; in other words, they let the child rule.

Other parents are overly demanding of the child when applying outer controls. They insist the child conform to their wishes and standards, without giving him the opportunity to make his own choices. The child who senses that his behaviors, activities, and feelings fall short of parental expectations becomes vulnerable and self-conscious. When denied the experience of autonomous functioning, the child may become compulsive in the need to master the environment. The child may insist that his toys be in a specific place or in a particular order, or that the daily routine be highly structured.

Unduly prolonged or intensive battles with the big 'me' of age two or three begin to sculpt the later character traits of unreasoning rebellion or blind obedience. The absence of a caring relationship, someone to want to please and to be like, can hamper the development of conscience and self-control, and yield a personality in which ego is king and impulsive satisfaction of the moment is the guiding rule (Rainer, Altschuler & Kallman, 1969, p. 367).*

Every child experiences some sense of autonomy, some early shame and doubt. But it is the mutual regulation of these feelings between parents and children that leads to the healthy resolution of this critical phase of development. If the child is able to gain appropriate control over the environment, to make choices and decisions, and to feel good about these new experiences, then autonomy and pride develop. If, however, the child is unable to develop self-control, and if others attempt to make his choices for him, then he will be more inclined to become self-conscious and insecure in his dealings with the world. It is this stage, autonomy versus shame and doubt, that we see as the most crucial one in the deaf child's development. Let us consider why this is so.

THE WORLD OF DEAF CHILDREN

In Chapter 1, Meadow comments that professionals tend to rely on the ease of diagnostic labelling and classification when discussing emotionally disturbed deaf children instead of on the in-depth examination of behavioral symptoms and their meaning. Deaf children have traditionally been labelled as "rigid," "immature," and "egocentric." These labels have been overused and unfortunately, have become stereotypes rather than descriptions. As a result, they have lost their usefulness and need to be re-examined.

What does "rigid" mean? What specific group of behaviors has led to the development of the term "rigid" in relation to these children? How can we better understand the child's use of maladpative behaviors to cope with the environment? We cannot look at the child isolated from the environment. Significant people and

---

*Reprinted with permission from Rainer, J., Altschuler, K., & Kallman, F. Family and mental health problems in a deaf population (2nd ed.). Springfield, Ill.: Charles C Thomas, 1969.

real-life situations continually interact with and influence the child's developing ego. In turn, each child's unique personality affects the surrounding environment. It is necessary to look at the interplay of internal and external reality.

A world of silence is a difficult concept for a hearing individual to comprehend—sound can never be blocked out totally. In order to understand why deaf children employ certain modes of behavior to cope with the environment, we need to examine the deaf child's world. Imagine that world, a place without sound, where people move about in response to auditory clues the child cannot perceive. What must it be like to have parents leave for a few days and return as suddenly as they left? What is it like to for him to find himself in a car filled with suitcases en route to an unknown destination? The deaf child frequently lives in a home where people are unable to communicate with him. The world can seem unbearably incohesive, like unrelated pictures projected rapidly onto a screen.

Unable to tolerate change well, the deaf child has often been labeled "rigid." We question, however, whether this "rigidity" is not a very sensible coping mechanism, a way to keep things organized in what seems like, and often is, a chaotic world. The deaf child wants to cling to routine; in this way, the future can be anticipated. This way, he functions without feeling scattered and unsafe.

Pejorative terms frequently used in describing the deaf child ("impulsive," "rigid," etc.) are also terms used by Erikson in describing pathologic states related to the second stage of development (Erikson, 1963). In our experience, most of the pathologic behaviors manifested by children in treatment are directly related to unresolved problems from this early developmental stage. Poor impulse control is a serious behavioral issue for deaf children. Typical is Marjorie, an 8-year-old child referred to our program for "poor control over her behavior." Her teacher reported that Marjorie had a difficult time delaying gratification. For example, when she wanted a snack at 10:00 and snack-time was not until 10:30, Marjorie screamed, kicked, and had tantrums until her wish was fulfilled. Children with impulse disorders act without thinking about the consquences. For instance, a deaf child may be angry with a friend over some misunderstanding. Without thinking that he or she may hurt someone and/or be punished, the child punches a classmate. A deaf child may strike out rather than talking things over.

Hearing people utilize language to channel their impulses. When angry, a hearing person may mutter or call out expletives. The limited language of the deaf child, however, often makes monitoring such behavior impossible. Unable to comprehend verbal explanation, he resorts to socially unacceptable physical means when he cannot get what he wants. Many deaf children get "nos" without the simple explanation naturally given to hearing peers ("Johnny, don't throw the blocks, you may break something," or "Ellen, don't push Judy, you'll hurt her!"). Inadequate explanations foster the deaf child's inability to relate cause and effect, to solve problems, and to make thoughtful decisions about his behavior. Coping mechanisms force the deaf child either to take control of the environment or to be controlled by it.

The deaf children we see for therapy are of varied socioeconomic backgrounds and have had different environmental advantages and disadvantages. Their common characteristic, however, is a tendency to meet basic emotional needs in antisocial or maladaptive ways. On one end of the spectrum, children are referred because of chair-throwing, fighting, stealing, tantrums, cruelty (often directed at animals), lack of ego controls, and poor judgment. These children are categorized as having impulse disorders. At the other end of the spectrum, overly dependent and inhibited children are less frequently referred for treatment. Although they confront many of the same issues as children with impulse disorders, they are not considered management problems in the classroom or at home. However, many of these children are in need of psychotherapeutic intervention.

The deaf child relies on only four basic senses to communicate with the environment. In a world permeated by auditory stimuli, these four senses cannot always supply sufficient information. Aggression against or withdrawal from this confusing world is common. In their extreme forms these reactions are considered pathologic and reflect the deaf child's unsuccessful resolution of earlier issues. To reiterate, successful coping with the second stage of psychosocial development, autonomy versus shame and doubt, is most critical for the healthy development of the deaf child.

THE PARENT'S WORLD: HOW DO WE COPE?

Although deafness may have been suspected earlier, it is most often when the child is between the ages of 1 and 3 years that the parents' suspicions of their child's hearing handicap are confirmed. It is well-documented that parents are emotionally overwhelmed at this time of diagnosis. (Schlesinger & Meadow, 1972; Mindel & Vernon, 1971). They face the sudden loss of their "normal" child. They experience feelings ranging from guilt over having produced a "defective" child and of being "inadequate" childbearers, to anger and hostility toward those professionals who make the diagnoses. They are depressed about the child's hearing handicap and mourn the loss of their "normal" child. There is anxiety over what new directions to take in the educational planning. They are inundated and overwhelmed by the mass of information they have been given. As a result, parental behavior changes. Parents who were formerly available to their children—physically, emotionally, and intellectually—are suddenly unable to "talk" to them. In order to cope with a recent diagnosis of deafness in their child, parents may tighten up, becoming overly demanding of the child and rigid in their expectations. Parents can become overcontrolling, insisting that things be done in particular ways. On the other hand, a parent may loosen up, becoming unable to provide appropriate and adequate controls and limits when the child most needs them. Parents may react to their hearing-impaired child with overprotectiveness, infantilization, and restrictiveness.

Charlie R. is a bright, highly functioning 3-year-old deaf child whose hearing impairment was diagnosed when he was 9-months-old, although it was suspected at 4 months. Charlie is capable of taking care of many of his own needs, but Mrs. R.'s fear of acknowledging his strengths prevents Charlie from utilizing them. A good example is Mrs. R.'s insistence that she continue to dress Charlie each day, although Mrs. R. is fully aware he can do this task for himself. Treatment eventually revealed Mrs. R.'s fear of having Charlie grow up. As long as he remained an "infant" she could continue to provide safety and protection for him. She was frightened that her deaf child would grow up and face a potentially hostile environment. Mrs. R.'s own unresolved guilt feelings around having produced a handicapped baby, manifested through her overprotectiveness, hindered Charlie from becoming an autonomously functioning child.

By squelching the child's functional autonomy through restriction and inhibition, parents can unknowingly lay the foundation for future power struggles. The hearing-impaired child receives more "no's" than "yes's." Directives and commands come without explanations. Rules and regulations seem arbitrary and illogical. In such situations, the child feels lost and confused. Some parents fluctuate between these two extremes, at times being rigid and demanding, at times being unable to exert limits and controls. These parents cannot provide their children with the consistency so vitally needed.

Until the reality of deafness is known, parents and child cannot cope constructively. Consequently, there is a huge discrepancy between parents' expectations and the child's achievements, which creates intense frustration for them both.

The frustration leads to an underlying stress and anger for which parents have no constructive outlets. As a result, they begin to avoid interacting with the child, and he begins to avoid interacting with them. Further attempts at child–parent communication become so stressful and frustrating that both the child and the parents understandably want to escape. Thus, the deaf child is often isolated in his own home, losing the emotional and educational benefits he needs and should get from close parental contact. The parents, in turn, lose the satisfactions of child-raising that they have a right to expect (Vernon, 1974, p. 97).*

Intuitively, the child senses that things are "out of control" for his parents and reacts by attempting to provide the needed controls for himself. He becomes overly manipulative and inflexible in order to establish a sense that he has firm controls over his environment.

Thus, we see that during this critical developmental stage for the child, parents struggle with precisely the same issues that face the child. Who is in control? When? How? With the resulting confusion and bewilderment, parents ask themselves and others "What can I expect?" They need professional support to deal with these feelings, to re-establish and strengthen the normal healthy flow of the parent–child relationship. Unfortunately, this help is not readily available. Few programs are designed to serve the psychological needs of handicapped children and their families. Mental health professionals later involved with the families

---

*Reprinted with permission from Vernon, M. Psychological aspects in diagnosing deafness in a child. In P. J. Fine (ed.): Deafness in infancy and early childhood. Baltimore: Williams & Wilkins Co., 1974.

recognize the inadequacy of services offered at the time of diagnosis and afterward. School personnel, often the only professional contact the parents have, are rarely trained to deal with the psychodynamic issues that face these family members. As a result, the parents do not have an opportunity to explore their attitudes and relieve themselves from the pressures and burdens of painful feelings. Thus, the child often becomes the target for the parents' confused emotions. As parents' conflicts remain unresolved, the autonomy issues with which the children must deal intensify. Parents and children become caught in a vicious cycle. Without the firm outer control the child needs to develop a healthy sense of inner control, the basic foundations for autonomous functioning are not established. This early conflict is at the heart of many emotional difficulties we have seen in our patients and in patients discussed throughout the literature.

CHILDREN OF "SHAME AND DOUBT"

The growing child rebels by taking control over those things mother and father can do nothing about—eating, toileting, and other bodily functions. As the child demands, threatens, and has tantrums to express frustration and anger, he makes the adult feel as powerless as himself. By rendering the adult powerless the child gains control over the situation and feels powerful. The adult feels forced to take control physically, by spanking or other means. The child grows immune to physical controls and, in the battle of wills, can and often does win. In this very complex psychological drama the child moves up and down the power scale. This is the child of "shame and doubt."

Parents often seek help in managing their children later when traditional methods of control have proven ineffective. Their children have not resolved developmental issues of Erikson's second stage and often need professional help in coping with their world. Many of the children who participate in our treatment program come for this reason.

In the initial therapy sessions, children are often bewildered at the lack of restrictions placed upon them. Only two rules exist in the playroom: children cannot break the toys, and cannot hurt themselves or the therapist. The therapist informs the children that what is said and done in the playroom will not be shared with their parents and teachers. Confidentiality is assured. It is often the first time the children have received this courtesy. Although the children have been given a minimum set of limits, it is anticipated that they will perceive the unstated message that the therapist believes they can control and be responsible for themselves, and the children perceive that the adult has respect for their ideas and feelings. The therapist wants to understand the children's world in the way they experience it rather than through the words or reports of others. Children test the integrity of the adult while also exploring their own feelings and capacities. The children's "work" begins to unfold.

The children often test the therapist by refusing to come into the playroom.

While refusing to enter the playroom is unusual behavior for hearing children, it is relatively common behavior for deaf children. Seemingly, through their rigid and immature behaviors, many of the deaf children are asking, "Who is in control?" With the perspective in mind that deaf children are often dealing with early unresolved issues of control, we expect them to refuse to enter the therapy room early and/or intermittently in the course of treatment. Deaf children challenge the therapist with this behavior—"let's see what you'll do now; there's no way I'm going into that room; I don't want to." This situation clearly recreates the power struggles that earlier existed and probably still do exist between the parents and the children. However, in this case, the therapist does not become part of the struggle, rather, he or she first explores whether a child is angry over something in particular. If not, the therapist simply states: "This is our time together. I would enjoy talking and playing with you. However, we cannot play out here. I will be in our room waiting for you. When you feel ready, come in. I hope you come in soon."

Children react with surprise when the adult in charge does not exert authority in a forceful manner. What has been avoided with this statement is the inevitable power struggle that would emerge if the therapist began to coax, bribe, or force the child into the room. These coercive methods and the ensuing struggles are usually long-standing family patterns. In the long run, the parents and the children both lose. The parents get angry and frustrated, exert negative controls, and the children become at once powerful and powerless. The therapist prevents the child from setting up the old patterns. No power struggle can begin with only one person. The therapist, unlike the parent, refuses to participate. In returning to the playroom and engaging him- or herself in other activities, the therapist lessens his or her own frustration and anxiety, thus remaining calm, productive, and therapeutic toward the child. Children have different styles for coping with the new experience therapy provides—freedom of choice and the opportunity to begin to develop autonomy and self-control. No one will force children to do what they say they do not want to do. They are given options.

Tony was hiding under the slide in the waiting room. As he saw his therapist approach he signed, "NO! NO! NO! NO!," then closed his eyes and rolled over. The message was clear that Tony would not go easily to the playroom. His face looked fierce. The therapist touched him softly and asked if something was wrong. He refused to look. She waited. Slowly he peeked out, saw her waiting, immediately closed his eyes, and signed, "No go, no."

Tony's parents looked on, feeling somewhat embarrassed at their "disrespectful" and unruly child, but also feeling good that the therapist was experiencing the behavior they knew well. Although many parents want to intervene when this behavior occurs, the therapist always asks them not to do so.

In time, with gentle prodding by the therapist, Tony looked at her: She let him know that she would be waiting in her office. She returned to the office and noted that 15 minutes of the session time had already passed. Sitting at her desk she left the door open.

After a few moments she heard someone running. Suddenly Tony flashed by the door.

He proceeded to run back and forth past the door for awhile. The therapist remained at her desk jotting notes. There was silence for some time. Then, a scraping noise. The therapist saw Tony scratching his fingers up and down the textured wallpaper of the hallways. When he knew she had been watching for a moment, he turned, glanced at her, and ran away. She returned to her desk. The situation was repeated many times. Each time Tony would look at the therapist, she asked if he was ready to come in. She repeated that she would continue to wait for him. On this occasion Tony never did enter the playroom.

The following session, Tony was again on the slide in the lobby when the therapist greeted him. He repeated his refusal to go to the room. She restated the message she would like to play and talk with him, but could not do so outside of the office. She would return to her office to wait for him.

Tony repeated the behaviors of the previous week in a quick run-through fashion. The therapist heard a knock outside the door; Tony was sitting on the floor next to the entrance. The therapist stated that she understood Tony's difficulty to come into the room. She repeated that she was willing to wait until he was ready. During this second session he entered the room with 10 minutes left to the session.

Tony needed 20 minutes to enter the room on the third session and 10 minutes on the fourth. When the therapist met Tony in the waiting room for the fifth session, he indicated he would meet the therapist in her office. He dashed off and was in the room before she was.

On one or two occasions Tony has preferred to stay in the lobby; however, it generally takes him only a few minutes to enter the playroom.

The preceding vignette illustrates Tony's ability to handle his behavior and impulses when provided with a supportive, nonpunitive, noncontrolling environment. Tony learned that he has behavioral choices that can affect his environment. He learned he can maintain his own behavioral controls. In addition, he has found in the therapist a person who respects his right to solve his own problems.

Tony is one of many children who have tested in this fashion. Each child has individual style and timing. For some children, only two sessions are necessary until they can enter the playroom. Other children need more time.

Another unique aspect of working with hearing-impaired children revolves around their ability to shut out the therapist by simply closing their eyes. With a hearing child the psychotherapist can reach the child by talking, whether or not the child chooses to respond. The auditory sense cannot be turned off—we are forced to hear even when we choose not to listen. The deaf child, however, can close his eyes and thus effectively shut out visual contact. This "weapon" can enrage any adult, stirring up strong feelings of impotence and rejection. A child determined to maintain the power struggle use this technique—one of the strongest means for a deaf child to keep control and manifest power over a therapist.

How does the psychotherapist handle this situation, which evokes such strong negative feelings? The sheer simplicity of the child's technique forces the therapist to taste the isolation of deafness, to feel the frustration engendered by it.

Sean is a 7-year-old deaf boy referred for negative, oppositional behavior at home and at school. He was described as a child whom no one could control, "the most stubborn and spiteful kid." For months, Sean tried to avoid his therapist. He refused to enter the room.

He hid or ran out of the building. After many similar incidents Sean finally came into the playroom. However, he let it be known that although he was physically present, he was not going to permit contact.

Week after week Sean walked to the room, crawled under a table or chair, and closed his eyes. He curled himself up, facing the wall. Sean reacted poorly to being touched. The therapist's challenge was to make contact without alienating him, violating his body integrity, or becoming involved in a battle of wills. The therapist sat close to Sean for a long period of time to let him know she was with him, attempting contact when possible. Slowly Sean began to relate through toys and games in the room. The process took months. After 2½ years of treatment, Sean began to communicate through formal language. Sean needed permission to be afraid, to cry, to feel anger. This child, earlier perceived as "powerful," had a most difficult time exposing his underlying painful feelings.

Another significant treatment issue with which deaf children cope is the emotional injury suffered by them in relation to the hearing handicap. This occurs throughout all developmental stages. Deaf children often experience separation anxiety in the initial treatment phase. The dependence fostered by oversolicitous parents, and frequently supported in the school setting, merges with children's lowered self-esteem to create problems for functioning autonomously. In stage 2, children attempt to gain control of their bodies and the world around them, to separate physically and psychologically from their mothers. Success breeds success; once children feel a certain level of achievement, they move on to more complex tasks.

During stage 2, children gain feelings of success from parents' praise and approval. As noted previously, it is at this very time that parents of hearing-impaired children suffer pain on many levels. To take pleasure in a child's small successes while confronting the fact of having a "damaged" child is difficult. The unspoken message to the child is that he is imperfect, unable to fulfill his parents' goals of and expectations for him. The parents and the deaf child notice hearing playmates utilizing verbal communication more and more. In addition, during this period it is probable that the deaf child receives his first hearing aid. For the hearing-impaired child and his parents, this becomes a period of noticing obvious differences and making judgments. As parents continue to react to their own intense feelings around their child and his handicap, they often are not emotionally available to the child, who does not receive the encouragement necessary to go out and experience the world about him. This is illustrated in the case of a family in which all the children but one, the deaf child, had two-wheel bicycles. The parents were too frightened to permit their handicapped child this freedom. The parents' unstated message to the deaf child was, "You are not as competent as your hearing brothers and sisters. We will take charge by protecting you and making decisions for you." Such a message devastates a child already having to cope with a bruised self-image. This deaf child felt trapped. He expelled his pent-up energies, anger, and frustration through tantrums. The growing child's natural desire to take over his environment was frustrated under these circumstances. As a result, feelings of competency and self-assurance diminished. The child's desire to reach out independently—to separate from mother—became overshadowed by fear. Fear of failure prevented autonomous functioning.

Danny entered the playroom. He looked frustrated. His mood fluctuated between anger and sadness. Finally, toward the end of the session, Danny took the chess set down from the shelf. He carefully lined up all the black pieces on one side of the table, the white pieces on the other side. He indicated that a river lay between the two "armies." The therapist asked who the "armies" were, why they were fighting. Danny replied, "War." The white pieces were the "strong, brave, smart, and hearing soldiers." He indicated that the black pieces were "dumb, weak, sick, and deaf." When the battle ended, not one white piece had fallen; not one black piece was left standing. The deaf army had lost the war. Danny stated that the deaf were "no good, can't do nothing."

Danny vividly described the deaf child's self-image. In treatment he eventually learned that he had many assets and strengths, but he would always remain deaf. A year later, Danny had different feelings about himself. In a discussion with his therapist, he signed "Some deaf smart, some dumb; but hearing same, some smart and some dumb—same."

SUMMARY

Adults are frequently bewildered with the behaviors manifested by children dealing with unresolved stage 2 conflicts. This bewilderment stems from the wide variations in these behaviors—stubborness, clinginess, compliancy, rigidity, compulsiveness, etc. If one views these behaviors through the Eriksonian perspective, it is possible to see them as inherent issues of the development of autonomy within the individual personality. Tony's, Sean's, and Danny's behavioral symptoms, though very different from each other, reflected each child's unique handling of basic stage 2 conflicts.

Throughout this chapter our efforts have been toward elucidating the theoretical basis that underlies our clinical work and its practical application with hearing-impaired children. With the knowledge that children referred for treatment have difficulties stemming from early unresolved issues of control, Erik Erikson's theory of normal psychosocial development has helped us to define our roles and tasks as therapists. Erikson has provided a workable model from which the psychotherapist can create practical, concrete therapeutic interventions for hearing-impaired children and for their families.

What does this mean from a preventive angle? With testing procedures now available to definitively diagnose deafness in infants and toddlers, we need to examine parent–infant and early intervention programs. Beginning at the time of diagnosis, it is of crucial importance that parents be offered a therapeutic setting where they can express, share, and begin to understand their feelings and concerns. In this way, not only can the bonds between parent and child be maintained but also insured and strengthened. A more global approach must be utilized by professionals working with families of deaf children. We emphasize that deafness is much more than an educational issue or an academic problem of language. If we are to develop a program for deaf children and their families that will be of optimal benefit for all involved, we must recognize the social, emotional, and psychological effects of deafness upon the individual and upon the family.

REFERENCES

Erikson, E. H. *Childhood and society*. New York: W. W. Norton, 1963.
Mindel, E., & Vernon, M. *They grow in silence*. Silver Spring, Md.: National Association of the Deaf, 1971.
Rainer, J., Altshuler, K., & Kallmann, F. *Family and mental health problems in a deaf population* (2nd ed.). Springfield, Ill.: Charles C Thomas, 1969.
Schlesinger, H. S., & Meadow, K. P. *Sound and sign: Childhood deafness and mental health*. Berkeley, Calif.: University of California Press, 1972.
Vernon, M. Psychological aspects in diagnosing deafness in a child. In Fine, P. J. (ed.): *Deafness in infancy and early childhood*. New York: Medcom Press, 1974.

SUGGESTED READINGS

Altshuler, K., & Rainer, J. *Mental health and the deaf: Approaches and prospects*. Washington, D.C.: U.S. Department of Health, Education and Welfare, 1969.
Axline, V. M. *Play therapy*. New York: Ballantine Books, 1947.
Davis, H. & Silverman, S. R. *Hearing and deafness*. New York: Holt, Rinehart, & Winston, 1961.
Erikson, E. H. *Identity: Youth and crisis*. New York: W. W. Norton, 1968.
Fine, P. J. *Deafness in infancy and early childhood*. New York: Medcom Press, 1974.
Gesell, A., Halverson, H., Thompson, H., et al. *The first five years of life*. New York: Harper, 1940.
Meadow, K. P. Parental responses to the medical ambiguities of deafness. *Journal of Health and Social Behavior*, 1968, *9*, 299–309.
Meadow, K. P., & Schlesinger, H. S. The prevalence of behavioral problems in a population of deaf school children. *American Annals of the Deaf*, 1971, *3*, 116.
Miller, S. *The psychology of play*. New York: Jaxon Aronson, 1974.
Moustakas, C. *The child's discovery of himself*. New York: Gallantine Books, 1966.
Myklebust, H. *The psychology of deafness: Sensory deprivation, learning, and adjustment* (2nd ed.). New York: Grune & Stratton, 1964.
Naiman, D., Schein, J. D., & Stewart, L. New vistas for emotionally disturbed deaf children. *American Annals of the Deaf*, 1973, *118*, 480–487.
Olshansky, S. Chronic sorrow: A response to having a mentally defective child. *Child Social Casework*, 1962, *43*, 190–193.
Reivich, R. S., & Rothrock, I. A. Behavior problems of deaf children and adolescents: A factor-analytic study. *Journal of Speech and Hearing Research*, 1972, *15*, 84–92.

Schein, J. D. Deaf students with other disabilities. *American Annals of the Deaf,* 1975, *120,* 92–99.

U.S. Department of Health, Education and Welfare *Psychiatric diagnosis, therapy and research on the psychotic deaf.* Washington, D.C.: Rehabilitation Services Administration, 1969.

Vernon, M. Psychological Aspects in Diagnosing Deafness in a Child. *Deafness in Infancy and Early Childhood* (Peter J. Fine, ed.). New York: Medcom Press, 1974, p. 97.

Williams, C. E. Some psychiatric observations on a group of maladjusted deaf Children. *Journal of Child Psychology and Psychiatry,* 1970, *11,* 1–18.

Eugene D. Mindel, M.D.

6

Therapy in the Office or Classroom?

For changing many of the behavior problems of deaf children, the classroom has more therapeutic potential than the psychiatrist's office. Children generally, handicapped children in particular, and children with communication handicaps specifically, are often best helped in places most natural and familiar to them. This seems to be a quantitative matter: the handicap reduces access to the cognitive resources available to the child for processing environmental information. and, an emotional matter: a handicap enhances a child's dependence on family and school. Such dependence can be the cause of anxiety in novel situations such as being in a psychiatrist's office. Deaf children usually have no advance knowledge of what to expect or what is expected of them there, not even the common conceptions within the ken of most hearing people. Turning to a psychiatrist for help in what seems like an alien place may occur only after many months of familiarization or never at all. There are times, therefore, when psychiatric assistance may be better directed at improving the climate in the life situations most natural for deaf children: home and school.

School personnel need assistance in understanding the psychodynamic significance of the deaf child's deviant behavior, especially as it manifests in the classroom. (The term "deviant behavior" is not used here with pejorative implication but only to suggest nonconformance to expected norms.) That behavior is a product of internal and environmental facts that can be discovered and explained. Placing behavior in a psychodynamic context enhances the capacity of school personnel to work more effectively with difficult deaf children. Understanding certain behaviors, like the often seen overly aggressive thrusts, reduces the tendency to react against them. Without feeling inclined to react, a teacher can approach a child with empathy and creativity. The following partially fictionalized case history is offered in demonstration of the above.

CASE HISTORY: ROLAND

Eleven-year-old Roland comes from a family of modest economic and educational attainment. We met because, according to his teacher, he was getting more
than a deserved share of classroom attention. He did this in an aggressive manner
often seen in deaf children: shoving and pinching, acting silly in the classroom,
doing his school work only when and if he wished to.

"What can I do about this behavior?" the teacher asked her supervisor, who
in turn asked me.

I explained to both that I couldn't offer an immediate solution because the
behavior sounded so similar to that of many other deaf children. I wanted the
opportunity to get more facts.

First, an interview with Roland was planned. After that, I met with the school
social worker, Roland's teacher, her supervisor, and the school psychologist.

Since I am only moderately fluent in sign language, being especially unfamiliar
with signs indigenous to his school, and since I had not been continuously exposed
to his speech, my first meeting with Roland was awkward. What I knew of his life
was second-hand. I was left with having to open our discussion by referring to his
aggressive behavior. This immediately aligned me with his parents and teachers.
I had to tell him—after he offered a quick promise not to do these things again—
that it was not my job to punish him; that it was up to other people to decide about
punishments; that we would just talk about the trouble he was having and about
some other things.

Ordinarily, in first meetings with children, I will spend some time defining
my role in relation to them, saying such things as "I'm a kind of doctor who talks
to kids about their worries."

It is necessary to spend time in helping a child understand that this meeting
with an adult will be a neutral nonpunitive experience. When I am asked by teachers
to see a child who is acting-out in the classroom, the potential neutrality of my
position can be defeated from the outset. And when the child fears that his or her
private thoughts will become public through me, the potential for a trusting relationship is diminished.

I tried to shift my discussion with Roland to some of the things he enjoyed
doing and some questions about his home life. I wanted to obtain a sense of the
vitality of his relationship with his parents. I could get none. Roland mentioned a
few of the things that he did with his father but he didn't know even what his
father's work was.

At the end of our first meeting, I felt as if I didn't really understand Roland
much better, and I looked forward to hearing more about him from others. But
since I had at least met him, he was no longer just an acting-out entity, but a child
fully endowed with all the typical human qualities.

The meaning of his impish smile, his slightly stooped shoulders, his difficulty
in looking directly at me might become clear as I listened to others talk about him.
I could not make sense of these minimal behavioral cues without additional data.

When our staff group met, and I listened to others speak about him, I first had to decide what was being asked of me. My identity in this group, on the surface, seemed rather clear. I was the one who would have some ideas about how to make Roland behave differently—better.

In my reading of it, Roland's behavior did not seem to be too far outside an expectable range of behaviors. I was puzzled about why I was being asked to consult on this particular child. Did the teacher intuitively believe that something more needed to be done?

Good psychotherapy is partly a science of intuition. I was on comfortable ground there. My role became a little clearer: help the staff reach below the surface in defining their relationships with Roland by helping to clarify and make more explicit interpersonal and intrapsychic factors that are now vague but disturbing to them. Once that was done, perhaps we would be able to see our way more clearly to some real cooperative efforts and planning.

The social worker had visited Roland's home several times. His mother was described as a pale woman who appeared downtrodden, overwhelmed, and defeated, but she didn't seem to be asking for help. The appearance of needing help is no small matter: seeing it in patients is an important motivator to many people in the mental health treatment sciences. Many want to feel that their services are really desired when they reach out to help others.

To Roland's mother, her son seemed to be just another hardship in her life-long struggle to survive economic and emotional barrenness. The social worker met Roland's father briefly, only once. He also seemed uninterested in the contact. He was known to be a reliable, low-level wage earner, but he seemed emotionally unavailable to his son.

The social worker saw herself as an unwelcome intruder in the parents' home. Neither Roland's mother nor his father seemed to offer much information that would help explain his aggressive behavior.

The psychologist's report indicated average intellectual functioning. Typically, for a deaf child, Roland's performance test scores were superior to his verbal scores. Variations on the subtest scores are helpful classroom guides for academic presentations, but they are not necessarily so for understanding emotional status. Projective tests such as the Rorschach and the Thematic Apperception Test were not performed for two reasons: they do not provide information ordinarily considered to be of use to a classroom teacher, and it is difficult to obtain projective data from deaf children because of the language barriers.

Several questions crossed my mind about the home atmosphere. Did the mother's defeated demeanor and apparent unresponsiveness really mean that she would not respond to guidance, or was this her typical face to the world? Had she always been an untrusting person? Did her lack of trust mean that in most or all previous contacts with mental health workers or school personnel she had felt as if nobody gave her what she was looking for? Did she know what she was looking for? Or, did she have a gnawing life-long hunger, deep and threading back to her own infancy?

I could get no picture of how Roland's father related to his son. They had done some things together—like camping in the summer time—but what was the quality of their communication? Roland's accounts of their interactions were dry and unenthusiastic. To a clinician, this suggests that real involvement and warmth were lacking in the father-son relationship; that the remoteness seen by the social worker was not just resentment of her intrusions into their family life, but went far beyond that. Was this inherent in the father's personality? Did it stem from the minimal-care kind of communication Roland and his father had? Or, had the father felt that having a deaf son was further proof of his own inadequacy?

I wondered about the specific meaning of Roland's aggressive behavior apart from it seeming like typical behavior for some deaf children. Sometimes, children use this kind of behavior to stimulate unresponsive parents. This pattern may be learned very early in a child's life; when an infant's crying or sham rage serves to alert the environment to his internal needs. The less responsive the environment, the greater the intensity these aggressive thrusts into the environment must be. That certainly seemed a possibility in view of the passive demeanor of Roland's mother and the remoteness of his father.

My initial attempts in working with the staff were directed at enhancing perspective and objectivity. Although the available clinical information was still limited, I thought that perhaps we could relieve some of the tensions Roland was creating and propose further steps that might prove helpful by directing the group toward conversation on the worth to Roland of the troublesome behavior at home and at school. In other words, we had to determine what the provocative behavior was worth to Roland such that he was willing to sustain punishment and disdain to preserve it.

I believed that the teacher was angry at Roland and at his parents' unresponsiveness to her presentation of the problems Roland had caused. She didn't think she could rely on the parents to bring pressure on Roland to modify his aggressiveness while in school. The parents retorted that Roland was not a troublesome child at home; they did not seem able to understand his provocative classroom behavior.

Roland's behavior had begun to affect the other classroom teachers as well. They were coming to Roland's teacher with complaints that he was provoking children in their classrooms.

Many teachers feel that their personal anger does not belong in the repertory of satisfactory classroom emotions—controlled annoyance maybe, but deep gut-splitting anger, no! Confronting a teacher with her or his anger may be a necessary task for a psychiatrist, but the psychiatrist should do so only if he or she can speak empathically and has a plan to follow the confrontation immediately in a direction away from the anger back toward the more constructive attitudes that teachers cherish.

The teacher, having felt provoked by Roland, fell neatly into his schemes for relating to adults. Roland can understand provoked people. Helpless rage, which probably describes his parents' life-long condition, had left Roland feeling up in the air. He needed to see an adult angry at him to know where he stood.

The parents, though they didn't verbalize it, probably felt considerable guilt over their angry outbursts toward Roland. We learned about their periodic outbursts only months later, after the mother had reluctantly consented to go to a family service bureau for counseling. This latter experience, though novel, proved quite satisfying to her. She had never felt unselfishly given to.

To Roland, the teacher had become the stand-in parent. What she needed was help in understanding that she was very closely identified with Roland's feelings and point of view. Just as his parents' unresponsiveness left Roland perplexed and helpless, so his teacher felt perplexed by Roland's refusal to change his provocative patterns. Roland made his teacher feel as his parents made him feel.

I proposed a series of meetings with Roland and underscored my availability to the teacher to discuss the classroom management. The social worker made regular telephone calls to the mother, relieving the teacher of the burden. The continued frustrating and nonproductive contacts with the parents had only further solidified the teacher's close identification with the frustration that her pupil Roland was feeling. Such an identification in and of itself is not a bad thing. From it develops the empathy necessary for an effective teacher of handicapped children. But with difficult children, the very things that help create the empathy can become a burden.

The social worker made several more home visits. She finally achieved some small sense that the mother was beginning to trust her; trust her in the sense that the mother believed that the social worker could do something that would make her feel as if she were being helped. She was able to admit to the social worker that she felt having a deaf child was life's final slap; that his birth had deprived her of any further hope that her situation would ever improve. Following this, the mother was able to accept the referral to a family service bureau. The father, however, continued to maintain his distant stance.

DISCUSSION

The foregoing story illustrates the operation of what I would like to call the *dynamic classroom*. It is a modified view of the traditional classroom concept, a place to develop academic skills and acquire knowledge with development of social skills a side benefit. The dynamic classroom should be well-differentiated from classrooms employing behavior modification. The implications of behavior modification classrooms are discussed in this volume by Lennan (Chapter 7). My own position, as a psychoanalytically oriented child psychiatrist, is that specifically designed behavior-modification classrooms may be the best we have now to offer disturbed deaf children—children who are too disturbed to function in regular classrooms but not so disturbed as to require inpatient treatment.

The behavior modifications I am referring to requires changing our notions of how to handle difficult deaf children at home and school by understanding what their behavior means to them and those whom it directly affects. The regular classroom becomes a dynamic classroom: filled with lively human social systems that bring teachers and children into active and knowing exchange. The classroom's vitality is enhanced by the infusion of information on interpersonal systems for teachers and auxiliary personnel, and information that will help them understand, with objectivity, who and what is influencing them and why, and what happens as a consequence. This kind of information will enable the classroom teacher to find creative ways around the child's difficult behavior—in ways that those of us without classroom experience cannot possibly do.

For the psychiatrist, a closer relationship with an established educational setting offers the advantages of seeing and evaluating the child in a real-life context.

In traditional office psychotherapy, a therapist strives for many months to achieve an empathic position with regard to the patient's life—seeing things through the patient's eyes. Communication problems with deaf children limit the development of that empathic position. It is often best achieved by the psychiatrist becoming a more active participant in the life contexts of the child, a direct observer in active ongoing communication with the parents and the teachers.

There are real cognitive and emotional limits on the extent to which children can objectify about their lives. A therapist working in his or her office must depend on descriptions of the child's functioning by the parents and by the teachers. Descriptions of the deaf child's behavior, and the opportunity to gather additional data as questions arise, are necessary for the psychiatrist to apply knowledge to the solution of some of the problems he or she is asked to participate in solving. The psychiatrist never solves these problems alone. As with most rehabilitation activities, he or she is more appropriately considered a member of a team.

Our ability to predict whether or not Roland and most other deaf children are going to be maladapting adolescents or young adults is very limited. The problem now is to help troubled deaf children adapt to their classroom life. If children achieve reputations as being difficult they will cooperate with their environments in building identities that can adversely affect their careers for many school years and sometimes beyond. Now is the time to help these children to alter their behavior in a milieu they already know well.

One phenomenon I have observed while participating in therapy with deaf people: some problems that might be treated and thus not progress far in hearing people may progress to bizarre and unmanageable proportions in deaf people. However, if these problems were dealt with at the appropriate time, they would not be progressive.

It is appropriate, therefore, that the psychiatrist's greatest participation should be when problems are forming, not later on when they are well-crystallized. And most often, the psychiatrist can best deal with such problems in environments natural to and comfortable for the deaf child—such as the classroom.

Robert K. Lennan, Ed.D.

7

Behavior-Modification Model in a Residential Setting for Multihandicapped Deaf Children

A review of the data obtained in the 1972–1973 Annual Survey of Hearing Impaired Children and Youth conducted by the Office of Demographic Studies at Gallaudet College, Washington, D. C., revealed that 3,438 or 7.8 percent of the 43,946 students included in the survey had educationally significant emotional/behavioral problems. The students in the survey represented approximately 80 percent of an estimated total population of 54,000 students receiving special educational services related to hearing impairments. It is important to note that these data include only those hearing impaired children with emotional/behavioral problems who were enrolled in educational programs. Naiman, Schein, and Stewart (1973) reported that 10 percent of eligible deaf students in a suburban New York county were not enrolled in school because they had behavioral problems, and the school system had no classes for emotionally disturbed deaf children. Thus, one might expect the incidence to be significantly higher if data on children who are not currently enrolled in special education programs could be obtained.

The reliability of the data on the incidence of emotional/behavioral problems among deaf children is somewhat suspect, due to the fact that respondents to the Office of Demographic Studies questionnaire are not provided with definitions of the additional handicapping conditions listed. In fact, Jensema and Trybus point out that

"No independent verification of reported handicaps was possible nor was any attempt made to determine the process by which a given reporting source decided to report an emotional/behavioral problem for a particular student. That there were differences among programs in this regard is clear from the fact that the proportion of students reported as having emotional/behavioral problems varied from 1.6% to 28.0% in schools of comparable size."*

---

*Reprinted with permission from Jensema, C., & Trybus, R. J. *Reported emotional behavioral problems among hearing impaired children in special educational programs: United States, 1972–73*. Washington, D.C.: Office of Demographic Studies, Gallaudet College, 1975.

Despite the questionable reliability of the data obtained, the fact remains that many teachers of hearing-impaired children believed that a significant number of their students had emotional/behavioral problems. In their reporting of these students, teachers would seem to be indicating the need for help in dealing with the emotional/behavioral problems confronting them. Schein (1975) suggests that only about half of the multihandicapped deaf children in school are receiving needed special attention.

Many teachers of hearing-impaired children look forward to the establishment of specialized classes and programs that will meet the needs of their students with emotional/behavior problems. While it is true that many states are responding to the need for educational programs for severely multihandicapped hearing-impaired students under mandate of Public Law 94–142, which requires states to formulate master plans for special education, it is highly doubtful that all hearing-impaired children with emotional/behavioral problems will, or should be, placed in such specialized programs. Thus, there will continue to be a need for a viable approach that teachers operating in a variety of settings can apply in dealing with the emotional/behavioral problems confronting them, whether it be in the so-called regular class, in a special class, or in a specialized program for the severely multihandicapped.

POSSIBLE APPROACHES

A basic consideration in planning and carrying out educational programs for hearing-impaired children with behavioral/emotional problems is the selection of an appropriate approach to use. Hewett (1968) describes three possible approaches to dealing with emotional/behavioral problems. The first of these, the psychodynamic interpersonal strategy, is concerned with the meaning and origin of behavior. The second, the sensory neurologic strategy, is concerned with the possible underlying organic causal factors related to behavior. The third approach is the behavior-modification strategy, which views behavior in terms of its adaptive function. The selection of one of these three possible strategies will determine the selection of goals and the procedures or methodology to be used in attempting to attain these goals.

Because both the psychodynamic and sensory neurologic approaches to dealing with emotional/behavioral problems are derived from medical approaches to illness (MacMillan, 1973), the data provided to the teacher by professionals operating from this perspective, while interesting and valid, may be of little help to the teacher in his or her search for an educational prescription for the child (MacMillan, 1969).

This point is illustrated by a story about Mrs. Jones, a teacher of the deaf, who had a boy in her class who concerned her. One day she chanced to meet the school psychologist in the hall and said to him, "Oh, I am so glad to see you, Mr. Brown. I have a boy in my class, Billy Smith, who has many problems and I need some advice on how to work with him." "Oh," said Mr. Brown, "What problems does he seem to have?" "Well," said Mrs. Jones, "his attention span is very short and he is a very active child, never seeming to be able to sit still for any length of time. He has great difficulty with reading. He also has difficulty in getting along with the other children. He accuses them of talking about him and picking on him." "That sounds pretty serious," said Mr. Brown. "I'll arrange to have him tested."

About 2 months later, Mrs. Jones met Mr. Brown again and eagerly asked him about the test results. Mr. Brown said, "I'm certainly glad you referred that boy to me, he has serious problems." "Oh," said Mrs. Jones, "what did you find out?" "Well," said Mr. Brown, "the neurologist who examined him reported that the results of the EEG indicated the possibility of mild central nervous system dysfunction and said that Billy is hyperkinetic. The results of testing I did indicate that Billy is dyslexic and has paranoid tendencies." "My goodness," exclaimed Mrs. Jones, "what does all that mean?" "Well," said Mr. Brown, "I think you will find that Billy will have a short attention span and will be a very active child; that he will have difficulty in sitting still for any length of time. He will have great difficulty with reading. He will also have difficulty in relating to other children because of his feeling that they are talking about him and picking on him."

Mrs. Jones sought help in the hope that she could get a specific educational prescription for Billy, but all she got was a set of esoteric labels which had little meaning or relevance for her. Mr. Brown may also have inadvertently lowered Mrs. Jones' level of expectation for Billy by labeling him as having mild CNS dysfunction, being hyperkinetic, dyslexic, and having paranoid tendencies.

The labels we attach to children in special education generally imply a deficit, and there are indications, as reported by Rosenthal and Jacobson (1968), that the labeling process can have a significant effect on teachers' expectation of children, which, in turn, affect the children's level of achievement. This phenomenon has come to be referred to as "the self-fulfilling prophecy" (see also Meadow, Chapter 1 of this volume).

The above is not meant as a blanket criticism of neurologists and psychologists. Many neurologists work closely with parents and teachers in prescribing and adjusting medication for children to help them function more effectively, and this makes it possible for the knowledgeable teacher to apply the appropriate strategy to shape adaptive classroom behavior with the eventual goal of reducing or eliminating the need for medication.

Psychologists can and do interpret information from psychological test results for teachers, which can be used to develop an educational prescription for the child. Hopefully, this sort of working relationship, which provides practical input for the teacher, will become more widespread as Public Law 94–142 is implemented.

A further constraint in the use of the psychodynamic approach with deaf children with emotional/behavioral problems is the lack of mental health services for the deaf and the shortage of professionals in psychology and psychiatry who are qualified to work with the deaf. Levine (1974), in her national survey of psychological workers with the deaf, found that 83 percent of the respondents had only on-the-job learning as their preparation for psychological work with the deaf, and 90 percent of the respondents were unable to communicate effectively, if at all, in sign language with a manually oriented clientele. This has serious implications when one considers the critical need for meaningful communication between therapist and client in the psychodynamic approach to dealing with emotional/behavioral problems.

THE BEHAVIOR MODIFICATION MODEL

Behavior modification, as its name implies, is primarily concerned with the modification and controlling of behavior. It "concentrates on bringing the overt behavior of the child into line with the standards required for learning" (Hewett, 1967). It does not consider behavior as being symptomatic of some underlying illness or disability. It operates on the premise that behavior is learned and is subject to change according to principles of learning demonstrated in laboratory research (MacMillan, 1969). Because behavior modification applies the principles of learning and learning theory (Skinner, 1953), it places the teacher in the role of the learning specialist, a role he or she is qualified to fill. According to Ullmann and Krasner (1965), the teacher employing the behavior modification approach is concerned with three basic questions:

1. What behavior is maladaptive; that is, which of the subject's behaviors should be increased or decreased?
2. What environmental contingencies currently support the subject's behavior (either to maintain undesirable behavior or to reduce the likelihood of performing a more adaptive response?)
3. What environmental changes, usually reinforcing stimuli, may be manipulated to alter the subject's behavior?

Behavior modification has been used with children with a wide range of handicapping conditions in a variety of special education settings with impressive results. Experience in our unit at the California School for the Deaf, Riverside, and in the Nassau County Board of Cooperative Educational Services program in New York (Naiman, Schein, & Stewart, 1973) has shown that it can be used effectively with deaf children with relatively minor modifications to accommodate for the child's hearing loss.

We first began using behavior modification in our federally funded Pilot Project for Emotionally Disturbed Boys in 1966 (Brill, Davis, & Lennan, 1969). Thirteen of the 21 boys who were subjects in the study over a 2-year period were later accepted into "regular" educational programs for the deaf. Since 1969, 61 children have made the transition from our Deaf Multi-Handicapped Unit into the regular program at our school or in their local school districts.

THE DEAF MULTI-HANDICAPPED UNIT AT THE
CALIFORNIA SCHOOL FOR THE DEAF

At the present time, we have an enrollment of 110 students with a wide variety of combinations of handicapping conditions. Mental retardation and emotional/behavioral problems are the predominant additional handicapping conditions. We have a ratio of 4 students to 1 staff member in our dormitories and classrooms. Our staff consists of 2 principals for the 2 subdivisions within our unit, 27 academic teachers, 2 physical education teachers, a dormitory staff of 30, and a psycho-educational consultant. Our psychoeducational consultant functions as a consultant to our staff. He has a doctorate in special education with specialization in behavior modification and learning disabilities. He had no experience with deaf children prior to joining our staff. He does not carry out psychological testing of children (this is the function of our school's psychometrist), nor does he engage in counseling of students. The major portion of his time and effort is spent in providing in-service training for staff members and parent education in behavior-modification principles and procedures, and in consulting with staff members and parents to design, implement, and evaluate behavior-management programs for individual children. We maintain behavior-modification programs both in our classrooms and in our dormitories.

BEHAVIORAL ANALYSIS

Behavioral analysis is the procedure we use in designing behavior-modification programs for individual children in our unit. It is a procedure common to all programs using a behavior-modification approach.

Our first step in behavioral analysis is the selection of a target behavior to be modified. We ask staff members to list, in order of importance, each of the behaviors that appear to be interfering with the child's functioning in a classroom and/or dormitory setting. Behaviors are described in terms that are both observable and measurable. We avoid the use of terms that are open to a wide range of interpretations, such as "hyperactive," "lazy," "aggressive," or "disobedient." Through this process, a single target behavior is selected that will be the focus of our efforts in working with the child. Having selected a target behavior, we next describe the alternative goal behavior toward which the target behavior will be modified. The goal behavior is stated in the form of a performance or behavioral objective that specifies the observable/measurable behavior the child will demonstrate, how well he or she will be expected to perform the behavior, and under what conditions.

Having selected a target behavior and specified an alternative goal behavior, we next observe and record the frequency of the target behavior. This collection of baseline data is carried out before a behavior-modification intervention is instituted and provides the basis for later objective evaluation of the effectiveness of the intervention. It also provides an objective basis for determining whether the target behavior is occurring as frequently as subjective observation has led us to believe it is occurring. Experience has shown that our perception of a particular maladaptive behavior can be distorted if we have a negative attitude toward a child. Objective observation may reveal that the behavior is not occurring as frequently as we thought it was, or that it is no more serious for the particular child in question than it is for other children in the same group.

We have found that teachers and dormitory counselors are resistant to collecting baseline data on behavior because they perceive it as too time-consuming and as interfering with their primary function. Once they are convinced of its importance and provided with practical technical assistance, they conscientiously observe and record data on behavior. This acceptance of the importance of data collection and recording usually comes about as a result of technical assistance and regular consultations provided by the psychoeducational consultant in designing a program for the child.

At the same time we are observing and recording data on the frequency of a target behavior, we observe and identify "antecedents" and "consequents." Antecedents, as the name implies, are the events that precede the target behavior, that seem to trigger it. Consequents are the events that follow a behavior, the environmental contingencies that support and maintain the target behavior. Observation of antecedents and consequents provides us with valuable information that we can use in restructuring the child's environment to bring about changes in behavior.

Once we have selected a target behavior, specified an alternative goal behavior, observed and collected baseline data on the frequency of the target behavior, and identified antecedents and consequents, we are ready to design an intervention program. This involves the selection of the particular behavior-modification procedure(s) that will be used and the identification of an appropriate reinforcer. We have used a wide variety of interventions in our unit. These have included behavior shaping through the use of primary reinforcers such as candy, soda pop, or crackers awarded on a continuous reinforcement schedule for such basic "readiness" level behaviors as making simple matching responses and maintaining eye contact with the teacher. The most common intervention used in our unit is the token economy in which children are provided with secondary reinforcers in the form of "happy face" tokens, pennies, or marks on a checkcard on a fixed interval reinforcement schedule. These secondary reinforcers are then exchanged for primary reinforcers at the end of time periods ranging from once an hour to once every 2 weeks, depending on the child's level of behavior and maturity. Recently, we have begun to shift from a fixed interval reinforcement schedule to an intermittent reinforcement schedule in some of our classrooms and dormitories and have noticed a significant improvement in the maintenance of levels of adaptive behavior. With some of our higher-functioning children, we have entered into contingency contracting (Homme, 1970), which is the application of the Premack (1959) principle that proposes the use of high-probability behaviors (activities that the child enjoys) to reinforce low-probability behaviors (activities that the child dislikes). In contingency contracting, high-probability activities (rewards) are provided for a predetermined period of time, contingent upon the satisfactory completion of a predetermined number of tasks (low-probability activity).

In all behavior-modification interventions, we pair social approval and praise with the awarding of extrinsic reinforcers, such as tokens and checkmarks. This pairing is designed to help the child reach the point where his or her behavior will be maintained at an acceptable level by such traditional reinforcers as letter grades and teacher praise alone.

We are conscious of the importance of moving children up on the continuum of reinforcers proposed by MacMillan (1970) to more mature levels of reinforcement so that we will eventually be able to wean them from a highly structured behavior-modification program (Fig. 7-1). In line with this goal, we also work at extending the length of time between reinforcing events as the level of the child's adaptive behavior becomes more stable. That is, we provide less and less frequent reinforcement for the child as his or her level of adaptive behavior increases and becomes more stable.

The final step in our behavioral analysis is the evaluation of the effectiveness of the intervention. Once again, we observe and record the frequency of the target behavior over a period of time and then compare the data collected with the baseline data obtained before the intervention was instituted. This provides objective evidence of the effectiveness of the intervention and indicates the need for possible changes in the intervention and/or reinforcer.

Thus, our behavior analysis involves

1. Selecting and specifically describing a target behavior
2. Stating an alternative goal behavior in the form of a performance or behavioral objective

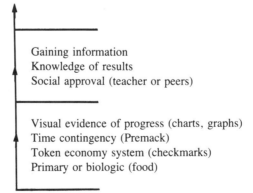

Gaining information
Knowledge of results
Social approval (teacher or peers)

Visual evidence of progress (charts, graphs)
Time contingency (Premack)
Token economy system (checkmarks)
Primary or biologic (food)

Fig. 7-1. A hierarchy of reinforcers (adapted from MacMillan D. [1970, p. 71]).

3. Observing and recording of baseline data on the target behavior
4. Observing and identifying antecedents and consequents
5. Designing an intervention and identifying an appropriate reinforcer
6. Evaluating the effectiveness of the intervention by comparing data obtained after the intervention has been in effect for a period of time with the data obtained during the baseline period.

ADVANTAGES OF THE BEHAVIOR-MODIFICATION APPROACH

We have found that behavior modification offers many advantages as an approach to helping children with emotional/behavioral problems. Some of the advantages follow.

1. Behavior is dealt with in the environment in which it occurs.
2. Minimal verbal communication is required. This is a significant factor in working with nonverbal or low-verbal deaf children.
3. The use of behavior modification promotes individualization by teachers in working with their students.
4. Behavior modification focuses attention on increasing or decreasing specific behaviors rather than on labels that tend to categorize and stigmatize children.
5. Behavior modification places the teacher in the role of learning specialist—the role that he or she is best qualified to fill.
6. Behavior modification has a significant effect on the attitude and behavior of adults working with children. We have found that the use of behavior modification has helped our staff to become more objective, consistent, and positive.
7. Behavior modification brings to the education of the deaf a new approach, developed outside of our profession, which can be used in working with deaf children with emotional/behavioral problems. Our experience has shown that psychologists with a behavior-modification orientation, who have had no prior experience in working with deaf children, can provide meaningful and practical input for teachers of the deaf. This input can help them to deal more effectively with the emotional/behavioral problems confronting them.
8. Behavior modification provides children with regular positive feedback from their teachers and dormitory counselors at frequent intervals during the day. This, as I see it, is the key factor in the success of the behavior-modification approach.

The reaction of many teachers when they are first introduced to behavior modification is that there is nothing new about it, which is certainly a valid observation. Effective teachers have applied these techniques informally since the beginning of time. The significant factor in using a behavior-modification approach is that it provides a model for teachers that helps them apply learning principles more systematically and effectively.

Behavior modification is not a panacea. It does not tell teachers what to teach or how to teach. It can be misused by teachers who are more interested in controlling children than in helping them to learn. It is, however, a tool that can help us to become more objective and effective in helping children with emotional/behavioral problems, if we use it wisely and ethically.

Given the large numbers of hearing-impaired children with educationally significant emotional/behavioral problems, a corresponding lack of mental health services for the deaf, and the shortage of psychologists qualified to work with the deaf, we have found behavior modification to be the most viable approach to help the deaf child with emotional/behavioral problems.

ALTERNATE APPROACHES

If we consider the development of the deaf learner with emotional/behavioral problems as a continuum with an absence of basic readiness behaviors such as attending and responding at one end and the ability to function independently and effectively in social and vocational settings in the community at the other end, then there is a need to consider alternative approaches as an adjunct to the highly structured application of the behavior-modification model in a controlled environment. For teachers and dormitory personnel working with the deaf learner who has serious emotional/behavioral problems within the structure provided by a school setting, the behavior modification model is a pragmatic and effective strategy to help the child develop the readiness behaviors that are essential prerequisites for functioning in a learning environment. Goal behaviors and contingencies are clearly specified and communicated to the learner and contingencies can be manipulated within the controlled environment of the school.

Objectives for learners in a behavior-modification oriented program have, or should have, as their basic goals the development of increasingly higher levels of adaptive behavior with a corresponding reduction in dependence on extrinsic reinforcers and structure within the learning environment. The achievement of these goals is dependent upon a number of variables such as the severity of the learner's emotional/behavioral problems, the learner's level of intellectual ability, the age at which educational intervention was initiated, and the competence of the professional staff to design and carry out an appropriate program to meet the learner's needs.

One of the basic challenges confronting those who work with deaf learners with emotional/behavioral problems in an educational setting is the issue of how to help the children they serve make the transition from the role of student in the protected, structured environment of the school to the role of an independent adult who can function independently and effectively in the community.

Counseling can provide a significant adjunct to behavior modification in efforts to achieve this goal. The goals of behavior modification and counseling are not incompatible in this regard. Both are designed to help the student make appropriate decisions or choices and to develop increased independence, responsibility, and self-esteem. Sussman and Stewart (1971) cite the development of responsible independence as a commonly accepted goal of counseling. Behavior modification, for its part, can help the deaf learner with emotional/behavioral problems develop the adaptive behaviors necessary to acquire the communication skills and level of cognition that are prerequisites to effective functioning in a counseling situation. The counselor, in turn, helps the client understand how his or her behavior and attitudes affect relationships with others. The counselor also helps the client develop an awareness of the need for changes in these areas, and assists in bringing about needed changes. Thus, the behavior-modifications and counseling models can be perceived as being complementary in their mutual goal to help the deaf learner with emotional/behavioral problems achieve responsible independence.

Finally, there is a need for cooperation between those staff members who employ a behavior-modification model in classroom and dormitory settings and the counselor. Together, they can identify those students who are ready to move into a counseling situation, and then later, as counseling proceeds, make decisions relative to the reduction of external controls concurrent with an increase in responsible independence in the school environment. Given these conditions, counseling can serve as a valuable adjunct to the behavior-modification model to help the deaf learner with emotional/behavioral problems develop the skills necessary for effective functioning in society.

REFERENCES

Brill, R. G., Davis, F., & Lennan, R. K. *Pilot program with emotionally disturbed deaf children*. Final Report Project No. G-2422 Grant No. OEG-4-7-062422-0208 U. S. Department of H.E.W., Office of Education, Bureau of Research, 1969.

Hewett, F. Educational engineering with emotionally disturbed children. *Exceptional Children*, 1967, *33*, 459–467.

Hewett, F. M. *The emotionally disturbed child in the classroom*. Boston: Allyn and Bacon, 1968.

Homme, L. *How to use contingency contracting in the classroom*. Champaign, Illinois: Research Press, 1970.

Levine, E. S. Psychological tests and practices with the deaf: A survey of the state of the art. *Volta Review*, 1974, *78*, 298–319.

MacMillan, D. Behavior modification: A teacher strategy to control behavior. *Report of the Proceedings of the 44th Meeting of the Convention of American Instructors of the Deaf*. California School for the Deaf, Berkeley, Calif. From the 91st Congress, 2nd Session, Senate Document No. 91-59. Washington, D.C., U.S. Government Printing Office, 1970.

MacMillan, D. L. *Behavior Modification in Education*. New York: Macmillan, 1973.

Naiman, D., Schein, J. D., & Stewart, L. G. New vistas for emotionally disturbed deaf children. *American Annals of the Deaf,* 1973, *118,* 480–487.

Rosenthal, R., & Jacobson, L. *Pygmalion in the classroom*. New York: Holt Rhinehart, & Winston, 1968.

Schein, J. D. Deaf students with other disabilities. *American Annals of the Deaf,* 1975, *120,* 92–99.

Skinner, B. F. *Science and human behavior*. New York: Macmillan, 1953.

Sussman, A. E., & Stewart, L. G. *Counseling with deaf people*. New York: Deafness Research and Training Center, New York University School of Education, 1971.

Ullmann, L., & Krasner, L. *Case studies in behavior modification*. New York: Holt, Rhinehart, & Winston, 1965.

PART II

The Deaf Adult

Kenneth Altshuler, M.D.
Syed Abdullah, M.D.

8

Mental Health and the Deaf Adult

The first mental health project for the deaf began in 1955 under the joint auspices of Columbia University and the Vocational Rehabilitation Administration. At that time, vocational rehabilitation personnel—traditional champions of the deaf—had become increasingly confounded: many of their deaf clients were educated according to the standards of the day but posed difficult behavioral problems for which there was no place to turn. Among the goals of the project, therefore, was a survey of all deaf psychiatric patients in New York's 21 state mental hospitals—interviewing and rediagnosing them with the aid of manual language—and the establishment of the country's first mental health outpatient clinic for the deaf (Rainer, Altshuler, & Kallman, 1963). Later the project developed an inpatient service where deaf people could be treated by a staff specially trained to work with them and also conversant in manual language. Discharged patients could be given psychotherapy in the outpatient clinic. Vocational rehabilitation personnel were on the premises to coordinate the clinical activities with activities and facilities of the Department of Vocational Rehabilitation (Rainer & Altshuler, 1966). Still later, a preventive mental health program at a school for the deaf and a halfway house were added. The latter was helpful in the patients' transitions from hospital to community (Rainer & Altshuler 1970).

In 1974, efforts were made to develop a three-tiered system of services to deaf children. In this plan, mobile teams deliver services to local schools, one of which has special classes for seriously disturbed children. The classes are staffed by a psychiatrist, a psychologist, and teachers. Supportive services are provided for the occasional youngster who is uncontainable in a classroom.

During the years from 1969 to 1973, a comprehensive study of deaf psychiatric patients and deaf adolescents in Yugoslavia and the United States (New York) was an additional development. The investigation was aimed at defining whether personality characteristics attributed to deafness, and certain of the clinical features observed in the deaf psychiatric patients in the United States were based on the handicap or were culture-related. As part of the same study, psychological test norms were developed for the deaf in both countries, and special facilities for Yugoslavian deaf patients were established (Altshuler et al, 1976).

As the New York group continued its efforts, others too entered the field. Among the first were the programs at the St. Elizabeth's Hospital, Washington, D.C.; the David T. Siegel Institute, Michael Reese Hospital, Chicago, Ill.; the University of California Center on Deafness, San Francisco, Calif.; and others in England, Norway, Sweden, and Yugoslavia.* Often in this chapter, mention will be made of procedures and data derived from the several studies of the New York group. This is solely because it has the longest coherent history and is the source of the authors' personal experience. Mental health workers in other centers have generally confirmed most of what will be reported and have made equally valuable original contributions (Grinker et al, 1971; Meadow, 1969; Mindel & Vernon, 1971; Robinson, 1968; Schlesinger, 1969).

HISTORICAL PERSPECTIVE

The beginning of psychiatric interest in the deaf corresponded in time with the first stirrings of a general revolution in methods of treatment for the mentally ill. Chlorpromazine (Thorazine®), the first in a new series of drugs called neuroleptics (major tranquilizers or antipsychotics) was introduced for psychiatric use in the early 1950s. The neuroleptics seemed to have specific effects on the cognitive and affective (emotional) disorganization that was typical of a large class of psychotic individuals. Chlorpromazine itself is a member of the group of drugs known as phenothiazines. Others of this group have since been found to have similar effects, and still other new, yet comparable drugs have also been developed. Somewhat later, imipramine (Tofranil®) and isocarboxazid (Marplan®), two other types of drugs, were reported to have specific antidepressant qualities, and these two prototypes, useful in treating depression, spurred the development of other substances with similar actions. Finally, lithium carbonate, a simple salt-like compound, was found to combat manic excitement and to be useful in the prophylaxis of recurrent depression as well.

---

*Editors' Note: As of this writing, there are mental health facilities for deaf people at the Mental Health Services for the Deaf, Santa Ana, Calif.; St. John's Hospital, Santa Monica, Calif.; Center for Family Living, Van Nuys, Calif.; Fort Logan Mental Health Center, Denver, Colo.; Gallaudet College, Washington, D.C.; Central State Hospital, Indianapolis, Ind.; Massachusetts Mental Health Center, Boston, Mass.; Boston School for the Deaf, Randolph, Mass.; Hawthorne Center and Northville Regional Psychiatric Hospital, Northville, Mich.; St. Paul-Ramsey Medical Center, St. Paul, Minn.; Maimonides Community Health Center, Brooklyn, N.Y.; Lexington School for the Deaf, Jackson Heights, N.Y.; Central Ohio Psychiatric Hospital, Columbus, Ohio; State Mental Health Program for the Deaf, Portland, Ore.; Dixmont State Hospital, Sewickly, Pa.; Austin State Hospital, Austin, Tex.; Baylor Psychiatry Clinic, Houston, Tex.; Mt. Vernon Center, Alexandria, Va.; Western State Hospital, Staunton, Va.; and Huntington State Hospital, Huntington, Va.

The effects of these discoveries have been dramatic. In 1955, New York State had close to 100,000 people hospitalized for mental illness in state facilities. Primary treatment had ostensibly been psychotherapy, with the adjunctive use of electroconvulsive or insulin coma therapy, which empirical studies had found to be of some benefit. But in fact, the overburdened state hospital psychiatrists were few and had little time for prolonged individual attention to any but the most acute of their patients. For the majority, the care was custodial, with an occasional emphasis on group recreation or cursory group therapy. Similar situations prevailed in states other than New York.

The new psychotropic drugs—neuroleptics, antidepressants, and antimanic agents—have changed this situation considerably throughout the country and the world. The state hospital population in New York alone is down to 30,000 patients. The projected goal for the near future is 20,000. It should be emphasized, however, that medication does not (necessarily) cure mental illness; rather it makes illness more containable. Thus the need for institutionalization has decreased (admission is required less frequently and the average length of hospital stay is reduced), but the prevalence of serious disturbance may not be markedly diminished. It follows, then, that there are far larger numbers of patients in the community than before, and, therefore, a burgeoning need for outpatient services and facilities such as group homes or hostels to care for those who, while not requiring hospitalization, can function only marginally on their own.

DEAF INPATIENTS

Perhaps the deaf would have benefited from these discoveries and changes regardless of other circumstances. The extent of such benefit, however, is somewhat open to question. When the surveys were done in New York, 250 deaf psychiatric inpatients were found in state hospitals alone. This figure excludes other institutions, and specifically the state schools for the retarded, which were estimated to house an additional 250 deaf persons. This number represents a frequency about three times as great as for the hearing, if fractions are made relating the number of deaf and hearing inpatients to their total number (deaf and hearing people) in the state. Reasons for this soon became clear: on one hand, psychiatrists confronted with mute persons gesticulating wildly were more liable to make mistaken diagnoses than with hearing patients whom they understood well. The most common mistake was the diagnosis, "psychosis with mental deficiency" (contributed to perhaps by the implicit confusion of such terms as "deaf and dumb"). On the other hand, diagnosed or misdiagnosed, the deaf patients continued to have a communication barrier that made their participation in treatment and the evaluation of their condition almost impossible. The result was that a far greater proportion of deaf patients had remained more than 5, 10, or 20 years on wards for chronic patients (Altshuler, 1964; Rainer, Altshuler, & Kallmann, 1963).

The hospitalized deaf patients as a group were more emotionally ill than the outpatients. Noteworthy also was that, wherever the hospital and regardless of the diagnosis ultimately assigned, the admitting doctor generally included the terms ''impulsive, aggressive, bizarre behavior'' in the list of presenting symptoms. The same was true in Yugoslavia where more than 70 percent of all deaf inpatients were described (in Serbo-Croation) in identical terms (Altshuler et al, 1976). Unlike the outpatients, most of the deaf inpatients were educational failures. Many had histories showing disturbances as far back as their early school years. Patients with useful speech and lip-reading skills were less common in the hospitalized group, and even the manual language of the hospitalized group was often severely limited. Rediagnosis, therefore, took time, patience, and help from the psychologists who, through experience, adapted their tests and interpretations for work with the deaf. Correctly diagnosed, the hospitalized group showed the full range of psychiatric illness found among the hearing. When allowances were made for excessive lengths of hospitalization among the deaf, even the disatributions were similar to those for the hearing in some of the major categories of illness. Data to compare outpatient frequencies accurately have been more difficult to come by.

TYPES OF MENTAL ILLNESS

Schizophrenia is the largest category of psychotic disturbances. It is typified by a loosening of thought processes, a blunted or otherwise inappropriate emotional expression often mismatched with ideas being expressed, and a high frequency of hallucinations or delusions. One half of the patients in both the deaf and hearing inpatients groups were schizophrenic. Psychosis with mental deficiency was a more frequent diagnosis of deaf than of hearing patients, even after correct diagnoses were made, since the causes of deafness (deafness secondary to retinitis pigmentosa or encephalitis, for example) can often leave brain damage and damaged intellectual ability in their wakes. Psychosis due to alcoholism seemed relatively rare.

One interesting finding was the relative absence of certain depressive signs found commonly among hearing patients with diagnoses of manic-depressive psychosis or with unipolar psychotic depression (often a recurrent disease that occurs without a manic phase). This is not to say that depression, even of psychotic proportions, is necessarily less common among the deaf; when present, however, its manifestations are generally different. A slowing of movement (psychomotor retardation), depressive mien, and delusions of guilt and self-recrimination are common among hearing patients with psychotic levels of depression but rare among the deaf. Severe depressions in the deaf are more likely to show a good deal of anxious agitation, activity levels near or above normal, and often somatic bodily preoccupations.

Occasional hospitalized patients in our survey presented a strange clinical picture. They were primitive, underdeveloped personalities who had been kept hidden at home, were made excessively dependent on their parents, and were blocked from experiences that would have enabled expansion of their intelligence and maturation. Human capacities, however, seem to be limited to a certain range for the expression of emotional illness, and most deaf patients were found to fit the usual diagnostic categories once the alterations in life experiences and symptomatology imposed by deafness were taken into account. The major psychoses have already been mentioned in this connection. Among the nonpsychotic disturbances occasionally found among the hospitalized patients were childhood behavior disorders—a group of illnesses that are usually reactive disturbances to family conflicts, excessive pressures to achieve, or internal physiologic difficulties. These are common among the deaf, in part, because the inevitability of parental confusion, guilt, and ambivalence, and, in part, because minimal brain damage or perceptual motor problems are common accompaniments of deafness, further interfering with adaptation. At times, such patients remained hospitalized after modest improvement occurred in their clinical condition: discharge was often impossible, since family interest had disappeared and foster placements were unavailable in light of the multiple handicaps.

The adult equivalent of the child's behavior disorder is situational maladjustment, a reaction to conditions of temporary psychological overload. These too are not infrequent among the deaf. In the early survey, an occasional patient was found who, once hospitalized, remained long after the causal situation had passed and recovery been achieved, simply because of difficulties in evaluation and post-hospitalization placement.

Neurotic symptoms and neurotic character disorders, rarely a cause for hospitalization, are also comparable in deaf and hearing patients, with the exception that impulse-ridden characters and impulse-control problems are more common among the deaf. Obsessional characteristics, such as meticulousness, punctuality, and minute attention to duty or assigned roles, are relatively infrequent. In theory, this stems from the roles of audition and language in early development, particularly as they are involved in conveying emotions and developing relatedness—major channels for learning disciplinary codes and establishing internal behavior controls. Similar theoretical considerations tie the relative freedom from obsessionalism to the absence of psychomotor retardation and guilt as manifestations of depression among the deaf (Altshuler, 1964, 1971, 1974).

PROJECT SPECIFICS

A teacher of the deaf was included as a permanent project staff member from the beginning to enhance and capitalize on the patients' remaining intellectual and communicative potentials. Also from the outset, the same professionals treating patients during their hospitalization later continued to work with them as outpatients, to maintain continuity of care. In addition, special arrangements with the Department of Vocational Rehabilitation were made to open a patient's case early in the course of hospitalization and do all testing and paperwork expeditiously; thus, training programs were ready for the patient on discharge and long waiting periods were avoided.

Such requirements, in addition to the fact that deaf, mentally ill patients—

even in remission—require closer supervision and staff availability than comparable hearing cases, necessitated a somewhat higher than normal professional staff to patient ratio. Persons attempting to establish similar facilities should bear in mind that the type of professional who provides the outpatient follow-up is less important (providing psychiatric consultation is available for medication review and evaluation of symptom recurrence) than the existence of timely follow-up at home and on the job, and in emergencies.

In other respects our unit was organized to give services normally offered in any good acute treatment facility: group and individual therapy, milieu therapy, occupational and recreational therapy, and pharmacologic therapy. Since the unit was coeducational, both male and female therapy aides were employed. Except as noted above, the pattern of overall staffing was similar to other acute treatment units.

PROJECT RESULTS

Given this setting, the deafness unit has been able, since its inception, to reduce the number of deaf patients hospitalized throughout New York state's hospital system from 250 to somewhat less than 50 at a recent estimate. This is considerably better than the reduction over the same time in the state hospital population as a whole (100,000 to 30,000), and supports the idea that such special services continue to be advisable.

As the back wards have been cleared of their deaf patients with the help of our unit, and as the number of patients maintainable in the community has been increased, the inpatient mix of persons treated at the special facility has undergone a gradual change. Currently, there are fewer acute cases (since they are often capable of being handled as outpatients) and more young individuals with still other handicaps combined with deafness and emotional disturbance, e.g., organic brain damage, mild mental retardation, social disadvantages (homelessness). Therefore, if state centers are to be established, planners should be ready to shift from an acute inpatient treatment emphasis to a larger outpatient population emphasis and to more multiply handicapped and chronic, socially, and therapeutically difficult inpatients.

ADMISSIONS AND PLANNING PROCEDURES

Along with the therapeutic revolution already referred to, there has also been a change mandated by the courts in regard to patients' roles and rights. Patients are better protected now against incarcerations against their will and are less subject to haphazard care. They have the legal right to reasonable treatment and to participate in its planning to whatever extent possible. Concurrently, chronic custodial maintenance of patients certified for hospitalization by the courts has given way to more active treatment of patients admitted on a voluntary basis, and the criteria for involuntary commitment have been strictly delineated.

These criteria are similar for both deaf and hearing patients. They include the bases that the patient has a diagnosable mental disorder and that he or she is more likely to respond to hospital treatment than to care in an outpatient facility, nursing home, or other setting. Minimal indications for hospitalization, in addition, are (1) the likelihood of patients injuring themselves or others; (2) illness of such severity that they cannot participate in treatment programs outside of a hospital; and (3) an unavailability of social support systems so that patients are unable to care for themselves or receive adequate care outside of the hospital.

When deaf patients present themselves for admission or are referred from any source in the state, they are evaluated, their rights are explained to them (insofar as possible in the face of what may be limited communication skills) and they must agree to voluntary admission. Their difficulties are formulated, problem by problem, and within a week, a plan is developed with therapeutic approaches directed at each problem area and with specific staff members assigned to direct responsibility for implementing each aspect of the plan. The treatment plan is designed with as much participation by the patients as possible, its short- and long-term goals explained to them and the patient's agreement and cooperation enlisted. As deadlines for achieving the goals are approached, the patients' progress is reevaluated, and new goals, treatment plans, and deadlines are established for whatever therapeutic goals remain.

As patients improve and time for discharge nears, a similar postdischarge treatment plan is designed. The special vocational counselor who is involved with all patients from the early phases of hospitalization participates as well, and all outside agencies—in addition to the outpatient after-care clinic of the special unit—that will have some part in the patients' subsequent rehabilitation are asked to sign on to this discharge plan.

Treatment is possible for deaf patients with any of the conditions for which hospitalization is a necessity. In the early years of the inpatient unit, it was not uncommon to have patients discharged and working in the community in 6 months, after up to 25 or 30 years of hospitalization elsewhere. Such apparent miracles have diminished as our sweep cleared the system of poorly evaluated patients. But the treatment possibilities remain as optimistic as for the hearing. Given appropriate diagnosis first, and then a knowledge of therapeutic techniques (and the modifications required by deafness), the skills to apply them, a working team, and stubborn patience, equal results are achieveable.

PSYCHIATRIC THERAPIES

In general, a division is made between psychopharmacologic and somatic treatments on one hand and the interactive or interpersonal treatments on the other. Both are directed toward altering feelings, and hence behavior, but the first group has its impact on the body while the second relies on some kind of communication and personal relationship.

On an empirical basis, we know with some certainty which medications or somatic treatments to use, though their mechanisms of action are only slowly being elucidated. We are more clear in theory, though not necessarily always correct, about how the interpersonal, psychotherapeutic techniques work, but less certain of the specific circumstances dictating the choice of one technique over another. In practice, patients who are hospitalized almost always require the use of both types of approaches, while patients with lesser degrees of illness are more likely to receive one or the other, with the usual emphasis being on a form of psychotherapeutic work.

Psychoses

In terms of psychotropic drugs, the primary antipsychotic group includes the phenothiazines. These and certain related drugs (the thioxanthenes, the butyrophenones, and the dihydroindolones) seem to have specific therapeutic effects on the disorganization of personality that is typical, for example, of schizophrenia. Thus, they are useful in the treatment of both acute and chronic forms of schizophrenia and as maintenance therapy for schizophrenic patients in remission. They are also useful in tranquilizing pathologic excitement states in other disorders as well (e.g., delirium tremens, acute mania). With regard to acute schizophrenia, there is a general timetable of response, with symptoms of excitement, aggressiveness, and insomnia subsiding in 2–3 weeks; those of anxiety, depression, and withdrawal being affected in about 2–5 weeks; and the perceptual and cognitive symptoms (of hallucinations, delusions, and disordered thinking) taking up to 6 or 8 weeks. Longer response times are required if dose levels are inadequate, and up to 30 percent of schizophrenic patients are not responsive to medication.

The general availability of these medications has altered prognosticiation in schizophrenia. Acute onset, negative family history, a rich emotional flavor to the illness (as opposed to an emphasis on cognitive deterioration), and early treatment were formerly considered indicators of a likely favorable outcome. The effectiveness of medication has reduced the prognostic importance of such features considerably, and recent studies affirm that the best predictor of rehospitalization is a history of prior hospitalization. Similarly, the best predictor of the ultimate level of function and social adjustment, with treatment, is the level of function attained before the advent of illness (Mintz, O'Brien, & Luborsky, 1976). A current view of deaf schizophrenics yields virtually identical results (Altshuler et al, 1976). Similarly, there seems to be little advantage in long-term over short-term hospitalization. With deaf patients, the primary reason for the former is, increasingly, difficulty in finding a suitable social network in which to place a patient ready for discharge but still in need of further support.

Affective Disorders

In the group of affective disorders (manic-depressive illness, unipolar depression), two types of medication are available and have proven useful in both deaf and hearing patients. The tricyclic antidepressants (e.g., imipramine) are most popular in this country and are effective in about 80 percent of psychotic depressions. Monoamine oxidase inhibitors (e.g., isocarboxazid) are also useful, but since they require special dietary precautions to avoid crises of high blood pressure (which can be induced when the drug interacts with organic substances present in certain foods), they are less frequently used in the United States in general and with the deaf in particular. On adequate doses, response to antidepressants is evident in about 3 weeks. The neuroleptics or major tranquilizers previously mentioned are also useful in cases of agitated depression, where extreme nervousness and excitement are prominent.

Lithium carbonate, as noted earlier, was recently rediscovered to have a calming effect on certain types of excitement. Research has confirmed its usefulness as a specific antimanic agent. It is used in cases of acute mania, often in combination with a major tranquilizer in the initial phase of treatment, and then alone and continuously as a prophylactic agent. It has also been shown to have a prophylactic effect in cases of recurrent depression. The several medications available thus have also altered the outlook for persons with affective disorders. Frequency and duration of recurrences may be reduced, and peaks and valleys of excitement or depression can be smoothed out and diminished.

Since most deaf patients requiring hospitalization present with clinical agitation, the major tranquilizers are the most common medications employed within this population. There is also some evidence that lithium may be an effective adjunct in selected cases even among those diagnosed as schizophrenic or those with personality disorders, when episodic excitement is present (Altshuler et al, 1977).

Behavioral Disorders

For minimally brain damaged youngsters, often misdiagnosed as primary behavior disorders, amphetamine or methylphenidate is useful if organic brain damage is present. If the child truly has a primary behavior disorder reactive to family or other conflicts, psychotherapy is the treatment of choice. Occasionally, one of the tranquilizers may also be utilized, either from the group already mentioned or from among such antianxiety agents as the benzodiazapines, if acute or chronic anxiety requires control. The benzodiazapines are also useful as adjuncts to psychotherapy in the outpatient treatment of adult and child neurotics when anxiety is prominent. Long-term outlook for the minimally brain damaged patient is uncertain, in part being dependent on the extent of organic involvement. For patients with reactive and neurotic disorders, prognoses hinge on the effectiveness of psychotherapy— often offered to families as well as to the symptomatic member.

Treatment Relationships

With or without medication and regardless of the level of illness or the inroads made by it on the patients' personality, the doctor–patient relationship and its psychotherapeutic effect remain central as treatment modalities (Altshuler, 1968).

One may note that people in pain approach the doctor or therapist in different ways. Expectations about the relationship and their own roles vary with level of maturity, sophistication, and the extent to which illness or suffering has eroded each person's natural potentials. The following hierarchical range can describe various attitudes of patients seeking help (Rado, 1953). At the "magic-craving" and "parentifying" levels, patients hope for miracles or view the doctor as children might see their parents, anticipating powerful parental interventions. On these levels, patients do not seek real learning or maturation and may even be incapable of achieving it. At the "self-reliant" and the "aspiring" level, patients expect to cooperate in learning how to help themselves in matters of everyday life or even, through insight and self-change, to use all their potentials for adapative growth.

In practice, people vary in the mixture of attitudes that characterize their treatment relationships, with one level or another in the ascendance at different times in the course of work. With some, the therapist's job is to point out the lower levels (and their sources) when they intrude, so as to make possible greater self-reliance and growth. With others, who may not be capable of such strides, the parentified or magic-craving hopes are utilized by therapists to guide, direct, and support the patients' steps toward self-care under the powerful though illusory protection of the doctor–patient relationship. In many patients with early total deafness, especially those who are severely ill, direct intervention may also be required with families, landlords, employers, and training and helping agencies to pave the way to better social adjustment.

The psychotherapeutic cabinet has a variety of tools with which to help patients at different levels of capacity. The direct relationship with a skilled therapist is the most important. It goes without saying that the ability to communicate easily in the natural language of the patient is a prime prerequisite for such a relationship to take hold and be effective. Group therapy is an adjunct wherein feelings and behavior can be shared with peers and identified as common to the group or shown to be outside the normal range. The group also provides a forum for peer review, advice, support, and friendship. A therapeutic milieu for inpatients, within which support is given for constructive efforts and all activities are planned with therapeutic intent, is also important; such techniques as behavior modification and the token-economy can be invoked to carry this type of reinforcement to a still further degree of refinement.

Psychotherapy, of course, is the art of creative listening. One listens with an open mind to what is said, what is implied, and with an eye as well to what is omitted. If one is open to surprise, patients will oblige with unexpected bits of knowledge, fantasies, and wishes, and sometimes even capacities to integrate new insights better than had been thought possible. This is true for all patients, deaf and hearing. With the deaf, however, some particular precautions are in order.

Stereotyping in Therapy with the Deaf

Efforts to work with, communicate with, study, and to provide services for *the deaf* all contribute to the dangerous tendency of stereotyping the deaf. The communication barrier, the common qualities of relative silence and limited language capacity, the apparent concreteness, are all factors that make deaf people particularly good targets for such propensities. Once embedded, the stereotypes serve at least two functions for the helping persons: it protects them from the discomfiture of close contact with others and the possible arousal of emotions of their own, and it serves as a convenient rationalization with which to protect themselves from the recognition of personal failure. While it makes their jobs safe, it also makes them dull.

For the patients, the stereotype maintained by the world about them can become a self-fulfilling prophecy: they are walled off from others by it and unable to break through without help. Many of our deaf patients have never had the opportunity to explore their ideas with another person. They have not been drawn out, pressed with questions, and stimulated to think. Though influenced by their emotions, they have seldom stopped to identify them, to label them, and to authenticate them by comparing what they feel with what the situation demands. The adolescent or college bull session of the hearing, designed to sharpen ideas and consensually validate feelings, has rarely been available for the deaf psychiatric patient. It is the therapeutic relationship that often provides such opportunities for the first time. Examples from hospital files show what can happen when stereotyping is avoided and the therapist capitalizes and builds on what he or she sees.

S.B. was a 26-year-old congenitally deaf man who irritably insisted that his roommate was selfish and inconsiderate and that it made him mad. He was listened to sympathetically. Over time, his other relationships were talked about: at home before his hospitalization, in school, at work, and in the community. It became evident that he had poor relationships in all these areas. As he repetitively recounted the events, the therapist nailed the situation down with a sympathetic, "He made you mad, too?" With such reflection, the form of exchange altered slowly. The doctor's comments began to be accompanied with questioning smiles and to be received with an increasingly curious and embarrassed ones. The unspoken question of the patient's own role and behavior took the foreground and he was able to begin to give up blaming others for everything unpleasant that happened to him.

A.D. was 20, deaf since 1 year of age, and recovering well—with the help of medication—from an acute psychotic break. He went home for a visit and returned later the same day looking depressed and irritable. Asked about the visit, he replied that it was fine, the train was O.K., the food was good, and that he'd had a good time. As to why he looked sad, he just shrugged his shoulders. The therapist recalled that the patient had left the ward with a suitcase full of clothes, and he asked about it. Only then the patient said he had expected to stay for the weekend, but he couldn't because his mother had said that there was not enough room for him. From this he was able to identify, talk about, and share the feelings of hurt and rejection that the home visit had stirred up in him. He was also able to link these feelings to the sadness and irritation he had felt since his return. Some time later, he was able to open the whole area of parental rejection from early on, and he developed a rather astounding—and useful—level of insight about the displacement of anger he had shown over the years. His impulsive acting-out diminished; he was able to forgive his parents, improve his relationships with them, and rise above his former angry and clinging dependence.

These illustrations show how an alert therapist can help a patient to break through compartments in the mind. In the first case, there was a denial by the patient of his own role, or an isolation of cause from effect. In the second there was also a compartmentalization, a separation of the events of the day and the past from the emotions they induced. By helping the patient to label his feelings, the doctor also enabled him to abort the move from amorphous and inchoate displeasure into immediate irritable or angry reaction. The patients slowly were able to recognize their feelings, identify them, evaluate their appropriateness, and decide how best to respond.

These vignettes, taking only moments to recount, summarize long months of work. Opportunities for contemplation of the self are not always seized upon eagerly, and deaf persons—no less than the hearing—can use language to rationalize rather than understand. Some of what must be admitted is painful or goes against pride. Our impression is, however, that such resistances are somewhat more easily overcome in the deaf than in the hearing. Whether it is a matter of naive honesty, or the attraction of the pleasureable surprise that someone could be really interested, is not clear.

Therapy with "Difficult" Patients

The patients discussed thus far were reasonably apt communicators. With others, insight is sometimes possible despite poor communication skills. Other techniques, however, may be required in instances where the patient's level of personality organization limits the ability or interest in utilizing self-understanding.

A 25-year-old congenitally deaf young man spent most of his meager earnings to get his portraits painted by sidewalk artists. The patient, having never gone to a school for the deaf, and having spent much of his childhood in psychiatric hospitals, had very poor communication skills. Pantomines were about his only means of communication. He was encouraged to bring his portraits to the therapy session to talk about them. During one of his sessions, the patient demonstrated that he wanted to know how long these paintings would last? For many many years after he was dead? Might his grandmother cry while looking at them? Would she continue to hang it on her wall even after he was gone? It was evident that he was seeking immortality and a permanence of sorts for a life that was empty and unfulfilled. His need to belong and to be loved and remembered lead him to a compulsive preoccupation with portraits of himself, for which he was paying several artists weekly installments. Once he was able to give vent to these cravings, the compulsion eased, though he continued to keep his room full of portraits of him smiling down at him from all angles.

Among the many interesting ideas about this patient is the fact that, despite the primitiveness of his communication, he was able to express a series of complex thoughts and feelings once the therapist was receptive to them. Direct admonishments about wasting money or about the need to save money and support himself would not have been helpful, nor would it have brought out the underlying concerns that were driving his behavior.

Another patient, age 28, came to the hospital soon after the birth of her first child. She had an agitated postpartum psychosis, was anxious, tremulous, and depressed, was afraid she would kill her child, and had delusional ideas that perhaps some damage had already been done. After a few weeks on tranquilizers and antidepressents, her anxiety lessened, the delusions subsided, and she was able to talk more freely about her easy frustration and impulsive anger toward the child. It became evident that she felt angry and even a bit jealous of her infant's freedom to be demanding and needy, and that she herself felt helpless and in need of equal care. She had grown up motherless, in the care of an alchoholic and neglectful father, and she had transferred the role of parent to her husband—with whom she behaved as a spoiled child. Exploration of her feelings was of some help to this woman, but her capacity for growth through that route seemed limited and she remained rather childlike.

In this case the therapist capitalized on the patient's tendency to think of him as a good parent by arranging for her to get instruction in child care and by planning with the staff—also cast as parent figures—to reward her with praise and recognition for success in playing out such mothering under staff tutelage. At the same time, group therapy gave her a feeling of the support and interest of her peers. Medication held the psychotic process in check. The direct psychotherapy combined the illusory reward of her magic-craving with the use of what insight she could achieve. She was soon back at home, functioning with some ease as a mother, and being seen regularly in the outpatient clinic and during occasional home visits.

In still more severe cases an even greater emphasis may be placed on medication, direct guidance, and simple support through training programs that can lead to work in sheltered shops and to semi-independent living. For people who require them, both medication and psychotherapy are continued in the outpatient clinic after discharge. Some patients remain attached to the clinic indefinitely for the adjustment of their medication and for intervention and intermittent direct help when situations at home or work build toward crisis levels. For adolescents at the hospital, special classes are arranged at a nearby school for the deaf. The hospital supplies the transportation. The daily length of time in class is variable, depending on the patient's level of health and his or her attention span and tolerance for work. The goal is to transfer patients to regular classes as they improve.

CONCLUSIONS

In general, the principle is to use medication for its antipsychotic or antianxiety effect and to enable a psychotherapeutic relationship to be built; within the framework of this relationship, to seek to define the patients' strengths as individuals and their individual feelings; to formulate their problems with them, and identify and authenticate the emotions aroused in connection with their difficulties; to support gains by means of the therapeutic milieu of the unit and group therapeutic approaches; and to move what gains are made into life beyond the hospital, with the continuous connecting thread of the therapeutic relationship and support of ancillary staff. The mix of these tools and principles varies with each case. *Results* are, of course, the goal. That they can be achieved, and are, is the reward.

REFERENCES

Altshuler, K. Z. Personality traits and depressive symptoms in the deaf. In J. Wartis (Ed.), *Recent advances in biological psychiatry*. New York: Plenum Press, 1964.

Altshuler, K. Z. Reaction to and management of sensory loss: Blindness and deafness. In B. Schoenberg et al. (Eds.), *Loss and grief*. New York: Columbia University Press, 1968.

Altshuler, K. Z. Studies of the deaf: Relevance to psychiatric theory. *American Journal of Psychiatry*, 1971, *127*, 11.

Altshuler, K. Z. The social and psychological development of the deaf child: Problems, their treatment and prevention. *American Annals of the Deaf*, 1974, *119*, 365–375.

Altshuler, K. Z., Abdullah, S., & Rainer, J. D. Lithium and aggressive behavior in patients with early total deafness. *Diseases of the Nervous System*, 1977, *38*, 521–524.

Altshuler, K. Z., Deming, W. E., Vollenweider, J., et al. Impulsivity and profound early deafness: A crosscultural inquiry. *American Annals of the Deaf*, 1976, *121*, 331.

Grinker, R. R., Sr. (Ed.). *Psychiatric diagnosis, therapy, and research on the psychotic deaf*. Washington, D.C.: U.S. Department of Health, Education and Welfare, 1971.

Meadow, K. P. Self-image, family climate and deafness. *Social Forces*, 1969, *47*, 428.

Mindel, E., & Vernon, M. *They grow in silence. The deaf child and his family*. Silver Springs, Md.: National Association for the Deaf, 1971.

Mintz, J., O'Brien, C. P., & Luborsky, L. Predicting the outcome of psychotherapy for schizophrenics. *Archives of General Psychiatry*, 1976, *33*, 1183.

Rado, S. Recent advances in psychoanalytic theory. *Proceedings of the Association of Researchers of Nervous and Mental Diseases*, 1953, *21*, 42.

Rainer, J. D., & Altshuler, K. Z. *Comprehensive mental health services for the deaf*. New York: New York State Psychiatric Institute, 1966.

Rainer, J. D., & Altshuler, K. Z. *Expanded mental health care for the deaf. Rehabilitation and prevention*. New York: New York State Psychiatric Institute, 1970.

Rainer, J. D., Altshuler, K. Z., & Kallmann, F. M. *Family and mental health problems in a deaf population*. New York: New York State Psychiatric Institute, 1963.

Robinson, L. Group psychotherapy with hospitalized deaf patients. In J. D. Rainer and K. Z. Altshuler (Eds.), *Psychiatry and the deaf*. Washington, D.C.: U.S. Department of Health, Education and Welfare, 1968.

Schlesinger, H. S. The deaf pre-schooler and his many faces. In G. Lloyd (Ed.), *International seminar of the vocational rehabilitation of deaf persons*, Washington, D.C.: U.S. Department of Health, Education and Welfare, 1969.

Fred M. Levin, M.D.

9

Insight-Oriented Psychotherapy with the Deaf

There are many reasons why insight-oriented or psychoanalytically oriented psychotherapy may be the treatment of choice for the intelligent deaf adult with emotional problems. Deaf adults who are capable of insight and have good language skills often find themselves, either by choice or necessity, acting as leaders in their communities. These people, as is true of their counterparts in the hearing world, may wrestle with emotional problems that affect not only themselves but also others who look to them for support and guidance. The same holds true for a family's welfare where effective psychotherapy for the head of a household, for example, will positively affect the family sometimes even beyond one generation. Children of patients undergoing psychotherapy may respond positively to an emotional change in their environment and, in turn, grow up to become better parents themselves.

As do the hearing, the deaf have a capacity for healthy emotional growth through psychotherapy but often don't have the opportunity. There is a creative potential within the deaf community that will not become fully manifest until or unless neurotic or disturbed deaf adults with creative or leadership potential make efforts to gain insight into their own feelings through psychotherapy.

An additional problem for deaf adults capable of insight is the limited number of qualified mental health professionals attracted to working with emotionally disturbed deaf people. Although the past 10 years have seen considerable progress in the number of people being trained to provide counseling for the deaf, relatively few psychiatrists (Rainer, Altschuler, & Kallman, 1963) and psychologists trained in psychoanalytic techniques have entered professional work with deaf people. Efforts at recruiting professionals for training and clinical research should be continued. From a practical point of view, there should be increased study of insight-oriented or psychoanalytically oriented therapy for deaf people. In this way, ex-

113

perienced and motivated people already working with deaf clients can enhance their understanding of why some of their therapeutic efforts succeed or fail. I believe that psychoanalysis constitutes the most useful theoretical model we have for understanding psychological conflicts and motivation.

BACKGROUND

In order to discuss insight-oriented therapy, a few comments about psychoanalysis and social role theory are needed. Psychoanalysis represents the prototypical insight-oriented psychotherapy. Shakow (1967) wrote that psychoanalysis may be thought of as (1) a therapeutic method; (2) a method of investigation; (3) a body of observations; (4) a body of theory about human behavior; and (5) a movement going much beyond its scholarly aspects. In practice, patients meet with a psychoanalyst 4 or 5 times each week for 45-minute sessions, lie down on the couch, and direct themselves to the dual task of verbalizing all spontaneous thoughts, feelings, and sensations, and directing attention to the way these spontaneous productions are reported. Psychoanalysts listen to both the content and the form of the patients' communication. They observe and introspect, periodically making comments they feel will help patients obtain self-knowledge. The repeatedly proven assumption is that this process of self-reflection leads to insight in working through conflicting feelings. This in turn increases patients' range of intrapsychic and interpersonal choices.

The works of Parsons (1956), Spiegel (1957, 1971), and Grinker (1961) should be consulted for details on social role theory, but essentially the theory holds that roles are culturally defined sequences of behavior. They are either assigned by virtue of age or sex, etc., achieved by effort or training, or arbitrarily assumed as in children's play. Examples would be parent and child, teacher and student, therapist and patient. When two individuals have accepted and fulfilled roles that form a pair, then complementarity is said to occur, and they will feel comfortable in relationship to each other. When a two-party transaction occurs with one of the individuals either refusing or unable to accept the explicit or implicit complementary role assignments of the other, then the interaction will be characterized by some anxiety. The anxiety, if recognized and understood correctly, can then lead to "insight" regarding the nature of the role assignments. Grinker (1961) states, "the implicit shifting role functions made explicit in the reverberating transactions, enter into awareness, and are then (capable of being) modified or controlled." Such spiraling transactions occur particularly in insight-oriented therapy, and in a sense define it.

Accepting complementary role assignments, such as answering questions, becomes absolutely essential at certain times during any treatment as an aid in establishing a therapeutic or working alliance. At other times, however, these responses may actually hinder the attainment of insight. This is because the patient's self-observing capacity is stimulated only when it is called into action. To call the patient's attention to expectations and behavior in the treatment situation, e.g., to wonder with the patient why he or she is asking a particular question, is to sharpen the patient's powers of self-observation and introspection. At moments when one is briefly distanced from personal behavior and more nearly the observer than the participant, insight into one's motivations and conflicts can occur. These insights may occur rapidly, with a sudden feeling of "Aha, now I understand." More often, they occur only gradually. An example of an "aha" reaction from an insight-oriented therapy session might be helpful.

A hearing teenager and her deaf mother had both been in individual treatment with me for approximately 2 years. Each appeared jealous of the other's time with me. The daughter began her 50th session by explaining that she had made an arrangement to go on the first date with a male friend. Her mother, however, had threatened to call off the date if the patient did not have the young man come to pick her up at home rather than meeting at his place first as she had planned to do. The daughter asked for my opinion in a way that made me feel she wanted me to agree that her mother's position was unreasonable. Instead, I pointed out that since she already knew how her mother felt, I was surprised she had made such an arrangement, especially considering how disappointed she would be if she were not allowed to go. She smiled and said, "I think it's guilt." She then spoke of feeling uncomfortable about leaving her mother at home alone, and of the need to see herself as somehow responsible for mother's unhappiness. Also, and to her surprise, she became aware for the first time of her wish to have me side with her against her mother and became more aware of her hesitation in beginning to date.

At this point it is important to distinguish between empathy and what is quite a different and less useful process for a therapist, namely, identification. A capacity for empathy implies a high degree of emotional maturity, which allows the therapist to experience vicariously the feelings of the patient, not confusing these feelings with his or her own. The therapist's knowledge of the meanings of one's own fantasy life and feeling states, as these occur periodically in relation to the patient during sessions, then becomes a tool for understanding the patient's emotional life.

In identification, which with novice therapists all too often occurs instead of empathy, the therapist's own problems intrude into the therapy. If therapists confuse their own and the patient's feelings, or are unable to deal with feelings or fantasies that are aroused during therapy, they may suppress or become overly involved and thus lose emotional and/or intellectual objectivity.

An example of identification in the case cited above would be if I had agreed with my patient that her mother was totally insensitive and told her that she should pick up her boyfriend if she wished. Had I identified in this way with her position, she might not have gained the insights she did. Knowledge of the psychoanalytic distinction between identification and empathy may help us help patients toward insights. Clearly, this patient was capable of developing insight into her behavior and feelings, given the opportunity and help to do so, but just as insight-oriented psychotherapy is not useful with all neurotic, hearing persons, it is not necessarily the treatment of choice with all neurotic deaf persons.

Deaf adults should be given a thorough screening evaluation before being offered psychoanalytically oriented therapy. Some deaf adults, though intelligent and skilled in language use, will not have the capacity or motivation to participate in this kind of treatment, quite aside from their deafness. To bring a person into such treatment, one who does not have the emotional capacity for self-reflection, would create a situation that might be worse than no treatment at all. The patient would not be able to meet the therapist's impossible expectations, and this could revive painful childhood memories of similar experiences with parents or teachers.

Originally, at the Siegel Institute, our referrals were often markedly regressed schizophrenic persons or those with borderline personalities or other illnesses requiring supportive psychotherapy or inpatient hospitalization. Later came more upwardly mobile, independently functioning people with more narcissistic or structural conflicts. By "structural conflicts" is meant that a person diagnosed according to the *Diagnostic and Statistical Manual* (1968) as neurotic (either hysterical, depressive, or obsessive-compulsive, etc.) is understood in terms of what Freud called the structural model. In this model, the mind is divided into id, ego, and superego. In practical terms, neurosis implies a fairly high degree of psychological maturation in terms of theory of origin; adult neurosis is thought to reflect a difficulty originally experienced in childhood between the approximate ages of 3 and 5, the so-called oedipal period. Such individuals are usually considered candidates for insight-oriented treatment.

In addition to careful selection of appropriate treatment techniques, we recommend that hearing therapists for the deaf learn sign language and acquire skill in the subtleties of this language. Language plays a vital role in emotional growth and development. When the therapist makes an effort to communicate in a deaf patient's preferred language, most often the language of signs, much is done toward setting the stage for later working through infantile or childhood feelings of helpless isolation, confusion, and despair. For persons who are born deaf or lose their hearing before language develops, a profound social isolation may ensue that is perhaps beyond the capacity of most hearing persons to imagine. In using sign language rather than choosing cumbersome note-writing or indirect communication through an interpreter, the therapist shows a willingness to help with the profound isolation and to understand these feelings as empathically as he or she can.

Having accepted patients after a screening evaluation and utilizing a developing but shared language system, we began to see encouraging progress in some of the first patients with structural conflicts referred to our program. Later, some of the more affluent members of the deaf community even referred themselves privately to staff members after seeing some successful results with the initial group of patients. We also found that some patients who were functioning at a low level of verbal communicative and sign language skills when first interviewed were judged more communicatively adept after a therapeutic alliance had been established. As hearing patients might learn to express themselves better as trust in the therapist develops, it seems that some deaf patients in treatment have enhanced communication with more and different signs as well as the same signs expressed more clearly.

INITIAL PHASE OF TREATMENT

As Mindel and Vernon (1971) point out, when a therapist is hearing and the patient is deaf there are prejudices to overcome on both sides. If the first moves in therapy are awkward for the therapist, he or she can be certain that they are even more awkward for the deaf adult, who is expecting only one more humiliation or at best, a waste of time. Yet, as in a game of chess, if these first difficult opening maneuvers are successful, there is a better chance of a good outcome.

In the initial phase of treatment, a therapeutic alliance is being established. This alliance represents a set of shared attitudes about the purpose and procedures of therapy. Many individual factors comprise the shared attitudes and successful therapeutic alliance. The patient must be able to utilize the treatment offered and have the motivation to be helped. The patient must be able to stay in treatment long enough for growth to occur. Concurrently, therapists must be genuinely interested in learning about other human beings, the patients. They must have the capacity to do this in depth, with tact. Finally, there are advantages in both parties liking each other and understanding that the therapy cannot be rushed and will take as long as it will take. Often a therapist is the first person in a patient's life willing to take the time needed for exploration, experiencing, and mastering of conflicting feelings.

Opposed to the therapeutic alliance are various psychological "resistances" that the therapist needs to understand and approach patiently throughout the treatment process. The term "resistance" refers to the patient's unconscious use of his or her own language, character, familiar emotional responses, and psychological defenses as protection against both anxiety and insight during therapy. Therapy consists, in part, of examining resistances in a tactful way so that the patient can understand how they serve as armor and against what anxieties and insights. Subsequently, emotional growth will make some resistances unnecessary.

Often, for deaf people, the first obstacle to establishing a therapeutic alliance is inadequate communication. Therapist and patient need to understand each others' words. Only in doing this can they later progress to an exploration of deeper level or covert meanings of verbal and nonverbal communications (e.g., language of signs, gestures, etc.). This obstacle is not necessarily a "resistance," but in specific clinical situations, sign language can be used in this way. At this point, some clinical examples will help the reader understand what this resistance may consist of. The examples given all deal with aspects of communication, which, in my experience, are often employed by deaf patients in the service of resistance.

Case 1

Ms. R. had always felt harassed by the hearing world. She was about to meet a psychiatrist for the first time. An incipient paranoia exploded in the waiting room, where she frightened the receptionist by signing with the fury of a boxer throwing punches. The receptionist did not understand signs and tried to indicate this, but to no avail! Ushered into my office, Ms. R. burst into even more rapid signing when she saw that I was a novice in sign language. Needless to say, her signing was beyond my comprehension, with one very interesting exception. She made it clear, in contrast to all the rest of her unclear signing, that she hated Jews, men, and psychiatrists! I am male, Jewish, and a psychiatrist. I quickly understood that the meaning of her communication was a request to immediately arrange for an interview with another therapist. I chose a social worker, a hearing-impaired woman with perfect fluency in the language of signs. However, I also made it clear to the patient that I was not removing myself from her treatment but would return at the end of the interview to reassess the situation. When I did so, I learned that things had gone well enough to reconsider offering myself as her therapist. The patient accepted the idea of working with me and we were eventually able to establish a working alliance.

My initial therapeutic maneuver addressed itself to the patient's anxiety; specifically, "Doctor, how can I talk with you about my deafness when you are not deaf, and when you cannot even communicate fluently in sign language?" The patient felt too helpless and humiliated to proceed in any other way. However, once a sense of trust was built on my first empathic response, the patient was later able to admit that she could not think of making things easy for me. Virtually all of her previous contacts with hearing people had been painfully confusing and humiliating. She had made me feel as helpless and stupid as she ordinarily feels in the hearing world. I had accepted her feelings rather than ignoring them. By returning at the end of the interview, I communicated my belief that I could help her (although I did not know sign language fluently) and my feeling that I wanted to help her if she could accept this. In this manner, a resistance was successfully dealt with and almost immediately it ceased to be a problem.

Case 2

A deaf adult with good speech, Mr. S. came hesitantly to his first interview. Although 30-years-old, he wanted his father to begin the interview for him. The parents had arranged the interview, rather than the patient himself, but I asked the parents not to come into the office. Slowly, but with increasing confidence, the patient began to explain his "confusion," including confused sexual identity. In the process, he periodically lowered his voice so that only his signs could be understood. Without the assistance of his excellent voice to facilitate communication I began to feel more awkward and helpless. This led me to an appreciation of how helpless and awkward Mr. S. felt in relation to me and the hearing world. By dropping his voice he made me a deaf person, and I did not like it. I decided not to comment on this, feeling it would make his helplessness seem even greater. After 12 months of work, however, I made a brief comment on his pattern of occasionally dropping his voice. For the first and only time in treatment his anger at being deaf emerged. Thereafter, he resorted much less often to lowering his voice, but the helpless rage at being deaf that had been touched upon scared him greatly and could not be contained by the therapeutic alliance. We met for yet another 6 months, dealing at times with his frustration at being deaf. He terminated treatment with only a vague plan to start again with me "later," and without ever fully working through the fear of his rage or the helplessness behind it.

Case 3

Mr. Z., a middle-aged man who lost his hearing at age 6, came to the Siegel Institute for marital counseling after his wife threatened to divorce him. He had been in psychotherapy previously, and a fuller discussion is reported by Dr. David Rothstein (Grinker, 1969).

In presenting himself to me, Mr. Z. signed in such an abbreviated way that he seemed to be saying, "I am not really deaf because I am not really signing." In other words, he signed in miniature. The patient's sign language was inconspicuous but understandable. This seemed to suggest low self-esteem and a wish not to be deaf. I wondered also about hostility toward me since I had to work extra hard to see his hand movements. At the same time, painfully embarrassed, Mr. Z. spoke of his disappointment in himself. He blamed his deafness for his sense of failure as a son, a husband, and a father. He seemed unaware of the significance of his signing in miniature and my difficulty in understanding it. Following two additional interviews, however, the signs spontaneously became more expansive, concurrent with an improved therapeutic alliance.

The alliance between therapist and patient to work on the patient's problems will sometimes occur almost effortlessly, as it did in this case. Mr. Z. rapidly idealized me. I also learned later that his small signs were meant to conceal disappointment in himself over his less-than-perfect knowledge of sign language. In his subsequent treatment I was able to see minor mistakes in his sign usage and his relative difficulty with finger spelling that he had meant to conceal from the start. To have commented on language and communication problems would have interfered, by reminding the patient of his inadequacies, with the rapidly evolving alliance.

Case 4

Ms. J. was a 29-year-old woman with a post-graduate degree. She had high verbal skills, although her tense and monotonal voice was not easily understood until one became accustomed to it. She knew no signs.

After an evaluation by another psychiatrist, Ms. J. began her treatment with me. During the initial phase of therapy, I usually asked her to repeat what I found unintelligible. She disliked this, but came to appreciate the importance of making sure we understood each other. Her speech was unusual, and I needed practice hearing it. Therapy with Ms. J. would have stayed on a very superficial level without this open approach to our communication dilemma. In Ms. J.'s typical relationships, she or others would sometimes pretend understanding that did not exist until the charade would break down in anger or disappointment in both parties. If this patient had repeated with me what had existed with so many others (including her parents), she would have avoided not only anxiety but also insight.

A second maneuver greatly facilitated progress and is described because of its general implications. The first psychiatrist to interview Ms. J. used total communication with her although she knew no sign language. I continued this practice so that now, after 3 years of treatment, the patient has become fluent in sign language despite previous failures. What sign language exposure and acquisition accomplished was to make the deaf world and her feelings about being deaf more accessible to her. For the first time she began to experience herself as deaf, but only after a long transition experience that she described as "feeling in between two worlds." Powerful feelings of sadness and rage over being born deaf were mobilized in a process that appeared to resemble mourning. It was as though she could not proceed with life until she made better peace with her wish to hear.

TRANSFERENCE AND COUNTERTRANSFERENCE

Transference connotes a process where unconscious reactions to important people in our past become displaced or projected onto others in our present life experiences. For example, we may treat older people in ways similar to those once used with our parents. Transference can occur in our daily activities as responses to others and in the therapy process as well. Although old reactions to parents, siblings, and other family members are often the most important sources of these current misperceptions of others, close relatives themselves may also be misperceived through transference distortions at anytime during our lives. So, for example, a particular adolescent may experience his kind father as critical and punishing because an earlier version of his father has been reactivated. In fact, the father may never have been anything but loving and sensitive but the patient may have habitually misperceived his father because of his own anger or rage.

The reader may wonder what these transferences accomplish for the patient. Primarily they are adaptive and defensive. They allow the patient to react or behave spontaneously rather than to remember and re-experience painful feelings. For example, if I treat you as my father and I behave as your son, then I can avoid recalling unhappy experiences with my father that might be stirred in my interaction with you. When I feel that "all fathers behave in a certain way, what can you expect?", then I am also telling myself that I will not upset myself thinking of a specific father (mine) and his son (me), and specific, painful disappointments. I may also avoid feelings of anger at my father, for being bigger, stronger, or for having a special relationship with my mother, etc. This is one way that we can avoid many kinds of feelings when they threaten our psychological equilibrium.

The concept of transference is not an easy one to understand even for the psychologically sophisticated. One of my teachers, Dr. Roy Grinker, Sr., traveled to Vienna as a young man, to be analyzed by Sigmund Freud. Grinker (1975) writes:

"I sometimes expressed to Freud my difficulty in understanding transference. One night my wife and I were invited to the house of young Dr. Sippy, who was being analyzed in Vienna. His wife, who I found out later was being analyzed by Freud, was at the party. We had quite a social evening and at an appropriate occasion I told a joke that Freud had told me. Well, at the next session Freud said to me, 'I thought we decided that this analysis was confidential.' I had thought the confidential part was on his side, not on mine, but at any rate, to my surprise, I burst out into tears at his criticism, and he said, 'Well, now you know what transference is.'*

Clearly, Grinker was reacting to Freud's clarification as though his own father had criticized or chastised him. His reaction tells us of his own sensitivity at the time to criticism. Freud was a father figure not only for the young Dr. Grinker but for a substantial part of the intellectual community of the Western world.

Countertransference, feelings of a therapist toward a patient, can be a significant problem if unrecognized. But, when recognized, these same reactions become the fundamental tool for the therapist's or psychoanalyst's gaining understanding of a patient. I believe that patients with handicaps generally arouse powerful countertransferences in their therapists. Some therapists may even begin their work with handicapped clients out of an identification with the damaged patient. Feeling damaged themselves, such therapists will struggle internally to "cure" others of problems that in some way remind them of their own. For instance, I know of a hearing patient who grew up in a household where the virtue of selfless caring for others was praised, while at the same time, individual family members could be unbelievably insensitive to each other's feelings. Partly out of a conviction that her father and mother had always been deaf to her, she developed an abiding interest in sign language and deaf education.

Patients in insight-oriented psychotherapy need therapists who are empathic but who do not overly identify with them. If the patient is complaining and the therapist is commiserating, then there are two participants but no observer. What grows out of this is a perhaps friendship but not a psychotherapy. The patient's observing ego fails to develop to capacity. Unfortunately, this sort of mock therapy can and does occur frequently.

It is important to alert novice therapists to some of these traps to help them help themselves toward emotional growth. In any thorough, insight-oriented therapy, attention must be given to transference/countertransference issues, that is, to the projective or role assignment aspects of the patient–therapist interaction. When treatment fails because the therapist has not considered such issues, the patient will become bitter and, understandably, may stay away from other therapists and health professionals. Also, some professionals develop stereotypes, as for example, that

---

*Reprinted with permission from Grinker RR, Sr.: Reminiscences of Dr. Roy Grinker. *Journal of American Academy of Psychoanalysis,* 1975, *3,* p. 216.

deaf clients have insurmountable communication problems or that they are only capable of concrete rather than abstract thought. While concreteness of thought, inability to abstract, and communication problems exist with some deaf patients, these are unfair generalizations for the vast majority of deaf individuals. It is important that the therapist avoid, through these generalizations, expressing exasperation at a therapeutic process gone awry.

Another common countertransference problem is for the therapist to avoid speaking openly with the patient about deafness. Especially at the beginning of my work, I would sometimes neglect to ask during evaluations about the origin and history of a patient's deafness. A patient's private fantasies about the cause of deafness can easily be ignored as though these issues were not meant to be exposed or explored, and yet the fantasies can have great significance. In fact, the mere asking of a question about ordinarily private matters may communicate, for the first time, permission for some patients to think about important experiences or behaviors. This in itself can relieve guilt and shame. To paraphrase a patient's thoughts, "If the therapist feels comfortable asking, maybe it's not so bad after all." When I began to ask patients about their deafness, I learned, for the first time, how much my own inhibitions about asking interfered with the patient's readiness for telling.

The therapists who characteristically jump into exactly what they are afraid of will have problems as well. They will inquire about matters such as the patients' reactions to deafness before there is a therapeutic alliance to support a useful interchange on the subject, or before the subject has actually occurred in the sequence of the treatment process. Therapists who need to be appreciated and praised or need to see some immediate results from the therapeutic encounter will also create problems by acting too hastily. Deaf people are so accustomed to not being listened to that they will probably seem overly demanding of attention themselves, and will necessarily starve a therapist "needy" for positive feedback. The patients' previous contacts with helpers who failed, may have convinced them that therapy is one more lost cause. It will take more time for patients under these circumstances to learn to trust or respect therapists.

In contrast, some deaf adults will start in therapy by offering their therapist lavish praise. Such praise may represent a way of defending against anger. The patient will need to become aware of that anger, to understand and to resolve it. Alternately, the praise may not reflect anger or be defensive at all. For example, such lavish praise may merely be the attempt by the patient to idealize the therapist. The therapist with limited self-esteem may interfere with such idealization by pointing out with false modesty his or her own "limitations" instead of quietly accepting the patient's praise. This is because the therapist's own unresolved grandiosity has been hyperstimulated by the praise. Unable to become attached to an admired therapist, the patient loses the chance to regain healthy self-esteem later on through a process in which the therapist is gradually seen more and more realistically. The detailed meanings of these points are elaborated further in the section on narcissism and narcissistic character disturbances.

Some deaf patients will expect or demand the therapist's participation in their lives, including such things as accompanying them to find a new apartment or a job. These requests may become traps for the novice therapist; they may really be covert invitations to stop the therapy by altering the therapist–patient relationship. The therapist needs to decide if agreeing to such requests will assist or interfere with therapy. Is the patient unable to perform these tasks alone and thereby making a reasonable request, or is the patient abdicating responsibility to avoid anxiety and ultimately insight? The therapist who needs to see all deaf people as helpless and tends to take over their lives may unwittingly stifle their autonomy and thus reinforce self-demeaning and self-depreciating postures.

An opposite extreme may be the instance of a therapist who loses empathic connection with patients, and does inappropriate things such as failing to help a deaf client with a crucial telephone call, intellectualizing that the patient "must do it alone." In these instances, the therapist may be disavowing personal needs to be nurtured and cared for. What the therapist disavows or defends against, as well as the defenses themselves, will become blind spots for both patient and therapist in the therapeutic process. Should this occur, the probability of the patient gaining an awareness of these issues becomes very slim indeed.

NARCISSISM AND NARCISSISTIC CHARACTER DISTURBANCES

Traditionally, "narcissism" in the psychoanalytic literature refers to a stage of development that is transitional between the autoeroticism of the infant and the object-love of the older child. Narcissism as used here refers to the sense of investment in the self as it becomes manifest in a number of precise ways in the therapeutic setting. There is currently some debate in psychoanalytic circles about how to understand the so-called narcissism of adults and children, but what follows generally represents at least one viewpoint, that elaborated by Kohut (1971, 1979). It is my belief that features of Kohut's thoughts on narcissism and narcissistic personality disorders have significant relevance to work with emotionally disturbed deaf people.

According to Kohut, the narcissism of children, demonstrated by their exhibitionism and grandiosity, is a normal part of development. He believes that optimal development tames this normal narcissism of childhood so that it becomes integrated into the adult personality and supplies "fuel for . . . ambitions and purposes, for the enjoyment of activities, and for important aspects of self-esteem" (Kohut, 1966).

The first phase in self-development is the formation of the sense of self. The infant does not spring full-blown like Pegasus from Medusa's blood with a stable, clear-cut self-sameness over time. The initial period of infantile experience is believed to involve unclear distinctions between self and nonself, inside and outside, infant and other. Only gradually do constellations of part-aspects of a person's self

and part-aspects of others come together into some (initially) unstable representations that we could call the "self" and "objects."

In the second phase, these representations of self and object undergo a process
of fixation or cohesion in memory. The cohesion of self and object representations
resist fragmentation in life or in therapy, and allow for the psychoanalytic treatment
of narcissistic personalities. Fragmentation should be understood as any gross disturbance in the sense of self or objects short of that seen most dramatically in the
psychotic states of schizophrenics. A human being's environment and genetic en-
dowment blend to assist in the development of a "cohesive sense of self." If a
solid sense of cohesion does not develop, an individual would not be considered
a narcissistic personality but rather a schizophrenic or borderline character. These
illnesses and some ways in which they can be distinguished from each other are
described in the next section.

The third phase involves self-development after the formation of cohesiveness.
Kohut refers to various forms of the self and considers their ultimate transformation,
when development is optimal into such things as true knowledge, humor, empathy,
and the ability to accept one's death. Considering the origin of the adult narcissistic
self from the child's normal grandiosity and exhibitionism, Kohut called the internal
representation in the mind of the earliest form of the self, the "archaic grandiose
self." He then added the idea of an "idealized parental imago." This internal
image of the parent's greatness as the archaic counterpart of the self then accounts
for the clinical observation of the narcissistic patient's ready idealization of therapist
comparable to the small child's admiration of a presumably perfect parent (Kohut,
1966).

The forms of the "archaic grandiose self" as seen clinically, constitute the
heart of Kohut's contribution. When they occur in therapy they can be viewed as
one would view transference. Kohut prefers to call them only transference-like,
and he designates three forms of archaic grandiose self: the merger, the twinship
(or alter-ego), and the mirror proper. The phrase "mirror transferences" has also
been used to refer collectively to all three of these therapeutically reactivated forms
of infantile narcissism.

The merger form of the grandiose self involves an experiencing of one's
greatness through feeling as if one is part of another person who, in turn, is seen
as perfect. Patients manifesting this merger-transference will, for example, fail to
distinguish between the therapist's property and their own because for them this
distinction does not exist. I cite the following example: A patient with muddy boots
dirtied the carpet in my office without feeling or demonstrating any remorse. She
was genuinely surprised when the incident was brought to her attention. To me her
surprise was an indication that her behavior represented a variation of the mirror
transference. Had she done this out of anger to me she would have felt guilty when
it was called to her attention. Instead, she was only surprised that I reacted. After
all, would I have been upset if she made her own rug dirty? For her, she *was*
making her own rug dirty, not mine. My acceptance of her behavior in that I did

not get angry, helped her to see more clearly how she had failed to differentiate us from each other.

In the twinship or alter-ego form of grandiose self, the other person is felt to be just like the self. The hidden greatness of the patient is then bestowed upon the therapist or other people. This shows itself clinically when patients have trouble because they have assumed, incorrectly, that someone else thinks exactly as they do. This is demonstrated by the actions of a patient who failed to call her therapist to cancel an appointment. When asked why she had failed to call, the patient seemed puzzled because she imagined the therapist could read her mind and did not need to be informed. In other words, the therapist knew what the patient knew and the patient certainly knew she was not going to keep the appointment.

This twinship form has an interesting variant, which I call a "nontwinship." It is seen clinically in the deaf patient's questioning, "How can you understand me? You're not deaf." In this case, the patient is expressing a manifestation of a twinship-transference of the grandiose self and has begun to question the twinship itself. "Maybe you are not like me" then suggests for the patient the possibility of not being understood. It also suggests the possibility of living in a world with others who are different from the self but who have something to offer the patient. Up to this point, understanding and empathic contact had been assumed on the basis of sameness between self and object. Now that sameness is opened to question and empathy is based on respect, affection and love are possible. It may be that from the standpoint of tolerance of separation, a crucial step in the development of self and object (as inner representations) occurs when the self and object are no longer seen as identical. For if others are like one's self, in one sense they cannot really be lost; but if the other person is recognizably different, then the loss of the object cannot be replaced by any increased attention to one's self, i.e., a real loss can occur.

Finally, in the mirror proper form of transference, the repressed or disavowed sense of perfection of the self is hidden from self-awareness by closeness to an admired person whose only function is to reflect back or echo one's own glory. We have all met such people. With them, we are made to feel as a nonperson because for them we *are* nonpersons. We are nonpersons in the sense of not being independent centers of initiative with our own thoughts, feelings, and wants. For such people. we are nothing more than a gleam in an eye or a loving smile. For people who have never passed beyond the stages of development implied in the series of merger, twinship, and mirror transferences, others are not real objects but, in Kohut's terminology, self-objects. They complete part of the subject's missing psychic structure. And when the self-object is not available, or even a minute failure in empathy from the self-object occurs, there is a mobilization of the patient's archaic grandiose self as seen by haughtiness, an experience of depressive isolatedness, and hypochondriasis. The therapist, armed with the knowledge that these feelings may reflect breaches in empathy or disturbances in a self/self-object relationship, can improve chances of being empathic and help the patient learn to understand how these feelings correlate with fluctuations in empathic connection to another person. When the patient's major problem is a need for such a mirroring/echoing self-object, he or she will feel particularly understood, and gradually, the therapeutically reactivated forms of grandiose self (previously repressed or disavowed) will be transformed and replaced; one might say they will be integrated with the adult personality. To make the correlations, as well as to provide the mirroring that I am describing, is the heart of the therapy for many narcissistically damaged patients.

My clinical experience suggests that many deaf adults appear to suffer from disturbances of the self. The hearing loss itself results in impotent rage at this assault upon one's body. It appears to be defended against by multiple layers of denial, disavowal, projection, and reaction formation. Judging from the reconstructions in therapy of the childhood of adult deaf patients, it is probable that these deaf children of hearing parents often failed to have the necessary echoing-mirroring experiences of normal hearing children. Without the mirroring, such children become arrested in their development. The archaic grandiose self remains repressed and too much energy becomes dissipated in the adult who must defend against narcissistic rage that could otherwise be available for work and love.

In referring to the repression of archaic grandiosity, I am not expounding an idea of narrow psychoanalytic relevance but the fact that a person's emotional growth may stop in an early phase of development. The greatest tragedy of these individuals is that often life for them is painfully boring due to a relative inability to respond to pleasurable stimuli, as well as more precarious because of their need to remain "connected" with certain key people. They also tend to bore or anger others because of their self-preoccupations.

A brief case history reported by the Brazilian psychoanalyst, Neto (1972) describes "an analysis of a deaf-mute" that by necessity incorporated sufficient modifications of traditional psychoanalytic technique to be more properly called psychoanalytically oriented psychotherapy. Some of Neto's data can be interpreted in terms of Kohut's self-object model.

The patient was a 21-year-old female, deafened at 15 months, who entered therapy because of feelings of isolation and difficulty establishing relationships with the opposite sex. In the beginning, Neto quickly learned that to have the patient lie on his couch as in traditional psychoanalysis was unsatisfactory. Not only was it often difficult for him to see her signing but it was impossible for him to communicate with her since she could neither see nor hear him. This made the analyst as "mute" as the patient.

The analyst and patient agreed to "talk" face-to-face. Their communication included her drawing pictures. An early one was of two buildings without any connections between them. The analyst interpreted this drawing in its transference implication as showing the complicated methods of communication the patient was obliged to use in order to communicate with others, especially with the therapist. Gradually, the therapeutic process deepened and the patient began to rely more on sign language. As Neto explains, she made it easier for him to see that she was afraid of harm, including harm from him. His use of sign language put him in contact with her imagination: "I invalidated her deaf-muteness as an obstacle to analysis. Consequently, she began to fear penetration by my interpretations." Neto considered this "penetration" solely in terms of its sexual implication. "She was afraid of being penetrated by my interpretations because she feared their fertile effort—a perception of her psychic reality which until then had been shielded by her deaf-muteness." This fear of penetration might also be interpreted as fear of getting closer to him and others to avoid interference with her narcissism. The self-object model of Kohut allows one to speculate that the patient's fear was that the analyst would be another in a series of insensitive, unempathic human beings.

A short time after the last session, after approximately 1½ years of treatment, the patient married, apparently having mastered enough of her anxiety over intimacy. Clearly she was well along in the task of growing emotionally. Treatment succeeded not only because of Neto's interpretations, but because he was empathic and intuitively understood her mirror-transference. This can be seen where he allowed himself to conduct an "analysis" sitting up which offended the view of traditional psychoanalytic therapy. Actually, however, it is not an absolute requirement of an analysis that it be conducted supine. He also modified the traditional approach by allowing time during which he and his patient could exchange pictures until she was ready to use sign language.

A second case history is of a man in his 40s who was deafened at age 6 due to meningitis. This clinical case, reported earlier as Mr. Z, case 3, comes from my own experience; however, Rothstein has reported on the same patient in "Office Treatment of Private Deaf Patients" (Rothstein, 1969). Although brief, this article deserves careful attention. In particular, Rothstein emphasized the patient's need to mourn the loss of hearing, which he feels is "universally unmet, even in reasonably successful, well-functioning deaf individuals," (also see case 4 earlier in this chapter). The opportunity to see the similarities and differences in the reporting of this patient by two different psychiatrists may also be of interest.

I began seeing the patient when his wife threatened divorce and he worried about harming himself. During the first week of psychiatric hospitalization, a kidney stone that produced mild back pain necessitated transfer of the patient to the urologic service for emergency surgery. The medical problem was actually suggested by the patient's spontaneous associations during the initial psychotherapy sessions. He spoke only of the medical aspects of the hospital. Because my suspicions were aroused, I asked for additional medical history. Finally he confessed that he had indeed had some chronic back pain. Years before he had been advised to obtain careful follow-up for kidney disease, which he had not done.

Two days after the kidney surgery, we renewed our daily psychotherapy sessions and uncovered an additional important bit of history. The patient's father had died shortly after surgery at the same hospital a decade before. It became clear to both of us that he had always feared surgery. Entering the hospital reminded him of a complex of losses that all had hospitalization as the common demoninator: the previous kidney stones that threatened the loss of kidney function each time they appeared; the father's illness, emergency surgery, and death shortly thereafter; and probably most importantly, the patient's early loss of hearing following meningitis.

The patient also told, for the first time, about his rage at his hearing siblings and mother, all of whom he accused of never having been sensitive to his feelings about being deaf. The lack of empathic connectedness with these people was shown, he felt, by their failure to have teletype telephone units in their households so that they could phone him or receive his calls.

The hearing loss appears to be the event around which the patient's pseudo-self-reliant personality became organized, leaving him with a distinct need to disavow many experiences, especially physical symptoms. During the hospitalization, he nearly lost a kidney because of his need to minimize the significance of his back pain. The need to disavow the significance of the kidney disease appears intimately related through an identical mechanism to a more profoundly upsetting loss still, his loss of hearing at age 6, which was equally out of his control.

After surgery, the patient went through a brief period of fear of his mother's "taking over." He was particularly worried that the therapist would listen not to him but instead to her. This seemed important both as a reflection of his regressive wish to be taken care of by his mother as well as a possible re-enactment of something that had occurred earlier in his life, possibly at the time of his meningitis. Unfortunately, this could not be pursued further but it seemed likely that the patient's earlier downplaying of his kidney stone was related to his ambivalent feelings about his mother whom he both yearned for and feared, and whose caring he seemed to experience primarily as humiliating.

This patient had a narcissistic personality disorder. The therapist became for him a mirroring, idealizable object with whom he did not need to fear humiliation. The significance of losing his father was primarily the loss of an empathic, admirable partner. The probability is that father was the much more sensitive parent, who provided better parenting in the sense of recognizing correctly when the patient needed help and when he was better left to his own devices. When the father died, this seemed to foreclose the possibility of forming satisfactory relationships with others. A vital self-object was lost. The patient felt as though he had lost part of himself, which he did in the sense that his father's abilities compensated for his deficits. In general, the creation of psychic structure or emotional growth occurs when one's losses are not too great. This means that the parent should only gradually be lost to the child in the sense of being seen more realistically in incremental and tolerable steps. The patient then gains back healthy self-esteem from what was previously his or her idealization of the parent. In this patient's case, the father was de-idealized too abruptly. The father was not able to keep the patient from getting meningitis and losing his hearing. He was unable to successfully manage his relationship with the patient's mother. And finally, he succumbed to a physical illness, creating for the patient a permanent loss at a time when he still was working through the de-idealization process.

NARCISSISTIC PERSONALITY VERSUS SCHIZOPHRENIA
VERSUS BORDERLINE CHARACTER DISORDER

Major confusion in making the proper diagnosis in deaf adults most often involves understanding the crucial differences between the various dysfunctional states of narcissistic personalities, schizophrenia, and borderline character disorders. According to Altshuler (1971), schizophrenia is no more frequent in the deaf population than in the hearing population. There are no reliable published figures of incidence of borderline and narcissistic personality disturbances in the deaf.

In general, the so-called fragmentation of narcissistic characters is more threatened than real, more transient than lasting. It is primarily defined by a surge of grandiosity, depressive isolatedness, and/or hypochondriacal concerns. Moreover, it will occur without associated formal thought disturbances and without hallucinations and delusions. The stimulus for this experience will most often be some break in empathy or another loss of a self-object.

Psychosis is frequently used as a behavioral term implying a psychological state in which the individual's coping mechanisms have failed in a massive way. Borderline characters at times of psychosis will seem to be exactly like schizophrenics. This dysfunctional state, however, will appear to borderline characters as more alien to their usual personalities, will often occur in conjunction with quantities of rage unmanageable by the defensive functions of the ego, and is generally of shorter duration than the schizophrenic psychosis (Grinker, Werble, & Drye, 1968). In schizophrenia, the fragmentation of psychotic proportions is usually due to overstimulation. It usually takes longer to resolve than the psychosis of borderline characters. It also can occur with delusions or hallucinations. When the schizophrenic is not fragmented, i.e., when nonpsychotic, there may still be evidence of a formal thought disturbance; without a thought disturbance, the diagnosis of schizophrenia always remains in doubt. Usually, such a disturbance in thinking shows itself by the patient's thoughts not fitting together. In extreme cases, the schizophrenic's thoughts may even seem bizarre, blocked, or so idiosyncratic as to be meaningless connections of words (word salad).

In summary, the disturbances in the sense of self are primarily only threatened in the fragmentation of narcissistic personalities in which, by definition, the self is cohesive (if only tenuously so) but is associated with profound alterations in functioning (a frank psychosis) in individuals without a cohesive self, such as borderlines and schizophrenics. In the latter two cases, therefore, the loss of functioning is sufficient to be designated a psychosis with gross disturbances in thinking, reality testing, and with symptoms such as delusions and/or hallucinations. Psychotic patients benefit from antipsychotic medication, so borderlines and schizophrenics will receive drugs such as chlorpromazine as an important adjunct to their supportive psychotherapy. Narcissistic personalities are felt to be treatable by insight-oriented care, including psychoanalysis, whereas psychoanalysts as a group generally view this to be highly inappropriate treatment for borderline and schizo-phrenic patients.

Deaf patients brought to psychiatric emergency rooms can present conflicting symptoms that may result in misdiagnosis and inappropriate treatment by an in-experienced clinician. Because effective treatment rests on accurate diagnosis, it is crucial to make the diagnostic distinctions between frankly psychotic and bor-derline disturbances. For the program at Michael Reese Medical Center, a social worker from our program who is hard-of-hearing and is an experienced therapist assists the psychiatric resident at routine evaluations of deaf clients in the emer-gency room. Her presence and assistance reduce the feelings of ''strangeness'' of the deaf client and contribute importantly to the differential diagnosis. For non-emergency evaluations, a multidisciplinary team approach is used, in which a psychiatrist and a social worker skilled in sign language see the patient, while a psychologist, also skilled in sign language, obtains a collateral history. In my opinion, this team approach is the most valid one for obtaining a workable diag-nostic impression for purposes of disposition.

TERMINATION

Some preliminary conclusions can be made on the termination phase of psy-chotherapeutic treatment with deaf adults. The decision on when to terminate has many variables and is almost never an easy matter.

Goldberg (1975) describes four personality changes of significance in identi-fying when termination is appropriate. These are (1) a re-experience and mastery of narcissistic injury; (2) a change in the response to interpretations; (3) a greater recognition and acceptance of one's lack of knowledge in general; and (4) an idealization of the treatment process. Goldberg is not suggesting that all therapy must end when these changes have occurred, nor that therapy should absolutely not end until these changes can be seen. Nor does this suggest that narcissism is the major issue in all treatment; however, most psychiatrists would accept that disturbances in the regulation of self-esteem are involved in all therapy to some extent. It is my tentative conclusion that the deaf population seems particularly vulnerable to disturbances in the sense of self, at least partly because of the bodily damage of the deafness itself and the problems this creates for deaf children ob-taining mirroring and echoing from their parents.

Re-experiencing and mastering narcissistic injury means the tendency for suc-cessfully treated individuals to restructure their lives so as to take into account their realistic abilities and limitations. Thus, a deaf adult might better master a work situation by choosing a job that takes his deafness into account or by acquiring the extra communicative skills needed for success. This is illustrated by a deaf patient who insisted upon becoming a lecturer at the college level in her chosen field despite the fact she was doomed for failure because of an inadequate voice. During the course of psychotherapy, she decided spontaneously to support herself instead by solitary work in creative art, at which she was truly talented. Through this readjustment of her work goals she increased her chances of success.

A change in the response to interpretations involves no longer experiencing the observations of others, including the therapist, as intrusive and disruptive of one's self. The improved capacity to attend to the thoughts and feelings of others also makes a person substantially more attractive to others. In addition, it provides for feedback, without which we cease to grow. When we are able to truly attend to each other, we can benefit from the observations and insights of others. To the extent that we function as complex information-processing systems, we depend upon new and accurate input in order to analyze correctly what is happening within and around us, and respond to others with appropriate behavior. It is also one of the biases of psychoanalysis that the more we understand the patterns of our feelings and behavior, the better able we are to make life plans that are fulfilling of our needs.

The recognition and acceptance of our general lack of knowledge is also crucial if we are to be open for new ideas. Unfortunately, there are many individuals who cannot tolerate the possibility that either they do not know something or that someone else does. Their rigidity and self-righteousness may further reduce their attractiveness. It is a wonderful thing to see this change as the result either of a successful integration of one's archaic, infantile grandiosity into the adult personality or the resolution of neurotic conflicts.

In successful psychotherapy, there is an idealization of the treatment process, which gradually subsides until therapist and therapy are seen more realistically. The patient is then able to perceive and accept that treatment does not create a perfected human being, although it can create a healthier one, provided the patient and therapist are suited to each other and motivated for work.

CONCLUSIONS

It has been shown that deaf people have the capacity for emotional growth but rarely have the opportunities to develop their capacities in productive therapeutic relationships. In the initial phase of psychiatric treatment, the major problem is establishing a therapeutic alliance. For the deaf patient with a hearing therapist, this is particularly difficult because of a number of factors. First are the years of mistrust built up in some deaf people from their perception of the hearing world. Second, the therapist may not be fluent in sign language or total communication. This skill is essential in order to set the patient at ease; otherwise, a communication barrier in the treatment reality may repeat past painful realities of an environment not equipped to understand the patient and to facilitate his or her growth. Third, there are specific transference and countertransference problems that will develop during psychotherapy with a deaf patient. The middle phase of treatment, especially, will involve identifying and working through some transference distortions, which I have attempted to define and illustrate. In particular, the therapist will need to be aware and make use of his or her own countertransference reactions to the deaf client so the therapeutic process does not founder in this phase. My clinical experience has been evidence to me that a working knowledge of Kohut's self-object model is vital to the successful understanding and resolution of the trans-ferences that are likely to occur in psychiatric work with the deaf. The deaf seem especially vulnerable to disturbances in the sense of self, and, for this reason, I have spent a significant amount of space in this chapter discussing Kohut's core concepts. I feel the reader who struggles with Kohut's theories will appreciate more exactly how they might aid psychotherapy with deaf adults, and that the theories offer some real hope for restoring a joyful and productive sense of self in these individuals.

REFERENCES

Altschuler, K.Z. Studies of the deaf: Relevance to psychiatric theory. *American Journal of Psychiatry*, 1971, *127*, 1521–1526.

Diagnostic and statistical manual of mental disorders (2nd ed.). Washington, D.C.: The American Psychiatric Association, 1968.

Goldberg, A. Narcissism and the readiness for psychotherapy termination. *AMA Archives of General Psychiatry*, 1975, *32*, 695–704.

Grinker, R.R., Sr. *Psychiatric social work: A transactional case book*. New York: Basic Books, 1961.

Grinker, R.R., Sr. Reminiscences of Dr. Roy Grinker. *Journal of American Academy of Psychoanalysis*, 1975, *3*, 211–221.

Grinker, R.R., Sr., Werble, B., & Drye, R.C. *The borderline syndrome*. New York: Basic Books, 1968.

Kohut, H. Forms and transformations of narcissism. *Journal of the American Psychological Association*, 1966, *14*, 243–272.

Mindel, E.D., & Vernon, M. *They grow in silence*. Silver Spring, Md.: National Association of the Deaf, 1971.

Neto, B.B. An analysis of a deaf mute. *American Journal of Psychotherapy*, 1972, *26*, 123–128.

Parsons, T. Boundary relations between sociocultural and personality systems. In Grinker, R.R., Sr. (Ed.): *Toward a unified theory of human behavior*. New York: Basic Books, 1967.

Rainer, J.D., Altshuler, K.Z., & Kallman, F.J. *Family and mental health problems in a deaf population*. New York: Department of Medical Genetics, N.Y. State Psychiatric Institute (Columbia University), 1963.

Rothstein, D. Office treatment of deaf adults. In Grinker, R.R., Sr. (Ed.): *Psychiatric diagnosis, therapy and research on the psychotic deaf, final report*. Chicago: Institute for Psychosomatic and Psychiatric Research, (grant RD-2407-S, HEW), 1969.

Shakow, D. Psychoanalysis. In *Schools of psychology, a symposium*. New York: Appleton-Century-Croft. Reprinted by the U.S. Department of HEW, National Institutes of Health (NIH-65084), pp. 87–122, 1967.

Spiegel, J.P. The resolution of the role conflict within the family. *Psychiatry*, 1957, *20*, 1.

Spiegel, J.P. *Transactions*. New York: Science House, 1971.

Larry G. Stewart, Ed.D.

10

Counseling the Deaf Client

Today, counseling with deaf adults is offered in a variety of settings. These settings range from rehabilitation agencies to community mental health centers. We may find counselors serving deaf clients in vocational training centers, postsecondary education programs, comprehensive rehabilitation centers, community referral and service centers, inpatient and outpatient clinics, and a variety of other locations. The contemporary scene indeed offers a strong contrast to time periods as recently as the 1960s, when the deaf client had to look far and wide to find a counselor capable of offering professional assistance in a form of communication readily understandable to the client. Even today, many deaf individuals have few opportunities to obtain such counseling, but the situation is much improved and getting better.

The past dearth of counseling services for deaf adults is both a cause and a reflection of the relatively limited research and professional writing dealing with the process, content, and outcome of the counseling experience with deaf clients. In the absence of sufficient numbers of qualified counselors, little research or sharing of experience was possible. With comparatively little organized knowledge of the counseling process with the deaf, educators of counselors for the deaf have faced obstacles in recruiting and properly training sufficient numbers of qualified counselors.

With the stimulus of federal funding for training programs, the 1960s and early 1970s witnessed a slow but steady growth in the number of counselors qualified to work with deaf people. Concurrent with this growth, a slowly increasing number of professional articles and research studies have reached practicing counselors and counselors-in-training. The reciprocal effect of increasing manpower and expanding professional knowledge has been a constructive contribution to the recent expansion of counseling services for the deaf people.

The field of counseling the deaf today is in no position to become complacent with its achievements, however. Far from it. There has been no major publication dealing with counseling the deaf since 1971 (Sussman & Stewart, 1971); there are currently no nationally accepted training and performance standards for counselors for the deaf aside from those of general counseling organizations (American Personnel and Guidance Association, American Psychological Association, etc.); there have been few research-based studies of counseling the deaf by the major training programs for counselors for the deaf; there are few practitioners who may be considered rigorous theoreticians who are involved in counseling the deaf; and, there are few articles or other publications dealing with methods and techniques of counseling with the deaf.

There are very real reasons for the current lag in the speciality of counseling the deaf when its development is compared with the general field. One of the primary reasons for the paucity of theory development and evaluation of methodologies in the area of counseling with the deaf relates to defining and describing the population "deaf people." Counselors who are experienced in serving deaf clients are well aware that, aside from hearing loss, there are very few characteristics of deaf people as a group that distinguish them from the general population. Hence, when we attempt to speak of counseling the deaf, we are often reduced to weak generalizations that in truth apply to some deaf people but not others.

A good example of this problem is the widely accepted generalization that nondirective counseling is not effective with deaf clients. A close examination of this issue would show that it is true for many deaf people and untrue for many others. There are deaf people who are completely unresponsive to a nondirective approach or, at worst, do not have the slightest idea what the counselor is doing when he or she asks open-ended questions such as, "How do you feel about (this or that)?" On the other hand, there are many deaf clients who make excellent progress in counseling with a counselor who uses nondirective methods and techniques. It is instructive to note that while nondirective methods work for some hearing clients but not others, we do not hear the same generalization that nondirective counseling methods do not work well with the hearing.

In facing the fact that the term "deaf people" often leads to invalid generalizations, we must recognize that an effective approach to dealing with the question of counseling methods and techniques with deaf clients requires that we specify the problems of different deaf clients that lead us to change our approach from the one commonly used with non–hearing-impaired persons. In doing so, we must admit that it is not always the deafness per se that mandates a modified approach but, rather the special needs of the individual. This perspective broadens our investigative horizons and necessitates that we ourselves understand why certain deaf individuals respond, while others do not, to a specific counseling approach. This question alone presents a major challenge, since all variables that impinge upon the success of the counseling relationship need to be controlled before valid statements may be made about the efficacy of different methods and techniques. Many counselor–researchers recognize the nature and magnitude of this problem and they, along with those who do not grasp why research is so difficult to carry out with "the deaf," retreat to the peace and quiet of nonpublication.

Yet, counseling with deaf clients goes on. Graduate students continue to seek guidance on how to counsel "the deaf" and look, most times in vain, for learned treatises that will provide them with clear-cut principles and procedures for ensuring success with a deaf client. In the face of mumbling from the old guard when asked "How?", the inquiring minds of youthful and not-so-youthful graduate students continue to seek—and rightfully so—answers to the question of what counseling methods and procedures work with deaf people.

ONE PERSON'S PERSPECTIVE

The pages that follow represent the perspective of one person—the author—on the issue of counseling strategies and techniques in the process of counseling with deaf individuals. In reviewing the literature, much can be gleaned of the "wisdom of the ages" in counseling deaf people. However, little light is shed on specific problems deaf people face *and* how these may be handled constructively in the counseling process. Consequently, I have chosen to present selected cases from my counseling experience, and to discuss specific problems experienced by the clients involved, as well as what was done in the counseling process to deal with these problems. This approach, I hope, will suggest some workable principles for use by other counselors as they approach the task of helping their clients. At this time no statement can be made regarding the effectiveness of my approaches to the problems presented, other than that I believe they were helpful. Others may wish to investigate these approaches to ascertain their efficacy.

I am deaf myself and I have been actively involved in counseling deaf people from all walks of life, of varied levels of intelligence and abilities, and of varied personalities and communication skills, for more than 15 years. I have written about counseling the deaf (Patterson & Stewart, 1971) and have been involved in research (Stewart, 1970a) and in graduate training for counselors with the deaf. In striving to achieve a greater degree of effectiveness in my own counseling with deaf people and communicating with others about my experiences and beliefs, I have come to believe that general theories of counseling are generally as applicable to counseling with the deaf as they are to counseling with other clients. The methods that stem from these theories are equally applicable. Many deaf clients experience no difficulty in participating in the counseling process exactly as a hearing client of comparable abilities would, *provided* the counselor possesses the communication skills and empathy level necessary for effective interaction with the client.

Some deaf clients are unable to participate in the counseling process because the counselor does not possess the requisite attitudes and communication skills. To be sure, there are deaf clients who cannot participate in counseling no matter how skilled the counselor is in the area of communication. Some severely retarded deaf clients without significant communication skills, for example, would be wasting their time in the counseling room. Yet, the same could be said of many hearing individuals, as, for example, those who may be severely or profoundly retarded. Hence, given that the deaf client does have some communication skills and some

ability to interact with another person, the counselor's skills become the key elements in effecting change in the counseling process. Deciding which methods and
techniques will work with a given client is a major task for the counselor.

CASES AND STRATEGIES

The following cases are presented to illustrate that effective counseling with
deaf clients depends not upon modifying theories and methods of counseling but
rather on implementing existing theories and methods through special communication techniques based upon a comprehensive understanding of the individual. As
we shall see, deafness per se has little bearing upon the counseling process itself,
but it *always* has a profound impact on the individual.

All identifying information in the following cases has been changed to protect
the privacy of the clients, including names and locations.

John

John was 36-years-old at the time of referral. Deafened at the age of 2 years
from spinal meningitis, he had attended three schools for the deaf in three states,
graduating at age 19. One of these schools had an oral orientation while the other
two had more or less "total communication" orientation. John had held a variety
of jobs over the years, and had lived in several different cities. He was married to
a woman who was also deaf and they had four young children ranging in age from
2 to 13 years. He was referred for long-term counseling after a psychological
evaluation had indicated the presence of a deep-seated anxiety disorder marked by
nervousness and irritability, somatic complaints, difficulty in getting along with
others, temper outbursts under job stress, and frequent job changes created by
interpersonal conflicts.

Initial contacts indicated that John was an exceptionally able "communica-
tor." He could express himself very well using Signed English, and could understand the counselor's sign language and finger spelling very well. In essence, there
was no communication problem between the counselor and the client. John's tested
reading achievement was at the 10th grade level, and his intelligence level was
above average. His hearing was essentially nonfunctional for speech, although he
used a behind-the-ear aid for sound orientation. His speech was stilted and generally
difficult to understand although those close to him could follow him with some
effort. John dressed çarefully and conservatively, and took some pride in his personal hygiene and grooming. He quite clearly was concerned about the impression
he made on others, and he generally wanted to create a favorable impression.

During the initial interview, John expressed indignation over his current employment conditions, where the other workers—some deaf, some hearing, all able
to use sign language—were "difficult to get along with and always making trouble"
for him. He was quite emotional when describing the slights and hurts he received

from others, and evidenced considerable hostility for those who in particular were causing problems through gossip and "squealing" to his supervisor. He felt others were unfair to him and made unnecessary problems.

Over the course of ten counseling sessions it became clear that John was suffering from many repressed anxieties and conflicts. He had "stomach problems," couldn't sleep well, became upset easily, had headaches frequently, and by his own self-description was generally "nervous." On the surface, he felt that others in his current life created his problems, and believed that if only his situation would improve he would be all right.

As the counselor–client relationship developed, John revealed considerable hesitancy and anxiety over self-revelation. In the past, he had had counseling at other locations, and in each case John felt that the counselor had destroyed his confidence by talking with others, who had in turn let information about him leak out to other deaf people. This had created much unhappiness for John, and at one point he challenged me by signing in a manner amounting to yelling, "How do I know you can keep your mouth shut! You counselors blab all over town!" However, over the course of several additional sessions John was able to resolve his distrust of the counselor and reveal many things about himself, much of which he was ashamed to talk about. Eventually, John was able to deal with many of the early, traumatic experiences he had lived through as a child. What these were has no bearing on our discussion; suffice to say that he progressed in counseling in a manner comparable to what we commonly see described by many textbooks on counseling with nondisabled individuals.

What were the special knowledges and techniques involved with John? In retrospect, the special features of the case seemed to be as follows:

1. Previously, John had received counseling services from a variety of professionals (psychiatrists, psychologists, counselors, physicians) who did not use sign language. He had left treatment disgruntled and essentially unchanged. His view was summed up in a statement made early in counseling: "Hell! I couldn't understand them and they couldn't understand me. It was a waste of time." It was clearly therapeutic in itself that John finally met a counselor who could interact with him with no built-in communication barriers. There were no, "Excuse me, can you please sign slower?" statements made by the counselor, nor were there repeated instances of "Wait! What does that sign mean?" The counselor and the client were both thoroughly acquainted with the slight shades of meaning of a signed variation here, a quizzical expression there, a significant pause at one point, a rapid string of expressions at another point.

2. Many dynamics common in the deaf community—as in any 'small community'—were operating to sustain John's maladaptive behavior. Gossip, group mores, factions and cliques, and the unavailability of social outlets among others who were unaware of John's problems closed him in and left no escape from social pressures and disapproval. The counselor's understanding of the pressures John had to live with facilitated a feeling on John's part that he was understood.

3. John, despite his good communication skills, was totally lacking in insight into his problems and their causes. He thought his stomach problems were sure signs of cancer. His headaches were just a problem inherited from his mother. He had no idea why he was so nervous. He couldn't understand why he had such a hard time sleeping. "Stress" was just an abstract word to him. His rapid heartbeats when he was upset meant he would surely have a heart attack any day. In short, he was abysmally ignorant of symptoms of anxiety. Through explanations provided by the counselor, John learned about these symptoms, and after a thorough medical examination (recommended to rule out real physical pathology), John was able to reach an understanding that there was nothing physically wrong with him; that his problems were created by inner emotional conflicts and stress; and that relief was to be sought through resolution of his repressed emotional conflicts and his maladaptive coping patterns.

To be sure, we may expect the same kinds of misunderstanding and ignorance among some hearing clients who appear for counseling. The only real difference in this case was that the clear communication via sign language achieved by John and the counselor permitted the latter to stay tuned in with John, to provide information when John was ready for it and not before, and to use the idioms, syntax, and colloquialisms of sign language to convey meanings that were understandable to John.

Recent research in the general counseling field (Rogers et al., 1968; Torrey, 1973) has indicated rather conclusively that the ability of the counselor to know the client, to be "with" the client, and to understand the client at a deep level is crucial to effective counseling. To a certain extent this means, for the counselor, a sharing in many aspects of the client's world. This sharing occurs more naturally among people who have a common developmental, cultural, educational, socio-economic, ethnic, and/or racial background. With deaf clients, it seems axiomatic that counselors long-acquainted with both sign language and its nuances, as well as the experience of deafness and its ramifications, will be ahead of other counselors of comparable abilities and skills in their ability to be "with" the deaf client. This seems to be one hard fact that counselors-in-training and practicing counselors will have to come to grips with: one cannot expect to be effective in counseling deaf people unless one has a genuine understanding of deaf clients and the form of communication they use. It must be borne in mind that we are not speaking of one type of background or one type of communication. At the risk of overkill, it must be restated that there are deaf people from all walks of life and possessing all kinds and levels of communication skills. A particular counselor thus may be better at counseling one type of deaf client (e.g., one with good oral skills and middle-income upbringing), whereas another will be better at counseling another type (e.g., one with only gestural communication, from an impoverished socioeconomic background.)

There are implications in the foregoing for counselor selection and training as well as for counselor self-expectations. The candidate for counselor training who has a background in communicating and interacting with deaf people may expect a more rapid progression in developing ability to counsel the deaf than the candidate who lacks this background, *provided* that attitudes, interpersonal relations skills, and general maturity are comparable. The counseling candidate who lacks this background with deaf people can expect a period of frustration while learning how to work with the deaf, even after completing course work and degree requirements. Beyond a classroom or a graduate program, it takes experience and time to acquire real ease and competence in communicating with many types of deaf people.

Ricky

Ricky was a 27-year-old adult who had been deaf since birth. His background included a broken home, an extremely neurotic mother, and an abusive father who ridiculed and shamed him in front of others. He had been in classes for the mentally retarded in public schools up until his 16th year, then attended school for the deaf for 2 years. After graduation (based upon his age rather than his achievement), he attended trade school to learn auto body and fender repair. He then worked for a period of time in a junkyard disassembling cars, and later as a laborer. His employment was unsteady, and he eventually applied for rehabilitation services. A psychological evaluation indicated that Ricky was a disturbed young man with a personality disorder marked by obsessive compulsive behavior, extreme nervousness, phobias, and sexual obsessions. Ricky presented as an extremely tense young man, moving stiffly, and exhibiting many nervous mannerisms. His intelligence was in the below-average range, and his reading skills were at the 5th grade level. He had a moderate hearing loss, and was able to use a hearing aid with some ability to discern spoken language. Although his speech was strained and high pitched, it was understandable. His sign language skills were excellent.

Signed English was used by the counselor, as Ricky readily understood others via this method. He was highly motivated for counseling and attended sessions twice a week for 1 year.

The counseling approach used involved several components: information sharing, emotional support, insight development, ventilation, relaxation therapy, and environmental manipulation.

Ricky was a very unusual young man. His enthusiasm for and dedication to self-improvement was phenomenal. For whatever reason, his trust in the counselor was total. He was not considered a dependent personality, yet he was entirely open to suggestions from the counselor for self-improvement. He was, in a very real sense, an ideal client. He came for each session ready to talk about himself, and if the counselor felt he was avoiding important areas, Ricky would seek to explore those areas. He worked diligently at relaxation therapy and carried over what he learned in counseling into his everyday life. The relationship between the counselor and the client was one of mutual respect and acceptance. Special care was taken to respect Ricky's prerogative in all areas of his life. He saw me as a resource, a person with ideas to help improve his life as he, Ricky, wanted to improve it. When Ricky would ask, "Do you think my idea is okay?" I would attempt to convey the idea—and it was a genuine one—that if Ricky felt that the idea would really help him to function better and feel better about himself, then it was definitely okay. When an idea was unclear, I would restate it and ask if that was an accurate description of the idea. Ricky then could clarify as he thought appropriate and examine the ramifications of the idea in his daily life. Eventually, Ricky learned that it was not for the counselor to determine how he should live his life, but only to help him to learn a process of determining what was right for him and to trust his own feelings.

Ricky's progress over the 1-year period when he was in counseling was remarkable. He mastered relaxation techniques to the point that he was quite relaxed under most circumstances. His nervous mannerisms decreased sharply, and returned, in greatly reduced manifestation, only under great stress. He came to regard himself as a person of worth rather than as the "screwed-up mess" that he considered himself to be prior to counseling. He also came to a status of independence where he could relate to his parents without letting them undermine his self-confidence. He attended a postsecondary training program and is still enrolled at this time.

How was counseling with Ricky different because he was deaf? In retrospect, the techniques of progressive relaxation, information sharing, and environmental manipulation were applied "intact." Methods and techniques were standard. Once again, the variations that developed were related to how these concepts and techniques were put into a form understandable to the client. Instead of strict English language structure at all times, many concepts were put into American Sign Language and pantomime. Much role playing was used. In describing relaxation techniques, demonstrations were paramount. A rubber band was used to illustrate what happened to muscles under stress and when calmness was present. A detailed explanation was used to show how stress and conflict during childhood, leading to emotional conflict and repression, could be translated into a constant state of bodily tension. Similar detail went into methods one could use to counteract this stress, tension, and repression. Bibliotherapy was used, as was the keeping of a diary describing his own dreams and feelings under various circumstances. Reassurance was used to support Ricky in times of dealing with feelings previously denied consciousness. Ideas were shared dealing with how to handle life circumstances. Communication was the key. A common language (sign language) and the safety of a counseling relationship marked by trust and confidence made growth and change possible.

Could approaches such as transactional analysis or psychoanalysis have been used with Ricky by therapists skilled in their use? I doubt it. Not with Ricky. His level of comprehension probably could not have dealt with the abstractions involved.

Billy

Billy was a strange young man. At 19, a graduate of a state school for the deaf, he had quietly escaped the notice of everyone and had slowly drifted into paranoid schizophrenia. His symptoms had been present for years, but only trained mental health workers or sensitive teachers could have spotted Billy's emerging maladjustment. He kept to himself, playing only with children much younger than he. He seldom communicated, and when he did it was to make demands of the younger children. Sometimes he hit them; sometimes he would force them to do errands for him or get him a soft drink or a piece of candy. If they did not oblige, he hit and/or threatened them. Much of his life was spent playing with toys, lost in a fantasy world. After graduation, he was arrested on a morals charge; he had forced a younger person, a minor, to submit to homosexual sex acts with him. Released on probation, he was referred for counseling in lieu of psychiatric help inasmuch as there were no physicians available with whom he could communicate.

Billy's intelligence was in the dull-normal range. Although he read at only the third-grade level, his ability to communicate via sign language was well-developed. His speech was poor and barely understandable, even to those who knew him. He was tall and raw-boned, with staring eyes that seldom blinked behind thick eyeglasses. He harbored many schemes to get even with those who had "wronged" him, and spent much of his days plotting elaborate scenarios for the demise of his tormentors.

Counseling with Billy was a long, complicated, difficult process. He remained unresponsive to open-ended questions. To direct questions such as "How are you feeling?", Billy would invariably reply, "Fine," even though he was obviously distraught or uncomfortable. He had a fixation about knives, and talked about them ceaselessly. "Do you like knives?"; "I want a large knife"; "Can I have a knife?"; "Why can't you give me a knife?"; "Look at this picture; Let me get a knife like this." The questions and statements continued intermittently during counseling and outside with others.

Billy was placed in a mental health treatment center in a security ward and remained there for 2 years. During this period, he participated in group therapy through the assistance of an interpreter, took part in other hospital routines, and was seen for two counseling sessions per week.

What was counseling like with Billy? First and most importantly, all counselor communications had to be direct and concrete, with no compound language structure. One idea at a time had to be presented. Insight development had to proceed extremely slowly as Billy struggled to understand the counselor. The following dialogue (translated directly from sign language) exemplifies this process:

Billy (B): Why me stay in hospital?

Counselor (C): Help you become well (healthy). (Pause) Your mind confused. Hospital help you think right, feel better.

B: Nothing wrong me. (Smiles, eyes take on crafty look) (Pause) When me go home?

C: You can go home when you become well. You said "Nothing wrong with you." Why you in hospital here? (This was an attempt to help Billy face the fact that he did indeed have a problem, since by facing this fact he could understand what behavior he had to change.)

B: (Smiles, shrugs) Sex problem. Not right pull down boy's pants. (Quizzical look) But what wrong, I like it. Nothing wrong!

C: You liked sex with boy, so you think it was okay. You think it is okay to do anything that you like, right?

B: Yes. Nothing wrong. (Smiles)

C: Billy, you said it was okay to do anything you like, anything you want. (Pause) Imagine (think picture) someone—maybe a big strong person—not like you. Imagine he decides to beat you up because he doesn't like you. Is that okay?

B: No! Can't do that. Not right. (Looks uncomfortable)

C: Explain why it is not right.

B: Man can't hit me. Hurt me.

C: It's not right for other people to hurt you, is that what you mean?

B: Right. Other people not supposed hurt me.

C: Billy, let's you and I agree . . . we think alike . . . have same idea . . . it is wrong to hurt people. Right? (Billy nods head affirmatively with vigor). Okay. Now I want to ask you . . . Is it okay for you to hurt a little boy? Is it okay to beat up a little boy?

B: (Hesitates, smiles) Why you ask me? (Billy was obviously living with one set of rules for himself, another set for others when it involved his feelings.)

C: You know what I mean. (Looks at Billy calmly)

B: (Shifts in chair) Do you like knife? (Smiles slightly)

C: (Ignores question) Is it okay for you to hurt or beat up a young boy? (Remains relaxed, as if there had been no diverting question from Billy)

B: (Shifts in chair, pauses, smiles slightly) It okay if he stubborn, won't do what I want. (Looks firm, intent)

C: You mean it's okay for you to beat up a little boy . . . but wrong for big person to beat you up. Right? (Same relaxed, noncommital posture)

B: (Smiles openly, becomes more animated) You silly. It not right for big man beat on me, me beat boy wrong. (Becomes slightly angry) But he refused sex me! (Billy was obviously referring to the incident that led to his problems with the law.)

(At this point the counselor veered away from this line of interaction, since Billy clearly could not deal with his needs and reality at this point.)

C: I see that you little upset, Billy. Let's stop talking about this problem now. Let's change . . . let's talk about how you are feeling now.

B: Feel fine. (looks irritated) Me mad you.

C: You are mad at me . . . did I upset you? (Again, calmly)

B: You stubborn talk about man, boy. Not like.

The nature of communication with Billy automatically ruled out many forms of therapy since their implementation hinges upon a particular type and level of verbal interaction and abstraction. Transactional analysis, psychoanalysis, rational-emotive therapy: these and others in classic form were automatically ruled out with Billy. To be sure, elements of each approach could be and were used, but their use in a consistent manner was not possible. As it turned out, and this is a retrospective analysis, the main strategies used were behavior-modification techniques, medication (under the supervision of a psychiatrist), emotional support, and the counselor's individual approach, which could best be described as eclectic with a heavy orientation toward reality therapy.

Billy's case was an extremely difficult one. There were scores of counseling sessions where his resistance and fragmented reasoning as portrayed above were even more pronounced. Eventually, however, he reached a point where he was able to understand and internalize some basic concepts of right and wrong, and he eventually developed other outlets for his strong sexual drives.

One may interpret Billy's problems from a variety of theoretical points of view; in the end, however, it was his behavior that was a problem to himself and others. ''Cure'' for him meant changing his behavior from the socially maladaptive to the socially adaptable and acceptable. Again, this occured via persuasion, support, interpretations, guidance, behavior-modification strategies, and retraining. Group therapy was helpful. The process involved not only interpreting during group meetings but also individual sessions afterwards where the events of the group were rehashed with him and suggestions made for his participation in the next session (i.e., how to let others know when he had something to say, how to use the interpreter, etc.).

Elizabeth

Elizabeth was referred to me by her Vocational Rehabilitation counselor, who expressed perplexity with regard to helping her. The referral information indicated that Elizabeth had graduated at the top of her class in a school for the deaf, with an overall achievement at the 12th-grade level. Reading comprehension was at the 9th-grade level, and math achievement was above the 12th grade. Her measured intelligence was in the superior range. Immediately after graduation she had attended summer school at a university that has a program for the deaf, then had attended a college for the deaf for 1 year. At the end of the year, she indicated to her guidance counselor that she wanted to attend a third college, this time to become a nurse. In preparation for doing so, she enrolled at this third college for summer school, only to drop out after 1 month. She indicated to her guidance counselor that she wanted to re-enroll at the first college to study teaching, but could not give a sound reason for her choice. At this point, she was referred to me for an evaluation and personal counseling.

At 22 years of age, Elizabeth was a plain-appearing, rather quiet young woman. At her initial evaluation, she seemed tense and wary. She was reticent during the clinical interview, answering questions briefly and, at times, evasively. She was noncommital about her family and personal feelings, and became uneasy when asked about her problems in setting firm educational goals. The evaluation corroborated the information regarding her intelligence and achievement, and further revealed a painfully shy, introverted person with a poor self-concept. Interest testing indicated low aspirations in all areas. However, her language skills and ability to communicate in Signed English were excellent. The findings led the examiner to recommend personal counseling for Elizabeth, along with a period of employment until she had achieved a better level of personal adjustment and clearer personal as well as career goals.

Elizabeth attended four counseling sessions where evaluation findings were discussed with her. She proved to be very defensive where her self-concept was involved, and at first rejected the possibility that her decision-making with regard to educational goals was based in personal adjustment difficulties. Initially, she refused to discuss her personal feelings with the counselor, but rather concentrated on asking questions about various occupational areas and educational programs for the deaf. Later, she became more open. The following is an excerpt from her second interview:

Counselor (C): Sit down Elizabeth. It's nice to see you today. (Elizabeth sits down, composes herself stiffly, and stares at the counselor with her face set.) Last week we talked about your test scores and your ideas about what they meant. We agreed that you would give this some more thought during the week, then today we would meet to discuss the various possibilities open to you for your future personal and career development. (Elizabeth nods slightly and remains quiet.) Perhaps we could get started by having you tell me what you think you would like to do now that you have the information provided by the tests you took.

Elizabeth (E): I don't know . . . I think I want to go back to (the college she first attended). (Pauses) I want to be with hearing students again. I don't want to be with deaf students all the time . . . our ways are different But [the third college] is too hard for me . . . there is no program for the deaf and I do need a little help because of my hearing loss.

C: Let me see if I understand you correctly. You don't want to attend Stratton College* [the second college] because you feel a bit uncomfortable with the social life there, since all of the students are deaf. (Elizabeth relaxes a bit; nods quietly in affirmation.) You also want to be around hearing students, yet [the third college] doesn't have special support services for the deaf and it would be difficult for you academically there. (Again Elizabeth nods, this time even more relaxed.) The [first college] seems to offer what you are looking for at a personal level: A program of support services for the deaf as well as opportunities to interact with both hearing and deaf students. Your

---

*Not the real name of the college.

reasoning seems to be sound in terms of your own desires, so I think you have it together on that score. It seems the next question is what you would like to study there. Your interest test—the Strong—didn't pick up any special area of interest on your part at this time of your life. What this basically means is that you like a lot of different kinds of work but up to this point in time there doesn't seem to be any single type of work you would like a great deal. Would you agree?

E: (Pauses) Well, I don't know . . . I want to become a social worker or teacher . . . I do like people . . . (Looks at counselor quietly).

C: (Pauses) Your Strong scores missed that . . . perhaps you have feelings about social work and teaching that were not picked up on the test . . . Perhaps it would help us if you could review your thinking about your career goals just before you went to [the first college], how your thinking changed, what your thinking was before you went to Stratton and how it later changed . . . this may give us better insight into your current perceptions . . . how you look at things now.

E: Well . . . when I went to [the first college] I wasn't really thinking a lot about the future. I did think about becoming a physical education teacher. I found out the courses were pretty hard there, and the interpreters were sometimes hard to follow. I thought about Stratton—all my friends were there— and I decided to go . . . . (Pause) At Stratton I thought about becoming a computer programmer . . . I'm good in math . . . but I didn't like the social life. I finally decided to come home and attend [the third college] . . . become a nurse. (Pause) I didn't like the courses I took this summer . . . they were too hard. I couldn't understand the teachers. (Pause) I think I will go back to [the first college] and become a teacher.

C: There are several things in what you have said we might talk about more and learn something from . . . Elizabeth, with so many opportunities available now I guess it is tough on a bright person like yourself to pick out one single career and pursue it. I note that your interests have ranged from physical education teaching to computer programming to nursing and then back to teaching. Your thinking pretty much is reflected in your Strong scores . . . you like a lot of things but nothing stands out as worth really hanging in there for. It seems that when anyone is really turned on by a career goal it is easier to put up with other things one might not like. For instance, if you really wanted to become a computer programmer perhaps you could put up with the social limitations you mentioned at Stratton College. Or, at least you would want to study computer programming at [first college] where you want to go now. Since you are changing colleges mainly because of the support services and social opportunities, it seems to me that career goals are secondary in your life now, and social, personal aspects are more important. Do you think this is an accurate observation?

E: (Considers what the counselor has said, pauses) Well . . . I don't know . . . I guess I have never thought of it like that . . . I don't know . . .

C: (Pause) Perhaps another aspect, Elizabeth, and I want to ask you to think carefully about this . . . another aspect is that there are personal and social concerns on your part now that kind of hold you back from really getting involved in a commitment to a career. . . . . Testing indicates that you have some personal feelings about yourself and other people that make you some- what unhappy . . . (Elizabeth slowly tenses up, mouth set). . . . I know this may be difficult for you to talk about, and perhaps I am wrong . . . but I do get the impression that you are not happy, that you have had a difficult time personally and in your interactions with others at the three colleges you have attended . . . and as a result you have not been able to really get into your studies and discover for yourself what you really want to do . . .

E: (Pauses) Well . . . I don't know . . . I haven't been happy, I had a hard time mixing with the other students at Gallaudet. I didn't like their ways . . . I had a boyfriend, and we broke up. . . . They said I was different, that I wasn't really deaf. (Elizabeth becomes sad, her eyes filling with tears.) I don't know what's wrong . . . there have been so many problems.

C: (Counselor waits; Elizabeth remains quiet, eyes filled with tears, face slightly flushed.) Well, Elizabeth, this is not an easy matter for you or anyone to deal with, but it is a common thing to happen. We sometimes get into pursuing goals that we aren't really committed to, and then lose sight of what is really important. You are a very capable person. You have excellent academic skills, and can expect to succeed at almost any career goal you set for yourself. You have to feel good about yourself, however, or any goal you set won't mean enough to you to really work at. Based upon our talks and test results, it's my impression that you will need to take time to deal with your personal feelings and values and goals before you can be productive in school or at work. As long as you have self-doubts and don't get good feelings from your relation- ships with your friends and acquaintances then the rest of it—classwork, book study, and other routines—becomes meaningless. Some people who find them- selves in this situation kind of tough it out and eventually work through their problems; others become dropouts and drift through life looking for they know not what. (Elizabeth is listening intently.) I guess at this point the thing you will need to do is sort through your own thoughts and feelings, consider our discussions, and decide for yourself what you want to do now and later. Perhaps returning to [the first college] will be just right for you . . . perhaps taking time out and working for a while and getting counseling will be really helpful . . . you have a lot of opportunities and options, and I am confident you can find the answer for yourself.

E: (Pauses) I will think about it and we can talk about it next week at our last meeting.

What was different here in the counseling approach used with Elizabeth? The counselor–client interaction is much as one might expect of any counseling session. Cognitive content is emphasized since Elizabeth was leaving on a vacation after the fourth session and thus time was very short. Signed English was used throughout by both Elizabeth and me, and this was rather important in facilitating under-standing. Elizabeth could read lips and had some usable hearing, and could con-ceivably have understood a nonsigning counselor or one who was not at ease with signing. However, the fact that we both used sign language naturally and effort-lessly undoubtedly was a factor in facilitating communication and progress in counseling.

Equally important was my understanding of Elizabeth's circumstances and background. I was familiar with each of the three college settings, and aware of the "no man's land" that hearing-impaired persons who are not deaf often find themselves in when interacting with all-deaf or all-hearing groups. At the same time I was aware that many individuals successfully resolve this sort of problem, and that those who fail to do so often have self-concept problems that make ordinary problems much worse.

Subsequent counseling sessions with Elizabeth revealed the basis for her self-rejection. Her parents disapproved of sign language and had never accepted her as a deaf person. They criticized her speech, her lip-reading skills, and her general personality. The father had a difficult temper, often striking Elizabeth and her siblings. A frequent mealtime theme in the home was how Elizabeth should not "handtalk" like other "dumb" deaf people, how she should never show others that she could not hear normally, how she should strive to behave as a "normal" person would.

The approach used in helping Elizabeth deal with her internalized self-rejection was basically client-centered therapy. The fact that I understood the nuances in-volved in her hearing loss, the flavor of being exposed to devaluation, and the nature of the communication barrier in many life situations undoubtedly helped Elizabeth know that she was understood when she spoke of her hurt and her rejection. At the same time, my failure to become upset by such rejection, my calmness when discussing the causes of her parents' behavior, and my focus upon moving forward to act constructively were perhaps more acceptable to her since I was not someone looking at the problems from an academic point of view but, rather, had in a sense "been there" and shared the experience.

This raises the question, "Is a deaf person more effective as a counselor for the deaf than a hearing person?" This is a moot question. How can it be answered from an empirical point of view? How does one define "an effective counselor"? How does one, via research, validate or invalidate the hypothesis in the face of difficulty in controlling other counselor variables as well as the client variables? I pass on this question.

Jim

Jim was 47-years-old when referred for counseling. Congenitally deaf, he attended college and had taught at a day school for the deaf for 24 years. He was married, had two teenage sons, and for years was involved in social and civic activities in the deaf community where he was perceived as a leader. Due to

recurring drinking problems, his performance as a teacher deteriorated to the point
where his supervisor asked him to leave. At the same time, his wife, weary from
years of frustrations due to Jim's problems, asked him to move out of the home.
Finding himself living alone in a run-down efficiency apartment, with no car and
little money, Jim went to the vocational rehabilitation office for assistance. The
rehabilitation counselor, unsure how to approach the question of Jim's vocational
future, requested a psychological evaluation and follow-up counseling as Jim made
decisions about his personal and vocational future.

Results of the psychological evaluation showed Jim to be an unusually gifted
man. With intelligence in the superior range, and academic achievement well above
the typical college graduate, Jim had a variety of options for future employment.
His strongest interests lay in the human services area, particularly teaching, social
work, and counseling. Although his personality indicated strong dependency needs,
no psychopathology was present. He was an open, caring person, perhaps too
concerned with the problems of the world for his own good.

A discussion of test findings was initially unproductive. Jim was quite negative
about himself, being deeply depressed by his change in life circumstances. Talk
about him and his woes was rife in the deaf community, and his shame over what
had happened was pronounced. Formerly a regular at bowling league meets and
social affairs at the local deaf club, Jim was avoiding any contact with old friends
and acquaintances. He had obtained a job as a mechanic's helper, and was earning
the minimum wage (then $2.60/hr) after having stepped down from a job that paid
$21,000/year. Sobered by the double blows of losing his job in disgrace and being
asked to leave by his wife, Jim was an abject figure as he entered the counselor's
office. He was convinced that his professional career was finished, his family would
never take him back, and he would become a derelict. He was positive that he
would have to remain in a low-skilled job all his life, and never again would have
close friends or be accepted as a valued member of the deaf community.

After observing Jim's depression during the first session where test results
were discussed, the counselor assumed a supportive role. Jim was encouraged to
talk about himself and ventilate his feelings of rejection, hurt, anger, and self-
hatred. This approach broke through Jim's fragile defenses and he wept openly for
minutes at a time as he poured out his frustrations and disappointment and despair.
It took four more sessions like this, with frequent teletypewriter (TTY) calls between sessions to lend Jim support during moments of profound despair and hope-
lessness. Finally, after 2 weeks of "mourning," Jim came in for his sixth counseling session. The following excerpt of that session illustrates the nature of the
counseling approach used with Jim. Jim was a fluent signer, using a combination
of Signed English and American Sign Language. His choice of the latter increased
during moments of high emotional content, and decreased with more cognitive
content. At all times he was alert, aware, and communicative.

Jim (J): Hello, Dr. S., How are you today?
Counselor (C): I'm keeping pretty busy, Jim. How are you doing?
J: Not so good, doc. (shakes his head) I never knew things could get so bad.

(Pauses) Well, what are we going to do about a job for me? This damn job I have is real joke. The guy I work with is unbelievable . . .

C: Yeah, I can imagine it's really something doing the work you are now at your age after so long as a teacher . . . you know, though, Jim, you don't have to keep working like you are now. You have a hell of a lot of ability. With some hard thinking on your part and some firm decisions, I know you can make something out of your life. (Jim looks unconvinced.) Let's be open about it, Jim. You made some mistakes and let drinking screw up your life. Your wife let you down at a time when you really needed her. OK, you found out that other people have their problems and their limits. You finally found out that you can't cut it both ways . . . you can't let your drinking get out of hand *and* expect people to live with what you do when you have had too much . . . . (Jim becomes flushed, shifts in his chair.) Hold it, Jim. I know you don't like hearing this, and you are getting upset. Just hear me out, ok?

J: It's ok. It's ok. I know what you're saying is right. Damn! I just hate being reminded what an ass I have been . . .

C: No, Jim. No. You are reading me wrong. You may think you are an ass. I don't. I see you as having made a mistake that a hell of a lot of people make. Some pay for it much worse than you have, and some get off easier. What is important is you did make a mistake, and you don't want to be stuck at where you are today. You feel like hell, and you have every right to feel that way. I'd be worried about you if you didn't. (Jim smiles ruefully.) But, you can pull yourself together and start over again. The cost will be a painful self-examination, decision-making, and hard, dedicated work.

J: OK, I'd like to believe you but this whole damn town is talking about me . . . . I don't see how it can ever blow over. My wife won't even let me see the kids . . . god! I'll be lucky if I can get a job in this town as a dog catcher. (Grins wryly)

C: (Smiles in spite of himself) OK, Jim, I know you see the worst now, but (sobering) believe me, while people can come down hard on a guy they are pretty forgiving in the long run. I am certain that as you pull your life back together again people will forget and, eventually, forgive. Things are not really that bad if we are talking about how others see you. People may talk a little, but I'll bet most of your friends are just waiting for you to let them approach you again. With you slinking off by yourself, how can they even say hello?

J: Ouch! That hurt. (Considers) You're right, though. I have been keeping to myself. I am so darned ashamed, though. Christ! Fired for drinking! Kicked out by my wife! Working as a grease monkey! Sleeping in a two-bit apartment! No car! No money! (Agitated) That SOB Joe Smith. . . . I saw him the other day at the bus stop and he really rubbed it in. I almost busted him when he smirked and said, "Hi, drinker! Heard your wife kicked you out." (Jim is really angry now.) I turned around and walked away but I don't know how much of that I can take. (Jim is now breathing heavily and shaking his head.)

C: Hey! That was a real dirty thing to do. I don't know this Joe Smith but I can't imagine many people like him.

J: (Beginning to calm down but still bothered) Right. He is a real bastard. (Considers) Yeah, you are right. He's the only one who really bothered me. (Long pause) Doc, this is shit for the birds. I am not going to let this talk business mess me up any worse than I am now.

Jim's reaction to talk in the community was adverse, but it was a real problem for him. The deaf community is comparable to a small town where there is little that does not get around sooner or later. This had been an especially difficult item for Jim for years; what he did in his personal life spilled over into his work life, and vice versa. As it turned out, he was not so much an addicted alcoholic as he was a deeply frustrated man who had few opportunities to make friends and associates of his own intellectual and interest levels. Attempting to become a "hail fellow, well met" type, he slowly retreated to drink rather than face his loneliness and feelings of boredom. It was especially galling to him to find that ultimately, he was not as sophisticated as he wanted to believe.

Jim was faced with a special problem, too, in that his rehabilitation counselor, who could not sign and who was not fully aware of Jim's potential, was encouraging him to undertake job training as a carpenter (Jim had taught carpentry in school). The following excerpt shows how this problem was dealt with during Jim's seventh counseling session, about one fourth of the way through the hour.

J: Oh, by the way, doc., Mr. L. (Jim's counselor from the vocational rehabilitation office) told me yesterday that he has a training slot open through CETA for me to work as a carpenter. Guess I will be starting 2 weeks from now. (Jim's face has a neutral expression as he relates this.)

C: (Looks doubtful) As a carpenter? That is surprising to me. I know you have skills as a carpenter but I sort of see you as eventually getting back into a professional line of work, either in teaching or, maybe, in counseling if you want to invest in graduate school. What do you think of the carpentry deal?

J: Well, it's a living. (Pause) I guess I haven't thought about it enough. I have been kinda coasting, getting myself together, figuring out what happened to me . . . trying to get a handle on it all. Working at the mechanic job just to eat . . . spending a lot of time walking and thinking, as you suggested . . . getting back in touch with myself and throwing away all the garbage I have collected in my head . . . I don't know (Reflective pause) I don't have much choice, do I? After all, Mr. L. is calling the shots.

C: No, Jim I don't think Mr. L. would want you to look at it that way. He isn't "calling the shots." You should be making your own decisions, especially now after you coasted so long not expressing yourself through all the years when you didn't really like the way your life was going. Mr. L. wants to help you, and perhaps gained the idea that you were interested in a carpentry job. Regardless, your decision about your future job will be one of the most important decisions of your life. Why don't you spend the next few days thinking back through you life . . . what kinds of things have you really enjoyed . . . what activities made you forget yourself and left you feeling good about yourself and what you did. . . . Forget about what you "can do" or "ought to do"; just think about what you enjoy now . . . then once you are clear in your own mind we can get together and figure out what careers offer what will give you enjoyment . . . then we can figure out how to get you into what *you* want to be doing.

J: (Looks interested) I've never looked at that way. Now that I think about it, why not? Hell, I don't even know why I got into carpentry work in the first place, let alone teaching carpentry. Now look at me! Thinking about working as a carpenter again! (Pauses) OK, let me think it over and we can talk about it next week. Can you tell Mr. L. I have changed my mind?

C: You want me to explain to Mr. L.? (Pauses) I wonder, Jim, is this something you would want to do yourself? It could be a good step toward your growing independence. What do you think?

J: (Looks thoughtful) Yeah, I guess so. I was just feeling a little uncomfortable since he worked so hard to set that up. I didn't know quite what to say to him about me changing my mind. . . . Do you think he won't mind?

C: Actually, Jim, I think Mr. L. would be happy to hear your ideas. After all, it's your life. No one else has to do the job that you get, and you are the only person who can decide if it's right for you. Frankly, I think you would be foolish to let someone else make that kind of a decision for you. You owe it to yourself to stand up and let everyone—Mr. L., your wife, your children, me, everyone!—know what *you* want to do with your life.

J: Damned if I don't think you are right, doc! How about that! (Looks wonderingly at counselor.)

One week later, Jim returned for his eighth counseling session. Appearing visibly stronger and erect, clean-shaven and clear-eyed, Jim began to recount how happy Mr. L. had been to learn that Jim wanted more time to consider career options and wanted to cancel the CETA plan. Equally important, during the week Jim had visited his family, and after talking it over with his wife, they had decided that he would move back into the family home. There had been a tearful reunion with his teenage sons. Jim was clearly bolstered by his family's support at this time. He talked about his future in the following segment.

J: I told you I would think over what I would like to do in the future. Well, I spent a lot of time this past week doing that. I talked about it some with (his wife) and she liked the way I was thinking about it. She thought I would like being a teacher of science, but I told her to hold on! That I would work it out. She accepted it pretty good. (Pauses, relaxed) You know, when I was younger I really got a kick out of working with deaf adults in a shop back home. I would explain about tools to them, and help some of them with their checking accounts, paying bills, and stuff like that. I have always liked people, and I like children but I like these older deaf people a little better. Lots of them are as sharp as a tack but their schools didn't teach them a lot of things. Do you think I might get some kind of a job working with deaf adults? (Jim looks at the counselor hopefully)

C: Jim, that idea sounds pretty exciting to me. Can you tell me one good reason why you couldn't get a job like that?

J: Hey! I asked you! (Smiles) OK, ok. I will make up my own mind, doc. I get the point! (Shakes head and smiles) Yeah, I think I can get a job like that somewhere. Dr. (Jim's former boss) told me when he let me go that he was sorry, that he would be happy to write a good letter for me if I promised to work hard on getting myself straightened out. I think I can get him to write on my behalf . . . a letter of recommendation. I have helped a few deaf people for Vocational Rehabilitation in the past . . . helped them apply for jobs, get a place to live, stuff like that. Mr. L. can write a recommendation for me, too. James Jones (president of the local deaf club) has said nice things to me about when I helped some of the deaf club members with their personal and family problems, so I think he will help me, too. (Considers) Do you think maybe I could get a job with the XYZ Rehabilitation Center? I heard they were looking for what they call a Personal Adjustment Teacher. I bet I could do that pretty well.

C: Jim, I think you are really getting your act together on this thing. I did hear that XYZ Rehabilitation Center was looking for someone, and they want a deaf person for the job.

Jim got the job. Today, 5 years later, he is coordinator of that rehabilitation center's program for the deaf, which serves approximately 20 deaf adults. His life has returned to normal, and he is once again respected in his community and active on its behalf. Jim continued in personal counseling for 6 months after he had started working at his new job. The day of his final session, he expressed something that counselors should remember:

J: You know, doc. I can't believe how my life has turned around. I have never been happier in my life. My wife and I, my kids . . . we are so grateful we have each other and our friends and our home and my job. I hit bottom in my life when I got fired from (school for the deaf). I thought about killing myself, but I couldn't do it. It would have ruined my wife and kids. I was in the wrong job for years and didn't know it. I didn't believe in myself, and I didn't know it. I was running away from myself, from my job, from my disappointment in myself for being in a life I hated. I wake up sometimes at night sweating and shaking, dreaming that I took that CETA job.

Jim's case is an example of the type of counseling and the level of verbal interaction that can occur with many deaf adults. No adaptations in methods and techniques were necessary. The form of communication used—sign language—was considered a crucial element to the total process. Writing would have been woefully inadequate. Speech and lip reading would have been too taxing of Jim's resources. The counselor's understanding of Jim's background, the deaf community, job horizons, and the dependency-provoking aspects of deafness, were also considered vital to an effective approach to guiding Jim.

Could other theoretical approaches work with others like Jim? Certainly. Jim is typical of many highly educated, highly verbal deaf individuals who could be helped by almost any approach *provided* that adequate communication methods are used. The counseling approach used—a combination of reality therapy and client-centered therapy—appeared to be highly effective. Whether psychoanalysis, transactional analysis, or another dynamic approach could have achieved the same results is highly debatable since their goals are quite different.

THE LOW-FUNCTIONING CLIENT

Thus far, all case illustrations have dealt with clients capable of communicating with a counselor in sign language, albeit the case of "Billy" was certainly illustrative of "difficult-to-talk-with" clients. However, there are large numbers of deaf clients who are almost totally unresponsive to the traditional dialogue-oriented counseling mileu. Such individuals, typically, are pooly educated, multiply disabled, and socially deprived. The multiple disability need not be a visible one; typically, it is poorly defined as "brain damage" or a "learning disorder."

Joe

The case of Joe is a good example. Orphaned at an early age, Joe had grown up in a home for orphans sponsored by a Big Brothers' organization in a mountainous midwestern state. He attended several years of public school as a "mentally retarded" individual, then enrolled at the state school for the deaf at the age of 10 years. "Graduating"—actually he left school due to his age—at 18 years of age, Joe returned to the small town where he had grown up and resumed living in the Big Brothers' home. He was employed as a sheet presser in a local laundry, earning only 65¢/hour, and came to my attention via a referral from the local welfare agency. I drove up to the laundry one day and went inside in search of Joe. The owner pointed Joe out, then left. Joe stood there, sweating over the ironing roller without looking up. I walked over, tapped Joe on the shoulder, and fingerspelled, "Hi. I am Larry Stewart. Is your name Joe?" Joe nodded, then returned to ironing. Another tap followed and I beckoned Joe to come along. Joe had other ideas, however. He pointed to his watch, shook his head, and resumed working. The boss finally came along and waved Joe away. That was my introduction to a man who turned out to be an intelligent, dependable, and yet totally nonverbal deaf adult!

Joe did not use formal sign language. He could not speak a word. Lip reading was meaningless to him. He couldn't write his name! His only means of communication were gestures, pantomime, and body movements. To this day, I do not understand how Joe could have attended a school for 8 years and not have learned *any* verbal language. Incidentally, his nodding upon meeting me was found to be Joe's way of ''getting along.'' He did not understand signs, but by nodding he was saved a lot of grief!

I quickly learned that Joe could not sign, and the gestural-pantomime process began. Below is a verbal description that needs to be seen to be believed.

> **Counselor (C):** You (counselor points to Joe) me (counselor points to self) go (counselor's arm and pointing finger sweep in arc to point toward the general direction of Big Brothers' lodging) car (hands grasp imaginary steering wheel and motion as if steering and nods head affirmatively to add a period to the statement).
>
> **Joe (J):** (Looks quietly at counselor, face immobile, eyes unblinking)
>
> **C:** Come (makes ''come on'' motion with hand and starts walking toward car).
>
> **J:** (Shakes head ''negative.'' Points to watch, points in direction of his ironing roller, points finger to self, taps finger on chest several times, then starts walking toward the ironing room.)
>
> **C:** (Hastily trots to Joe, waves him down, stops, composes self, smiles, draws self up) Boss (points toward boss, standing watching counselor's antics in amusement) says (holds hand in front of face, makes motion resembling duck bill opening and closing) okay (makes circling motion with thumb and forefinger) come (sweeps hand and arm in front and away toward direction of Big Brothers' lodging) me (points finger toward self, pauses, smiles, nods head affirmatively, waits).
>
> **J:** (Looks at counselor impassively, swings gaze toward his boss, who smiles and shakes head ''yes'' and makes ''go away'' motion with hand and arm. Looks at counselor, pauses, then nods head ''yes'' and starts toward door.)
>
> **C:** (Gives sigh of relief, hitches up pants, and hurries after Joe.)

It was humorous, and Joe seemed to pick it all up because he was smiling when I caught up with him. From that point on, Joe and I developed ways of communicating simple but important information. Joe soon was living in an apartment in a large city, taking on-the-job training as a dry cleaning presser. A deaf adult was employed to teach Joe how to get around town using local transportation; how to buy food and clothing; how to take care of a checking account; how to follow safety measures in getting around at night in the city; how to get to the deaf club and countless other things. Most important, Joe began to really learn sign language. Finger spelling came much later, but first efforts were to develop meaningful and useful sign language that did not hopelessly confuse Joe. After 2 years, Joe was fully employed at union scale wage as a top quality presser. He had his own apartment, which he shared with another deaf man, and was a regular at the local deaf club as well as athletic events involving deaf teams.

The following is an excerpt from one of my concluding counseling sessions with Joe. Formal sign language, minus finger spelling, was used.

C: Job good, fine?
J: Fine, hard work. Like much. Money fine (smiles).

C: Live home, o.k., clean, fine?

J: Good (nods head vigorously), D (name sign of deaf man who taught Joe so much) help, teach right clean, careful.

C: Good, ride bus back-forth (there's a sign for this!) fine, no trouble?

J: (Nods head ''yes'') Fine, no trouble. Easy. Cheap. Save money. Buy ticket (monthly pass).

C: Go deaf party, play games, fun, ok?

J: Fine, good time. Like. Friends many.

C: Body strong, sick none?

J: (Shakes head) Fine, sick nothing. Right eat, not foolish eat. Sleep good, drink beer nothing, smoke nothing.

C: Money how much earn weekly?

J: (Takes out check book, extracts pay stub, looks at it intently, holds hand up and makes numerals) $110.00.

C: Week, two weeks?

J: Week (smiles).

C: (Gapes. This was in 1965!)

J: (Laughs)

C: Wonderful. Proud me you (I am proud of you). Boss ok, nice man to you?

J: Fine, little hot-head, ok. Patience, tomorrow better.

C: You happy, happy move to (name of city where he was living)?

J: Much happy. Friend D, LS (sign of counselor), many many (many other friends).

THAT was counseling! Yes, Joe taught me a lot about counseling.

OTHER SPECIAL COMMUNICATION ISSUES
RELATED TO COUNSELING

There are often deaf clients whose preferred method of communication differs significantly from the counselor's. For instance, there are some deaf clients who refuse to use sign language and at the same time have very poor speech. Others have very limited verbal language but still insist on using speech in a garbled, incoherent manner. Others know neither sign language nor speech, and attempt to use nonstandard, idiosyncratic sign language that no one else understands. Some even use bizarre mouthings intended to resemble speech but actually amounting to grunts and wheezes. Some of these individuals actually have verbal language but lack insight into how poor their speech production actually is; others have no verbal language or sign language, and imitate the visual aspects of communication without really having any idea how to get their meaning across. These are exceptional cases, but they do exist.

The method of achieving effective communication in these instances usually amounts to the counselor patiently slowing the client down and indicating when he or she does not understand. At times this can be severely taxing on the counselor's and the client's patience, but with time there is usually an improvement in mutual understanding.

Still another type of client is the deaf man or woman with good speech who rejects sign language in an attempt to be "normal." However, their speech reception is often poor or mediocre, or the counselor is able to understand the client but unable to express himself! This is a highly frustrating situation for the client as well as the counselor, and sometimes the only solution is for the counselor to write. Chaos ensues, however, when the client rejects writing and insists that the counselor continue speaking!

The deaf counselor also may get his or her lumps! Sometimes the client may refuse to sign, and then both the client and counselor must read lips and talk to one another. Often this works fine. On occasion, however, one or the other fails to lip-read properly or misunderstands much of what is said. In these latter instances, those are two frustrated individuals indeed, who sit facing each other in the counseling room!

There are some clients who reject their own deafness so violently that they are unable to relate to a deaf counselor. Such individuals are rare; most can withhold their rejection and eventually come to feel better about the counselor. A few just cannot accomplish this. In such cases it is incumbent upon the counselor to recognize what is happening with the client, and initiate proper referral to a hearing counselor.

Finally, there are some instances where parents can be a problem in the counseling process. It is very common for parents of young deaf adults, and some older deaf adults, to accompany their "child" to the initial counseling session. This is especially true in the vocational rehabilitation office. When it does happen, the parent (usually the mother) quite often tends to take the lead and "answer" for the deaf client. This can present an awkward situation for the counselor unless an effort is made to prevent it. After having experienced several difficult sessions of this nature, I finally found a solution. This solution consisted of scheduling separate appointments, one for the parents and one for the client. The secretary, at the time of scheduling, is careful to indicate that separate appointments are scheduled, and when the time for the first appointment arrives, handles the situation accordingly. However, when the occasional snafu occurs and the counselor ends up in a room alone with the client and parent(s), the best thing to do is relax and watch what happens. A lot can be learned about parent–"child" relations and attitudes!

CONCLUSIONS

It is hoped that this chapter has given the reader a better understanding of the "state of the art" in counseling with deaf adults and that the case narratives have provided meaningful insight concerning some issues and strategies in counseling with deaf persons.

It should be apparent that the responsibility for developing knowledge and skill in mental health needs and treatment of the deaf has fallen to a relatively small number of professionals in this field. There has been substantial growth in recent years in the number of counselors qualified to work with the deaf and with this development, professional knowledge has expanded. In my own work and study, I have found that various therapy techniques used with the hearing population can be used or adapted for use with the deaf. The important question is "Does the approach meet the special needs of the individual?" It has been my experience that if the approach is viewed from this perspective first, the use of appropriate and effective sign language minimizes the effects of deafness. As a counselor who has impaired hearing, I may have an advantage in the subtleties of sign language and "first-hand" understanding of the "deaf world" and the social, vocational, and psychological impact of deafness. Nevertheless, the requirements of a professional worker with the deaf are the same as those for a worker with the hearing, with added requirement of specialized communication skills.

REFERENCES

Patterson C.H., & Stewart, L.G. Principles of counseling with deaf people. In A.E. Sussman & L.G. Stewart (Eds.), *Counseling with deaf people*. New York: Deafness Research and Training Center, New York University, 1971.

Rogers, C., Gendlin, E., Kiesler, D., et al. *The therapeutic relationship with schizophrenics*. Madison, Wisc.: University of Wisconsin Press, 1968.

Stewart, L.G. Perceptions of selected variables of the counseling relationship in group counseling with deaf college students. Unpublished doctoral dissertation manuscript, University of Arizona, 1970a.

Stewart, L.G. Some observations from counseling deaf students. *Report of the proceedings of the 44th meeting of the convention of American instructors of the deaf*. Washington, D.C.: U.S. Government Printing Office, 1970b.

Sussman, A.E., & Stewart, L.G. (Eds.), *Counseling with deaf people*. New York: Deafness Research and Training Center, New York University, 1971.

Torrey, E.F. *The mind game*. New York: Bantam Books, 1973.

SUGGESTED READINGS

Avery, J., & Youst, D. Counseling at NTID. In A.G. Norris (Ed.), *Deafness Annual III*. Silver Spring, Md.: Professional Rehabilitation Workers with the Adult Deaf, 1973.

Brick, L. The use of role playing as an educational and therepeutic device with the deaf. *Journal of Rehabilitation of the Deaf*, 1967, *1*, 53–58.

Collins, J.L. Counseling the post-secondary deaf student: Implications for elementary and secondary education. *Proceedings, Convention of American Instructors of the Deaf*, 1971, pp. 654–650.

Collins, J.L. The use of group techniques in counseling at the National Technical Institute for the Deaf. In J.D. Schein & D. Naiman (Eds.), *The use of group techniques with deaf persons.* New York: Deafness Research and Training Center, New York University, 1971.

Elliott, H. Marriage counseling with deaf clients. *Journal of Rehabilitation of the Deaf,* 1974, *8,* 29–35.

Fusfeld, I.S. Counseling the deafened. *Gallaudet College Bulletin,* 1954, *vol. 3.*

Goetzinger, C.P. Factors associated with counseling the hearing impaired adult. *Journal of Rehabilitation of the Deaf,* 1967 *1,* 32–47.

Johnson, R.K. Personal counseling. In R.L. Jones (Ed.), *The deaf man and the world.* Silver Spring, Md. Council of Organizations Serving the Deaf, 1969.

Johnson, R.K., Koch, H., & Werner, R. Counseling and placement at Gallaudet College. In A.G. Norris (Ed.), *Deafness Annual III.* Silver Spring, Md: Professional Rehabilitation Workers with the Adult Deaf, 1973.

Kane, J., & Shafer, C. *Personal and family counseling services for the adult deaf.* Final Report; RD-2560-S. U.S. Department of Health, Education, and Welfare, 1968.

Landau, M.E. Group psychotherapy with deaf retardates. *International Journal of Group Psychotherapy,* 1968, *18,* 345–351.

McGowan, J., & Vescovi, G. Counselor (with the deaf) selection, education, and training. In A.E. Sussman & L.G. Stewart (Eds.), *Counseling with deaf people.* New York: Deafness Research and Training Center, 1971.

Mueller, J. Vocational counseling and guidance of deaf college students. *Exceptional Children,* 1962, pp. 501–504.

Myklebust, H.L.R., Neyhus, A., & Mulholland, A.M. Guidance and counseling for the deaf. *American Annals of the Deaf,* 1962, *107,* 370–415.

O'Hara, M. A plea for coordinated guidance and meaningful help. *Deaf American,* 1968, *20,* 13–14.

Rainer, J.D. Group therapy at the New York State Psychiatric Institute. In J.D. Schein & D. Naiman (Eds.), *The use of group techniques with deaf persons.* New York: Deafness Research and Training Center, New York University, 1971.

Reddan, R. Counseling the severly handicapped deaf person. *Journal of Rehabilitation of the Deaf,* 1974, *8.*

Reddan, R.L., & Duggan, P.W. The role of the counselor in an integrated technical vocational program for deaf students. In A.G. Norris (Ed.), Deafness Annual III. Silver Spring, Md.: Professional Rehabilitation Workers with the Adult Deaf, 1973.

Robinson, L.D. Group psychotherapy for deaf psychiatric patients. In J.D. Masserman (Ed.), *Current psychiatric therapies,* (Vol. 6). New York: Grune & Stratton, 1966.

Robinson, L.D., & Weathers, O. Family therapy of deaf parents and hearing children: A new dimension in psychotherapeutic intervention. *American Annuals of the Deaf,* 1974, *119,* 325–330.

Rosen, A. Deaf college students' preferences regarding the hearing status of counselors. *Journal of Rehabilitation of the Deaf,* 1968, *1,* 20–27.

Roy, H. Vocational and counseling aspects of deafness. *American Annals of the Deaf,* 1972, *107,* 562–565.

Sanderson, R.G. A personal theory of counseling. *Journal of Rehabilitation of the Deaf,* 1974, *7,* 22–28.

Sarlin, B. Group therapy. In J. Rainer & K. Altshuler (Eds.), *Psychiatry and the deaf.* Washington, D.C., U.S. Department of Health, Education, and Welfare, Social and Rehabilitation Services, 1967.

Schein, J., & Naiman, D. (Eds.). *The use of group techniques with deaf persons.* New York: Deafness Research and Training Center, New York University, 1971.

Sharpiro, R.J., & Harris, R.I. Family therapy in treatment of the deaf: A case report. *Family Process, 15,* 1976. 83–96.

Steinman, H. Hearing impaired marriages: A counseling challenge. *Journal of Rehabilitation,* 1973, *34,* 12–13, 40.

Sternberg, M.L. Group counseling with the non-communicative deaf. In J.D. Schein & D. Naiman (Eds.), *The use of group techniques with deaf persons.* New York: Deafness Research and Training Center, New York University, 1971.

Stinson, M. Group communication for the deaf. *Journal of Rehabilitation,* 1971.

Sussman, A.E. The comprehensive counseling needs of deaf persons. *Hearing and Speech News,* 1970, 12, 13, 22, 24.

Sussman, A.E. Group therapy with severely handicapped deaf clients. *Journal of Rehabilitation of the Deaf,* 1974, *8,* 122–130.

Thompson, M. Group work with the hearing impaired. *Hearing and Speech News,* 1970.

Thoreson, R., & Tully, N. Role and function of the counselor (for the deaf). In A.E. Sussman & L.G. Stewart (Eds.), *Counseling with deaf people.* New York: Deafness Research and Training Center, New York University, 1971.

David Walsh, C.Ss.R.

11

The Role of the Clergy
Serving the Deaf

Although the majority of deaf people in the United States do not practice religion in a formal way, they, like most Americans, profess a belief in God. And most, when asked if they belong to a church—a word in more general use among the deaf than the word religion—will answer in the affirmative. This lack of a formal practice of religion seems strange in view of the intimate relationship between religion and the early education of the deaf in the United States. It is paradoxical that while there has been a dramatic increase in the number of persons attending religious signlanguage classes and volunteering to do religious work with the deaf, there has been a considerable decrease in the number of deaf persons going to church; a decrease, in my opinion, greater among the deaf than among the hearing. However, despite this low attendance, one can find in both larger urban areas and more sparsely populated sections of the country many small, well-organized deaf congregations with a dedicated clergy meeting weekly or monthly, enjoying well-prepared services in a friendly atmosphere.

Can today's clergy and other religious workers constructively assess the present religious situation of the deaf community, define their own roles, and discover ways of extending and strengthening their ministry to the deaf community?

RELIGION AND THE EDUCATION OF THE DEAF

There is an historical bond between religion and the education of the deaf. Giangreco in *The Education of the Hearing Impaired* (1970), writes, "The Rise of Christianity (30 A.D.) was the beginning of meaningful philosophical change towards the deaf." Aristotle (384–322 B.C.) expressed society's attitude prior to that when he taught that those born deaf were incapable of reason. Centuries after

161

Aristotle's death, his teachings were still reflected in the Code of Justinian (530 A.D.), which denied all legal rights to those born deaf, including the right to marry, and which specified that guardians appointed by law were to have complete charge over the deaf. No restrictions were placed on those who were hard-of-hearing or who had lost their hearing after birth.

Christianity, however, did not have any immediate influence on the education of the deaf. Little seems to have happened for several centuries. Stone and Youngs, in their *Catholic Education of the Deaf in the United States, 1837–1848,* describe St. Augustine's (354–430 A.D.) recognition of the innate intelligence of the deaf and the possibility of communication through a language of signs. Stone and Youngs also refer to St. John of Beverly's eighth century attempt to educate the deaf as recorded in Bede's *Ecclesiastical History,* published in 1723.

Little is known of efforts to educate the deaf until the 16th century, when two Spanish Benedictine monks led the way. Ponce de Leon (1520–1584) not only taught several persons, deaf from birth, to "speak, read, write and keep accounts but also to become proficient in Latin and Greek." Juan Pablo Bonet (d. 1629) was the first person known to have written on the education of the deaf. In the 17th century, a deeply religious layman, Johann Konrad Amann (1669–1724) of Switzerland, was a firm advocate of speech and speech reading for deaf students. In the 18th century was born the most famous person in the history of the education of the deaf, the French priest, Charles-Michael Abbe de L'Epee (1722–1789). In 1760, he established in Paris the first school for the deaf in the world and is considered the originator of the use of sign language in the education of the deaf.

In the United States, too, the deaf are indebted to a clergyman for the establishment of the first school for the deaf. In 1817, Rev. Thomas Hopkins Gallaudet, after whom Gallaudet College in Washington, D.C., is named, founded the American School for the Deaf in Hartford, Conn., and is considered the father of deaf education in America. Other members of the clergy, following in Gallaudet's footsteps, were to be involved in the establishment of 35 of the state schools for the deaf, considered by some educators to be the heart of the U.S. educational system for deaf children.

Not only did religion, through these pioneers, have a strong influence on the education of the deaf in the nation's public schools, but almost from the beginning, private religious schools have had a limited but important presence. The well-known St. Joseph's Institute for the Deaf in St. Louis was opened by the Sisters of St. Joseph of Carondelet in 1837, followed in 1859 by the highly regarded St. Mary's School in Buffalo; in 1869 by St. Joseph's in New York; in 1876, by St. John's, Milwaukee; in 1884, by Ephpheta in Chicago; in 1890, by Chinchuba Institute in Louisiana; in 1895, by St. Joseph's, Oakland, Calif.; and in 1899, by the Boston school at Randolph. Six more Catholic schools were to be established in the 20th century. The Missouri Synod of the Lutheran Church also opened two schools, the Detroit Lutheran School for the Deaf in 1873, and the Mill Neck Manor Lutheran School for the Deaf at Mill Neck, N.Y. in 1951.

THE ROLE OF THE CLERGY IN THE PAST

Powrie V. Doctor (d. 1971), who taught at Gallaudet College for many years and was, perhaps, after Thomas Gallaudet the best known teacher of the deaf in the United States, often spoke of the importance of clergy in the lives of the deaf because he recognized that the clergy were often the first people the parents of a deaf child and the deaf themselves turned to for help. Joanne Greenberg's novel, *In This Sign*, describes the strong stabilizing influence of the church and the clergy in the deaf community. While the Abel and Janice Ryder family was not the typical deaf family of 50 years ago, Greenberg's story points out that the weekly church service, with the opportunity to meet many other deaf persons, was the highlight of their lives.

Because I can reach back 30 years into my own experience and have close contacts with veteran clerics of many denominations, I have a perspective on the church and the world of the deaf that extends from the early part of the century to the present decade. Surprising information is available in the archives at Gallaudet College of the religion–deafness relationship in the 19th century, which led Carolyn Jones, Associate Librarian, Researcher, and Bibliographer at Gallaudet, to make this interesting observation, "From the very beginning religion was wrapped up with the education of the deaf in the U.S."

As early as 1853, services for the deaf were conducted at St. Ann's Episcopal Church, New York City, and in 1876, two deaf men were ordained to the ministry. The Gallaudet archives have the original text of a sermon given by the Rev. Thomas Hopkins Gallaudet at the American School for the Deaf in 1817. There is excitement in tapping these valuable sources.

Traditionally, clergymen were patriarchs—the "hearing" people who knew sign language, to whom the deaf brought their problems; economic problems that hearing people have, such as payment of rent, finding a job, collecting a pension, making payments on home, car, and furniture. These are the usual family and school difficulties but, in addition, there are problems that relate specifically to deafness, such as tensions in coping with hearing children, the need for an interpreter at the lawyer's or doctor's office, the unending conflicts with other deaf persons in the church society, in the local club for the deaf, or with a rival club. No one acquainted with the world of the deaf would disagree that ministering to a comparatively small deaf congregation may be a heavier work load than serving a larger hearing congregation. Veteran clerics of the past have been both amused and frustrated that a typical congregation of fewer than 200 people could require so many hours of service.

Family problems demand the largest portion of the clergy's time. The relationship of deaf parents to their hearing children has always been something special. The desire for the success of their children, a normal parental responsibility, is accentuated for deaf parents. They are anxious that their children achieve a prestige denied to them, and as a result, they exhibit a special determination that their children get ahead. They celebrate their children's successes with a special pride, yet there is frustration from lack of good communication with their children's teachers and with the parents of their children's schoolmates. Deaf parents meet most family and neighborhood challenges with serenity, but when the inevitable misunderstandings come they are brought to the cleric's door.

It has always seemed to me that the children of deaf parents develop, at an early age, unique qualities of responsibility and reliability, flexibility and independence, and sometimes aggressiveness. Naturally, much of this comes from the fact that their parents are "different," that the parents often have had to depend on their very young child to communicate with the neighbors, with salespeople in stores, and even with members of their own families—parents, uncles, aunts, etc., who had never attempted to learn the language of the deaf. Many of the children of deaf parents have also suffered the experience of having their parents and themselves made fun of. Theirs is the family on the block that is "different." In my years of home visitations, anyone could point out where the deaf family lived. These experiences help to form the determined, outgoing personalities that so many sons and daughters of deaf parents possess—the daughters especially. Interestingly, many highly qualified interpreters for the deaf are daughters of deaf parents.

One has to admire the dignified acceptance on the part of deaf parents of the frustrations peculiar to deafness, the realization that they and their children have sometimes been made fun of, that people think of them as different. A number of deaf families have told me that they seldom punished their children physically because if the children cried, the neighbors would think the deaf were cruel to their children—a fact not lost on the children. The great accomplishment of these deaf parents has been the transition from a childhood and youth in an institutional environment of a large state school for the deaf to the more intimate atmosphere of homes of their own, with attendant responsibilities.

Many of the characteristics of pastoral service to the deaf seem to transcend time limitations. We know that time is fluid and that the past can flow gently and often unnoticed into the present. There have been subtle changes in the ministry to the deaf, a more sophisticated approach, for example, but there are interesting peculiarities in ministry to the deaf in the past that are still observable today.

Routine activities of the clergy have always been to provide for worship services and to organize religious education programs; to officiate at weddings, baptisms, and funerals; to visit the sick and shut-ins; to provide counseling; and to participate in the life of the community. One vital function with many congregations is that of peacemaker. This is especially true in deaf communities, where it is an embarrassing fact of life that infighting, unnecessary divisions, and rival factions are common. Perhaps this is more true of the past than it is today, now that the automobile and television have given the deaf an escape from the closeness of the deaf world. Deafness fosters a unique unity, an interdependence and companionship unknown to most hearing persons. But it is a small world. The population of a given deaf community can be less than 100 people. Most of the adult deaf know one another quite well, often having attended the same state or city school for the deaf. Their handicap in communicating with the hearing world often limits them to the world of the deaf.

So far, deaf people have had few opportunities for leadership positions in the general society where they form such a small minority. The few leadership positions open to them have generally been in their own community, particularly in their own organizations. The most obvious areas of leadership opportunity are the local deaf clubs, which are managed by deaf persons and where the members can take pride in being elected officers. It is within these clubs that cliques, often led by life-long opponents, will quarrel over such matters as membership rules and, most commonly, financial accountability. Clerics have seldom been able to offer solutions to these problems, which are extremely important in the deaf community. Absolute neutrality has always been necessary; otherwise, the cleric would lose half of the congregation. Because of the difficulties in the social organizations of the deaf, I have always held the opinion that a religious organization for the deaf should be known as a church rather than a center or club. For example, the Lutherans always call their centers the Lutheran Church for the Deaf.

I wonder if the pastors of the deaf in the past and the present would agree that there is one unique element in our special ministry that has gradually changed. This is the mutual possessiveness whereby the cleric, often the only priest or minister for the deaf in an area as large as a state or several states, seemed to "own" the deaf, while the deaf community regarded the pastor as "theirs" alone. By "owning the deaf," I mean that as shepherd of this small flock, the cleric may often have dominated the deaf, generally acted as their spokesman, and sometimes considered the deaf world his or her own territory, to be protected from organizers and occasionally even other clerics, who were always attempting to establish new societies and associations. This possessiveness on the part of the pastor was often matched by a deaf community that did not care to see their pastor shepherding other "sheep," especially hearing people who already had easy access to clergy. Since their pastor was often the only cleric who knew sign language, the deaf felt that his or her time belonged to them and they resented any clerical gravitation towards hearing persons at any church or social gatherings.

Today there is less possessiveness on the part of the pastor; who no longer dominates the deaf community. However, deaf persons retain much of their possessiveness and are quick to notice and comment on a pastor's preference for the company of hearing persons. I have always felt the deaf community's resentment of such preference is justifiable, because to them it is an oblique though unwitting way of "putting down the deaf."

Another expression of possessiveness on the part of the deaf community in the past that has not changed is their insistence on a "full-time" pastor. It frequently happens that a small group of deaf persons, perhaps only a dozen families, will ask church authorities for a clergyman to serve them in a full-time capacity. This may seem to be just a status symbol, but the deaf know from experience that the pastor who, having other responsibilities, ministers to the deaf part-time will rarely learn to communicate effectively and will not understand the culture of the deaf. It is necessary that the pastor identify with the deaf community and be part of their lives. The deaf community will share their pastor with other deaf congregations. They will excuse his or her absences to travel to the state school for the deaf to conduct services, particularly if it is the one they had attended. But if they have to share their pastor with a hearing congregation, they know it will not be long before personal frustration in being unable to communicate fluently with the deaf, and a sense of failure in meeting their expectations, will lead him or her to ask for another assignment or to accept, without protest, a transfer to a hearing congregation. Once again, the deaf would be faced with breaking in a new pastor, submitting patiently as sign language is practiced on them. The constant turnover of clergy in some areas may be responsible for the definite decrease in church attendance. My own opinion is that ministry to the deaf is not a part-time clerical position; it is a vocation. This view parallels that of the famous Father Alvin Illich of Cuernavaca, Mexico, who stated that the best thing for Latin America would be for the American clergy there to go home unless they would cease to be ''lend-lease'' pastors (temporary helpers), and would identify with the Latin American community by dedicating their lives to its service.

Almost all members of the clergy I know have found this vocation a joyful and extremely satisfying one, although it has often isolated them from their colleagues who ministered to hearing congregations. Nevertheless, there is one negative factor that frequently in the past, and occasionally in the present, has saddened our apostolate. This is the 200-year-old controversy over methodology: whether it is more effective to educate deaf children by the ''oral method,'' which means the use of speech and speech reading, or through the combined use of speech, speech reading, sign language, finger spelling, and writing. There is no need here to go into definitions of oralism, the combined method, total communication, or cued speech. It is enough to know that most educators of the deaf, as well as the deaf themselves, feel that this unending controversy has seriously delayed the development of a universal optimum method for educating the deaf.

The debate was a very real part of my life for many years because while I was the pastor of the Catholic deaf in New Orleans, in Detroit, and in Chicago, even though I was the only priest serving the deaf, I was not permitted to be involved in the religious education of deaf children because I knew signs. Several highly placed ecclesiastical authorities felt that my pastorate should be limited, as one expressed it, ''to the older people who never learned to lip read.'' This was unfortunate because later on when these children left school they invariably became part of the adult deaf community. It would have helped greatly to have known them as children.

The clergy's position in the controversy has often been awkward and misunderstood. Many clerics in this country have felt that since the use of total communication is, in their opinion, a superior method of educating a deaf child, they had an obligation to lobby with educators and parents to support this method. Conversely, I have always felt the choice of method was the responsibility of the school administration and, rather than confuse both parents and children, the instructor in religion should adopt the policy of the school. Therefore, whenever I have the opportunity to conduct classes in religion for "oral" children I used speech and speech reading. However, the stigma was there that I was the priest who talked on his hands. I still feel today that the clergy should adapt to the immediate situation. My own home town, St. Louis, takes great pride in its two internationally famous oral schools, St. Joseph's Institute for the Deaf and the Central Institute for the Deaf.

There does seem to be more than an educational issue involved in this oral–manual controversy. Through the years, the strongest supporters of the use of sign language, those in administrative positions in the state schools for the deaf, have frequently been the children of deaf parents who have grown up in the culture of the deaf. Tradition is on their side since our first schools did advocate the use of sign language. This tradition enjoys the continued approval of the prestigious Conference of American Executives of the Deaf and of the Convention of American Instructors of the Deaf. On the other hand, to a cleric not tied to any philosophy, whose job does not depend on espousing any particular method, it is still quite obvious that few advocates of the oral method know sign language or have had much contact with the adult deaf world. It is equally obvious that few sign language advocates have ever taught in or been very much around persons from an outstanding oral school. We know that the method of total communication is now receiving wide recognition. (The Conference of Executives of American Schools for the Deaf has adopted the following official definition of total communication: Total communication is a philosophy incorporating appropriate aural, manual, and oral modes of communication in order to ensure effective communication with and among hearing-impaired persons.) Reading between the lines in professional journals, however, I sense that the controversy is far from over. The clergy must still see its priority as pastoral service, adapted to the needs of all the members of a congregation, regardless of their educational background. While it is a recognized fact that members of the clergy have had an important role both in the development and continued use of sign language in this country, they must be open to alternative possibilities.

ROLE OF THE CLERGY TODAY

Even though most of the deaf do not attend church on a regular basis, there is still a strong relationship between the deaf community and religion. Listed in the American Annals of the Deaf are the executive offices of major religious organizations serving the deaf including the Lutheran Church's Ephphata Conference of Workers among the Deaf and the Ephphata Service for the Deaf and Blind; the Episcopal Conference of the Deaf; the General Council of the Assemblies of God Ministries to the Deaf; Home Mission Board of the Southern Baptist Convention; the International Catholic Deaf Association; the Lutheran Church—Missouri Synod Board of Missions; the National Catholic Office for the Deaf; the National

Congress of Jewish Deaf; the National Council of Churches of Christ in the U.S.A.; and many others.

In the last 10 years, religious programs and opportunities for deaf people have grown at an astounding pace. Workshops, leadership weeks, bible camps, and fellowship and community programs are available at minimum cost. Many religious organizations of the deaf hold annual or biannual conventions. Paradoxically, as the number of these opportunities increases, the number of people attending church regularly decreases. Perhaps the words of the late Archbishop Hallinan of Atlanta concerning church work in general can be applied to programs for the deaf: "Less and less are receiving more and more; more and more are receiving less and less." The clerics of today, even though their work is the invisible work of God in men and cannot be analyzed or computerized in purely human terms, still require the help of professional evaluation to maximize their efforts.

In the last 15 years, the world of the deaf has undergone dramatic changes. The number of deaf persons attending college has tripled; the median income of deaf persons attending college has risen; the teletypewriter (TTY) has been adapted for use by deaf persons. There are now captioned films, sign-language interpreters for televised news programs, classes for learning sign language. All of these have contributed to the growing public awareness of deafness. The emphasis on the rights of minority groups has helped the deaf community achieve greater recognition of their own rights. While the overall picture of the deaf is brighter now than it ever has been, life has still not changed significantly for a large number of deaf persons who have no TTYs, who have the same low-skill jobs, who are employed below their potential, and who remain isolated in their neighborhoods.

Also contributing to the changing world of the deaf has been the rise of professional organizations: the American Deafness and Rehabilitation Association (ADARA; formerly the Professional Rehabilitation Workers for the Adult Deaf); The Registry of Interpreters for the Deaf (RID); the International Association of Parents of the Deaf (IAPD); the National Center for Law and the Deaf, to mention just a few of the more recently established organizations. Added to these new organizations is the increased activity of the American Athletic Association of the Deaf, the U.S. Deaf Skiers Association, and the Miss Deaf America pageant.

The change in the world of the deaf has also changed the position of the clergy in relation to the deaf community. The cleric is no longer the parent figure; nor is the church, in many areas, any longer the center of most of the social life of the deaf community. A sense of deaf pride, a growing awareness that deaf people have the competence to do things for themselves, coupled with a determination to be less dependent on hearing people, have all been gradually changing the image of the clergy.

The deaf community, while recognizing the value of the social aspects of the ministry, has reached a religious maturity that makes them expect well-prepared liturgies and challenging homilies as well as more structured religious education programs. As in the past, the deaf also expect their pastors to visit the sick and the shut-ins, to officiate at baptisms, weddings, and funerals, and to be available for counseling. They see the need for greater emphasis on youth work with its spiritual demands. Finally, the deaf community, once patient with a pastor's less than professional knowledge of sign language, now insists that he or she attain a high level of communication and possess both expressive and receptive skills for an effective pastoral ministry.

This last expectation is more difficult to meet than it may seem. As other factors in the culture of the deaf are changing, so also is sign language. Fifteen years ago, sign language was still rather limited in that its vocabulary was small, consisting of a few hundred words in common usage. This fact, however, did not prevent the deaf from expressing themselves in it; it was the everyday language of the deaf. I once heard the famous Father Daniel Higgins, author of one of the first sign-language dictionaries, show the flexibility of sign language by pointing out that there is nothing of the *Summa* of St. Thomas Aquinas, a compendium of theology, that, despite its depth and abstract nature, could not be expressed in sign language. However, the majority of deaf children are now in schools or classes where the philosophy insists on signing exact English; that is, language in which the word sequence conforms to correct grammatical structure rather than to the flowing picture language of American Sign Language (ASL). Many teachers are quite vocal in expressing their preference that the clergy and staff of volunteer helpers use the same method in religion classes that is used in their regular classrooms.

Will the deaf of tomorrow communicate only in signed English, or will they guard and perpetuate the traditional ASL? Many deaf persons have already expressed their resentment that most of the changes in sign language have come not from the deaf but from hearing people. It seems to me that signed English is having a definite influence on ASL; deaf persons who have been out of school for many years are beginning to sign differently from the way they signed 10 or 20 years ago. Will it all end up in a two-track system, whereby one track will be the everyday language of the deaf with its idioms and expressions, and a second track will be the more cultivated language of the classroom, the lecture hall, and perhaps the pulpit? The clergy faces the problem of deciding on the mode of communication best suited to each congregation. Congregations vary in their culture and educational background. In general, my personal choice has been the use of ASL with its natural beauty and dignity. Again, there is need to be open to alternatives.

Almost all clerics will agree that even if the facilities, the services, and the communication skills are all at a level of excellence, they are nonetheless ministering to a gradually decreasing flock, made up of the "old faithful," the "pillars" of the church. Is this a phenomenon peculiar to the deaf? The latest *Gallup Opinion Index* on religion in America, published in December 1977, shows that 49 percent of adult Americans attended church weekly in 1955, whereas in the period 1970–1975 there was a drop to 40 percent. It is encouraging that in 1976, attendance rose to 42 percent. Also, on the positive side, the index reported that in the same year, 86 percent of adult Americans placed considerable importance on their religious beliefs.

The 1977 Gallup poll did not make a separate study of deaf Americans. We do not have a national study on the religious habits of the deaf community. It is my opinion after considerable discussion with deaf groups, with deaf leaders themselves, and with religious workers for the deaf across the country, that between 20 percent and 30 percent of the American deaf attend church regularly. This estimate includes both areas where there are special religious services for the deaf and where such services are not available. Why is there such a considerable difference in church attendance between deaf and hearing Americans?

One reason might be that the practice of religion is generally a family tradition, and many deaf persons spent most of their childhood and youth in residential schools for the deaf, away from their families. In many such schools, the students were encouraged to attend church on Sunday with their fellow deaf students, and frequently the service was conducted in sign language or interpreters were present, but I doubt if this group activity had the same impact as that of a family worshipping together. On those weekends, holidays, or summer vactions when deaf students were home, they were inevitably faced with the reality that they could not participate in the service their parents attended because they could not join in the prayers or singing and could not hear the homily. There were no interpreters present. The question that parents have asked me most frequently over the years is what to do about church for their deaf son or daughter. And many asked if there was an obligation for a deaf child to attend church.

A second reason why a lower percentage of deaf persons attend church regularly than do hearing persons is the rather obvious one of inconvenience. For hearing people, the church is frequently in the neighborhood; for deaf people, the church may be many miles distant and often in an area where public transportation is poor, especially for older people and especially on weekends. Hearing persons often have a choice of churches and ministers of their denomination; deaf persons, even in large cities, will seldom have more than one church or minister of their denomination. Many churches are able to offer their members a choice of times for the service, often in the morning and in the afternoon. It would be most unusual for a deaf congregation to have the ministerial personnel to provide this convenience.

The literature on the education of the deaf is filled with references to the difficulty deaf people have with abstract terms and therefore with understanding abstract religious teachings (Getz, 1956). While conceding that ASL has a limited vocabulary and, being primarily a picture language, is concrete, I have always had difficulty in accepting the opinion that deaf people have problems with abstract thought. I believe that this is a textbook myth that has been handed down for many years without supportive evidence. However, even if this opinion is true, we must distinguish between theology and catechesis. As a scientific, systematic presentation of a body of religious teachings, theology does require a high level of abstraction and deaf people would experience difficulties in studying it, not because of their deafness but because of their vocabulary limitations, limitations that can be overcome by adequate education. Catechetics, however, is the art of reducing the abstract principles of theology to practical teachings, the theoretical to the realistic; of discovering in theology the intellectual and moral guidelines for life; and of applying religious truths to the concrete human situation. This need be no more difficult for deaf than for hearing persons. The practice of religion, viewed as a life experience rather than a learning experience, can profit from the use of sign language, a language that can so movingly express religious concepts, e.g., the beauty and nearness of God and the distinction between good and evil.

Although deafness limits the easy acquisition of language, deaf people, through their natural understanding of sign language, pantomime, and gesture, can learn the basics of religion easily and in depth. For example, in discussing the evil of sin, what more vivid and dramatic expression can we find than God's words to the followers of Moses, "You will not be my people and I will not be your God." Is there a more touching expression of God's care for us than the words of Christ when He picks the flower in the field or points to the bird in the air and teaches that if God is concerned with these, how much more does He care for us. The parables of the Prodigal Son or the Good Samaritan in the New Testament, which almost require pantomime to convey their lessons, are excellent examples of the superiority of visual language in teaching religion. For Christians, a catechesis based on the life of Christ is not abstract, not theoretical, but is a warm, human, living presentation of the love of God for people through Christ.

In continuing to discuss reasons why a lower percentage of deaf persons attend church on a regular basis than persons with normal hearing, I would repeat my opposition to the "abstraction theory," namely, that it is difficult to teach the deaf religion because abstraction is a problem for them. There has been little research into deaf people's understanding of religion. However, in 1974 the first major research on the religious thinking of the deaf appeared with the publication of *The God of the Deaf Adolescent* by Antony Russo. Father Russo's work was based on 4 years of careful research, including interviews with 150 deaf students. For some experienced religious educators, his monumental work has verified what they have always believed, that our religious education texts and programs have not been able to reach the deaf in depth, not because of any intellectual limitation on their part, but because we have not as yet developed religious education materials specifically designed for the deaf.

Because clerics and religious educators have often failed to reach the deaf in depth, we cannot assert that those who no longer attend church have lost their faith in God, in their church, or their temple. Many never understood their religion on a personal, individual basis. Therefore, there is little reason to criticize deaf people or their families or the schools for the deaf. The great challenge facing the clergy of today is to develop the content Father Russo describes in his book. Research is also needed to understand what motivates deaf people. Are deaf people moved by the same factors that influence hearing people, or are there distinctive mental and emotional forces within deaf people, the understanding of which is necessary to give direction to their lives? The pastors of the deaf know many who possess a loving intimacy with God, whose lives are an example and an inspiration to all of us. It is our responsibility to discover the secret of their gift that it might be shared with other deaf people.

If it is true that the decreased attendance of the deaf at religious services is due primarily to the fact that they can now find elsewhere the social and recreational programs that once attracted them to church, it is also true that deaf persons often realize the spiritual vacuum in their lives and will welcome a realistic ministry geared to their special needs.

THE CLERGY OF THE FUTURE

One certainty about the future is that we cannot predict what events and forces will shape our lives. So the clergy, already straining to cope with the present, can only attempt to discern the working of the Spirit in the People of God, and maintain an openness to new ideas, new movements, new moods. It cannot be foreseen, for example, whether the practice of religion will grow in the lives of deaf people in America, or decrease. The cleric with a deep personal faith understands that all depends on the grace of God and that his or her responsibility is to develop a spiritual flexibility that will permit the understanding and influencing of the future.

The development of the dignity of the individual, considered the dominant social characteristic of the past 100 years, and witnessed by such historical events as women's suffrage, the struggle for civil rights, the death of colonialism, and rise of labor unions, will most likely continue as men and women strive for total freedom. Karl Rahner, considered by many the most creative theologian of this century, in his chapter, the Theology of Freedom (1969), says "He is free who has *autopraxia,* that is, who can do what he wants." He considers full freedom to be "self-realization," which is possible only through God. Some writers are now using the word "personalism" to describe this demand by individuals to live their own lives, determine their own relationship to religion, form their own consciences, "do their own things." I frankly believe that this philosophy has arrived, and the clerics of the present and the future must learn to live with it. Ten years ago, Rahner noted this religious transition from religious conformity to personalism, "The Church in much of the traditionally Christian world is still on the way from being an established Church (that is, a social institution to which all more or less belong) to a Church of personal faith in a pluralistic society."

I believe that Rahner has said it all; he has a clear perception of where religion is today. In *The Christian of the Future,* he offers his insights into tomorrow's attitudes towards the practice of religion. His writings have had a deep influence on my own pastoral philosophy. I have come to believe in an extremely personal approach to people, a one-to-one apostolate. While much emphasis today is placed on the community, it seems even more important to focus on the individuals making up that community. Rahner powerfully expressed the individual's relationship to God when he wrote that everybody responds with an eternal yes or an eternal no to God's love. This response is strengthened by the unique freedom of each individual.

Because the deaf congregation is small and often scattered over a large territory, even an entire state, this philosophy of a personal approach is important to the pastors of the deaf. They must know their people intimately, on a first-name basis, know the names of the children and the rest of the family, even the name of the pet dog. They must be interested in where the people in their congregations work and what they do, in their background, where they were born, which school they attended, their hobbies, their recreations, their sicknesses. They should inquire as to the cause of their deafness (a topic I find deaf persons quite eager to discuss); whether they were born deaf or suffered an illness in early childhood that may have caused their deafness. It is my belief that it is only when you know the total person that you can minister spiritually in depth.

The personal relationship of a pastor to a particular person should avoid any amateurish professionalism, such as an insistence on too many details in a religious census (How often do you attend church?) or an exaggerated religiosity (Do you pray every day?), which can offend a church member's sense of freedom. In a person-to-person communication, pastors will reveal themselves, their family backgrounds, their work experience, their hobbies. A cleric might use, as a measurement of success, whether he or she has succeeded in building a deep, permanent friendship with the members of the flock. One of the gratifying aspects of the work with the deaf is that since the number of members in a deaf congregation is usually much smaller than in a hearing church, it is possible to know members in a very personal way. No organizational ability, no talent for preparing inspiring services, no power in the pulpit, can substitute for the impact of the pastor's warm, friendly home visits. An old Protestant adage says, "A house-visiting parson makes a church-going people."

In the special ministry to the deaf community, there is one area that is open to considerable debate at present and, I suspect, will be even more so in the future. As stated earlier in this chapter, clergy in the past were very much involved in social work for the deaf. Today, too, many pastors still spend much, or most, of their time in interpreting for the deaf; attending meetings at open homes for the aged deaf; helping to improve educational facilities; organizing seminars to study the meaning of the new legislation; planning summer camps; attending conferences on rehabilitation; etc. While religion is part of person's total life interests and must not be relegated to the pews on Sunday morning, a pastor can become exhausted in the activities just mentioned and have little time or energy left for spiritual ministry, for prayer, preaching, or teaching.

There is a growing number of agencies and resources available today to take care of the social, educational, and rehabilitation needs of the deaf, and it seems likely this number will continue to increase. If clerics and religious workers take over the responsibilities of these organizations, who will take over the responsibility of bringing the Good News of the Gospel to the deaf community? Years ago, I had to determine the priorities in my service to the deaf and, realizing my training was in religion, I have concentrated on that. Many clerics and church workers, convinced that the Gospel requires a living testimony of service to people's material needs, would not agree with this.

Is there a middle ground? A number of pastors have found there is, having often initiated projects to assist the deaf community and then have turned them over to qualified personnel within their own organization or to other agencies. Many pastors have been active in an advocacy role. While not accepting the responsibility for social or educational programs or projects, they have supported the personnel and agencies involved and have often served as catalysts in involving parents groups, social agencies, and the deaf community. An advocacy role is attractive to clerics because the dignity of their position contributes to the efforts others are making and is a source of encouragement to social workers for the deaf, who, often like the clerics themselves, feel isolated in their work.

A willingness to accept this advocacy role is most valuable, since the cleric will no doubt continue to be a very active source of referrals to the rapidly increasing number of organizations now assisting the deaf. Naturally the cleric must keep up to date with the services now available and must develop good working relationships with those who staff such organizations. Sometimes, he or she will be in a position to form a community team that will pool the community resources to speak as the unified voice of all those serving the deaf. Such leadership on the part of the pastor will continue the long tradition of the close relationship between the clergy and the deaf community.

Those readers of this book who have had only limited experience with the deaf may not realize that many services that hearing people take for granted, such as marriage counseling, mental health care, adult education programs, and vocational assistance, are still almost nonexistent for deaf persons. The present climate of concern for all handicapped persons offers the dedicated cleric a unique opportunity to assess the needs of the deaf community in the area and to initiate effective action to meet those needs. Clerics should have the confidence that they still possess a unique charisma through which they can accomplish much for the hearing-handicapped.

CONCLUSION

The theme of the world Federation of the Deaf Congress in Washington, D.C., in 1975, was "Full Citizenship for All Deaf Persons." This should include full *religious* citizenship as well, in order that deaf people may have the availability not only of the dedicated clergy now serving them but also of clerics and religious workers who are themselves deaf. At present, there are very few deaf clerics and religious workers; however, within the next few years, it is expected that religious training programs will be available to deaf men and women.

REFERENCES

Gallup opinion index 1977–78. *Religion in America,* 1977, *145,* 11.

Getz, S. *Environment and the deaf child,* Springfield, Ill.: Charles C Thomas, 1956, p. 139.

Giancrego, C. J. *The education of the hearing impaired.* Springfield, Ill.: Charles C Thomas, 1970.

Greenberg, J. *In this sign.* New York: Avon, 1977.

Rahner, K. *Grace in freedom.* New York: Herder & Herder, 1969.

Rahner, K. *The Christian of the future.* Germany: Herder & Herder, 1967.

Russo, A. *The God of the deaf adolescent.* Paramus, N.J.: Paulist Press, 1975.

Schein, J. D., & Delk, M. T., Jr. *The deaf population of the United States.* Silver Spring, Md.: National Association of the Deaf, 1974.

Stone, M. E., & Youngs, J. P., Jr. Catholic education of the deaf in the United States, 1837–1948. *American Annals of the Deaf,* 1948, *93,* 412–413.

PART III

Societal Issues

William C. Stokoe, Ph.D.
Robbin M. Battison, Ph.D.

12

Sign Language, Mental Health, and Satisfactory Interaction

The study of language, the study of mental health and illness, and the study of deafness have long existed as separate fields. Yet it seems clear to us, an anthropologist and a linguist, that the subjects of these three studies relate more closely than some of their students realize. In what follows, we will first try to show how an anthropological view can relate them, with strong implications for action, and then will treat in some detail specific instances of the interrelatedness of deafness and mental health with language, particularly with sign language.

Much can be said, of course, for an approach to solving problems presented by the paradigms of traditional disciplines: Medical study of deafness has led to restoration of hearing for some, but even more signficantly it has brought knowledge of what can cause deafness and of how some kinds of congenital deafness can be prevented. Linguistic study has provided understanding of sound systems in language and so has brought improvement in the way that those with hearing impairments can be taught to speak. But until very recently, few linguists have taken any direct interest either in the spoken language of deaf persons or in the gesture-based sign languages that the deaf use for communicating among themselves. Professionals in mental health have infrequently considered the difficulties that deafness imposes on diagnosis and treatment. For an account of early linguistic and psychiatric theory and practice related to deafness, see Lane (1976); for a

This study was made possible by grants from the National Science Foundation (SOC 741 4724) and the Gallaudet College Office of Research. The authors wish to acknowledge the help of Raymond Trybus, Dean, Gallaudet Research Institute, former Director of the Office of Demographic Studies, who made available both his data and his advice on its interpretation. Grateful acknowledgment is also extended to Harry Markowicz, Richard Meltzer, Eugene Mindel, Katharine Newman, Carol Padden, and James Woodward for stimulating comments on earlier versions of this paper. The authors remain solely responsible for any errors.

recent multidisciplinary consideration of language and hearing, see Kavanagh and Cutting (1975). Such difficulties stand out starkly in a study by Rimland cited in Tinbergen's Nobel Prize Lecture (1974). In the study, 445 young children with developmental disorders were diagnosed as having one or another of these 8 conditions: autism, infantile autism, childhood schizophrenia, emotional disturbance or mental illness, brain or neurologic damage, retardation, psychosis, and deafness. Each of the children was diagnosed twice, but, says Tinbergen, "If the art of diagnosis has any objective basis, there should be a positive correlation between first and second opinions . . . the diagnoses are practically random" (Tinbergen, 1974). Tinbergen has not exaggerated. The first opinion held 16 of the children to be psychotic, the second so diagnosed 10 children; but not 1 child was called psychotic by two doctors. Even closer to our topic, 12 children were diagnosed as deaf in their first examination, 13 children in the second; but these were 25 *different* children. Not one child in the whole 445 was diagnosed as deaf by two specialists. In the light of this, it seems reasonable to suppose that a new way of looking at deafness, language, and mental health together could do no harm.

AN ANTHROPOLOGICAL VIEW

Deafness, language, and mental health are included in the central matter of anthropology, because this matter, generally termed *culture,* includes every aspect of all the activities in which members of a society engage. But there are more specific ways of relating our topics to *cognitive* cultural theory. Culture, according to Goodenough (1967), "does not consist of people, things, behavior, or emotions," but can be described as "what people in a community have had to learn." He goes on to say that, "Linguists are able to produce elegant and accurate representations of what one has to know in phonology and grammar if one is to speak particular languages acceptably by native standards."

Using acceptability by (hearing) native standards as a point of departure, however, linguists, medical authorities, psychologists, and laymen have looked at deafness as pathology. Few if any profoundly deaf persons can learn to speak acceptably by native (hearing) standards. From this premise, nonprofessionals and specialists alike have formed the false opinions (1) that the deaf are deficient in language; (2) that the deaf have cognitive deficits; (3) that the deaf cannot think abstractly; and (4) that the deaf must be treated as sick people in search of a cure. Whole societies have sometimes accepted such false opinions, and social opinion can powerfully affect mental health. Deviant behavior, especially that labeled criminal, insane, or (in non-Western cultures) diabolical, comes as much from society's opinions as from any actions of the persons so labeled (Selby, 1974). Re-education of the public to regard as human those who cannot hear and engage in normal spoken interaction could well begin with the professionals who have taken too narrow a view of normality in behavior, especially language behavior.

A less prejudicial view of deafness can be derived from the principles of ethnoscience, or cognitive ethnography, as it is also known (Spradley, 1972). The ethnographer of this sort tries to find out what it is that a deaf person must learn, not only to use the particular language of the deaf by its native users' standards, but also to operate with full knowledge of the forms and organization of people, things, behavior, and emotions. The ethnographer looks for what makes being a member of deaf society different from being a member of one or another hearing subculture. But the deaf individual has to learn more, of course: how to behave acceptably by hearing standards. Looked at as part of the cognitive map, which integrates a particular subculture for its members, deafness is vitally related to language and to mental health. Some of what a deaf person has to know to communicate with those who are also deaf and those who are not is *language* by any pragmatic definition—but not necessarily one and the same language. Moreover, what one has to know to behave acceptably, by the standards of others, largely determines mental health. Conversely, unacceptable, unsocial, or antisocial behavior often leads to diagnoses of mental illness or mental deficiency.

For most people, just learning the cognitive map, i.e., the categories and forms and organization of people, things, behavior, and emotions, of their own societies has inestimable value. But deaf people, despite their own and others' unstinting efforts at learning and teaching, may fall short of native facility in the spoken language that decodes the cognitive map. When this happens, ignorance of even some of the rules for hearing society can lead to behavior that society judges aberrant. One result of such judgments is well known to professionals who work with the deaf: Deaf persons are placed in mental health institutions not because of illness or dysfunction but because they cannot hear and cannot speak or respond to those who do not know their language and their cognitive maps.

Language, then, does determine what is acceptable—if not to be mentally healthy at least to escape suspicion of abnormality by others—because language both provides members of a community with a means of judging acceptability and provides those growing up in a community with their major means of learning what they need to know.

THE GENETIC AND THE CULTURAL
BASIS OF LANGUAGE

Language is defined differently by the different disciplines that recognize its importance, but two points are insisted upon by most of the language sciences: (1) Language is part of human genetic makeup; and (2) Language has to be acquired through interaction with others who have it. Another way of stating this almost paradoxical double nature is that a capacity for language in the form of the cognitive power to operate symbolically is a human universal, but the particular language a human infant acquires is a function of its particular cultural and subcultural environment.

Deafness cannot help but change this relation of nature and nurture. The child who is born deaf or deafened early has inherited human capacity for language. However, there are only two possible language environments for the deaf child—this in contrast to the hundreds or thousands of particular language environments for a hearing child. The two—a *hearing-speaking* and a *deaf-signing* subculture—are not equally probable, however. Although nine out of 10 deaf children begin life amidst hearing speakers, the chances are small that they will learn the hearers' language and all its connections to persons and actions and ideas without great difficulty. (The British Ministry of Health, in 1966, for instance, found that both the intelligibility of speech and the ability to receive information by speechreading on the part of deaf teenagers (15–16 years of age) who had completed a course of education measured about 10 percent of normal [Lewis, 1966].)

One deaf child in 10, however, is born to and brought up by deaf parents. Such a child learns early all that needs to be known to sign parents' language acceptably—the usual standards imposed on growing children. Such a child, in fact, begins by making sentences of that language by combining two signs at about 1 year of age (Schlesinger & Meadow, 1974; Williams, 1976). The hearing child begins to make two-word sentences about 2 years of age (Brown, 1973). Yet, despite this striking difference in developmental timetables, it is still only 1 in 10 or more of deaf children who has this "normal" chance to acquire language by interaction with adult users. Part of the reason that other deaf children are not given a reasonable facsimile of a deaf, sign-language environment is simply ignorance: Too few professionals and parents know that when sound does not penetrate, a child's innate language capacity must be given a chance through regular visual–manual language interaction. But there is more than ignorance behind this failure to provide a real language environment. It is a condition known to anthropologists as ethnocentrism: hearing persons do not use their eyes and bodies directly and primarily to acquire and express language, and so they tend to believe strongly that no one else can do so.

THE STRENGTH OF THE GENETIC PREDISPOSITION

Striking confirmation has been found that deaf children, like all children, have full human capacity for language. Goldin-Meadow and Feldman (1975) studied 4 deaf children whose hearing parents wanted no signs used, but who were so young that they had not yet acquired any regular responses to speech. They found that these children did use gestures—at first holophrastically, as children's first words are used to take in whole situations or incidents. Later, the children used gestures differentiated into a noun-like class to name things and people, and a verb-like class to relate processes and actions to describe states. Still later the children joined gestures from these two classes to make utterances; i.e., they used their gestures syntactically.

The experimenters tested the possibility that the children were learning the syntactic use of gestures from their mothers. It turned out, however, that only some of the mothers did use gestures in meaningful arrangements, and these only a long time after the child had regularly been doing so. The implications of this are that some of the mothers learned this gesture language from the children, and that the use of gestures to represent noun ideas and verb ideas in combination came from the children's innate tendency to use language as a syntactic system even without any direct access to a particular spoken or signed language.

The children in this study are special, but not because of anything exceptional about their genetic makeup. Their early experience is typical in most respects of deaf children with hearing parents, even though we can see it in this light as deprivation of usable language experience. Their case is special because, despite the fact that the mothers did not know what the children were doing with their language capacity, these children had the great good fortune of interacting with intelligent human beings who took the trouble to understand their gestured utterances, who appreciated that they were saying what they wanted to say, and who recognized their behavior for what it was—language.

It is hard to overestimate the benefits to children's mental development and health that can accrue from their caretakers' paying attention to utterances, and acting as if what the children say (in speech or in gesture) makes sense and is acceptable. It is likewise hard to imagine anything more detrimental to mental health and development than a refusal or inability to treat and think of the child as making sense.

THE EFFECT OF APPROPRIATE INTERACTION

Still more fortunate than those few children whose spontaneous gesture language is recognized as following universal patterns of syntax acquisition are the fewer deaf children growing up in a small society of deaf family and friends.

First, we may consider the effects of familial deafness on mental health by looking at relationships between parental deafness and diagnosed emotional behavioral problems of deaf children. There is a large body of data available from the Office of Demographic Studies (ODS) at Gallaudet College which conducts an annual survey of hearing-impaired children and youth. In their questionnaire for the school year 1969–1970, the ODS included questions on the hearing status of each child's parents. The questionnaires were filled out by school personnel, not by parents. For each parent, the respondent noted whether the parent had normal hearing before age 6, a hearing loss before age 6, or whether data was not available. Additional handicaps (other than deafness) were also noted for each child, including the categories ''emotional problems'' and ''behavioral problems.''

Data were collected that year on 35,285 children between the ages of 3 and 20. If we exclude those for whom the data on either the parents or additional handicapping conditions were unknown, then we are considering 18,748 children.

If we further restrict our attention to just those children who either had no additional handicaps, or who had emotional/behavioral (EB) problems *only,* then we are considering 14,178 children.

We focus on EB problems separately to maximize the probability that they are not secondary manifestations of another disturbance, e.g., blindness, epilepsy, perceptual-motor problems, or mental retardation.

The groups of children with both parents hearing or only one parent with a reported hearing loss were combined because there was found to be no significant difference between them ($X^2 = 0.11$). As we see from Table 12-1, there is a significant negative dependence ($X^2 = 14.04, p < .005$) between the circumstance of having two deaf parents and the incidence of reported EB disorders. When both parents are deaf, the percentage of deaf children having EB problems is only 5.0 percent; when one or more parents have normal hearing, the percentage is 9.2 percent. The incidence of EB problems is thus 84 percent higher among the children who have one or more hearing parents. We reason that there is a lower incidence of EB problems when there are two deaf parents because of early and well-established communication patterns and language use with their deaf children. Between deaf children and their deaf parents, the quality and quantity of interaction is greater because they share sign language as a medium for interaction. A shared language between the generations enables the transmission of social norms, personal needs, fears, and reassurances, and the kind of communication necessary for self-expression and social integration (beginning at the level of the family). This is in addition to a host of other potentially beneficial factors, such as having a sympathetic and realistic role-model in the family.

Case Study

The child in Williams' (1976) classic study grew up in a home where American Sign Language (ASL) was used alternatively with English (expressed in signs and

Table 12-1
Reported Emotional/Behavioral (EB) Problems Occurring in the Absence of Other Handicapping Conditions, for Deaf Students as Related to Deafness of Parents (School Year 1969–1970)*

Category of Deaf Children	Number of Parents Becoming Deaf Before Child Reaches Age 6		Total
	0 or 1	2	
EB	1,237 (9.2%)	36 (5.0%)	1,273
Normal	12,223 (90.8%)	682 (95.0%)	12,905
Total	13,460	718	14,178

Chi square = 14.04, $p < .005$.
*Data from the Office of Demographic Studies, Gallaudet College, Washington, D.C.

finger-spelled words). In such an environment, his innate language capacity was revealed earlier than that of the deaf children of hearing parents who had to invent their own gesture lexicon and syntax. Todd's first two-sign syntactical structure (the question "Where spoon?") was produced at the age of 10 months (Williams, 1976, p. 37f), but the early appearance of a location–noun–question transformation is only part of the story. Equally impressive is the naturalness, indeed the joyfulness, of his growing up in a household where his signs and sign sentences were understood and where he could increase his understanding of the world through understanding the sign sentences used by others.

Consider this account of his curiosity about himself and the business of living:

. . . when he was three years old, he asked me at the table (in signs), "Where does the meat go?" I asked him what he meant, and he replied: "Look, I swallow the meat, and where does it go?" I then explained to him in details he could understand, and he was pleased and satisfied with the answer.*

It is our contention that being able to formulate and to express such a question about such matters and being able to elicit and understand appropriate answers gives a deaf child (and the parents) a far superior chance for mental health than being mute or being misinterpreted, or even being reprimanded or punished when gestures are used.

Even more basic to the mental health of the child is a feeling of acceptance, of belonging. Here is the eloquent opening of the Williams' study:

My husband and I had long expected that our children would have impaired hearing. Our genetic makeup showed this: Our parents, my uncle, and his four sons are deaf on my side, and four uncles on his side, and so are we. I was born deaf. My husband lost his hearing at the age of six months during an attack of whooping cough, which could be a sign that he was easily susceptible to deafness. When our son Todd was born, he showed so much alertness with his eyes and was so unresponsive to normal sounds that we knew he was like us.*

Into these words, "He was like us," a great deal of wisdom about mental health is compressed. In context, they refer to profound deafness, a condition that makes the vast majority of deaf children unlike their parents. Even worse, for the mental health of the whole family, the deafness causing the difference may be ignored in a well-meant attempt to force the child to use the spoken language. As a consequence, the child then shows a difference in general behavior that often gets classed as abnormal or defective, and the parents torture themselves with guilt about the difference.

Ethnography, as a study of just what people must learn in a certain subculture, may seem a long remove from the heartbreak in a hearing family with a deaf child, but it does call attention to the central issue for mental health in the majority of situations: "The baby is deaf; the baby is not like us!"

---

*Reprinted with permission from Williams J. S. Bilingual experiences of a deaf child. *Sign Language Studies,* 1976, *10,* 39, 37.

A deaf child in a hearing family may, but need not, grow up to be different, or alienated. But in early life, the difference extends only to the surface expression of language (and to insensitivity to language sounds). Human capacity for language is in the brain—genetically—and not in the end-organs of hearing or the machinery of speech. If that were not so, then no experience nor learning would be needed for speaking and understanding. For all hearing babies, learning to speak requires a long period of interaction: first through touch, then through gesture and rhythmical body actions and facial expressions, and only later through vocal sounds shaped more and more closely to acceptable adult standards—this is the normal progression. In all the earlier stages of this multisensory apprenticeship in human communication, a deaf child is or can be quite like hearing children. But this is so only if his caretakers have no fear or embarrassment about communicating—very naturally— with touch, gesture, bodily rhythm, and above all facial expression (Sarles, 1977, p. 200). The experience of deaf children in deaf families (e.g., Williams, 1976) shows that differences may be a matter of surface expression of language only and that interaction with other beings can be satisfying interaction, uniting not dividing.

CODING SOCIAL INFORMATION

Many studies relating language and deafness have stressed only the communicative aspects of language. But as the above figures on EB disorders of deaf children suggest, when mental health is at issue, the social aspects of language are important too. It is not enough to simply express ideas to other people with language; one must constantly allow for the social context and the social consequences. One must express ideas in certain ways, must monitor the effectiveness of the communication, regulate the ensuing social interaction, provide one's own personal stamp on the conversation, and define the in-group or out-group status of those in the conversation (among many other language-mediated activities).

Language must fit the social situation, and its user must learn (in a given culture and even subculture) what is considered rude, witty, boorish, tactful, banal, pleasant, hostile, friendly, and respectful for a number of situations involving a great variety of people and places. In this extended sense, language includes a variety of cultural codes, or sets of rules, which people must master and use skillfully if they want to have satisfying social and personal relationships. And of course most people want to; how else can they feel in harmony with their society?

Code-switching, i.e., control of all these social and language rules, is really one part of general communicative competence, and is usually held to be a function of age and maturity. All of us can remember things said by children that made adults blanch, turn green, reach for the spanking paddle, or roll on the ground with laughter—things said in complete innocence, but which were somehow inappropriate. Experimentally, Krauss and Glucksberg (1969) have shown that some aspects of fitting the language to the person you are speaking to is a function of age; you get better at it as you get older.

In a general sense, one language may include a whole range of codes, but a single individual generally masters no more than a few of them. We are speaking here of regional, ethnic, and sexual (male/female) variation in language—matters of voice, pronunciation, lexical choice, and sometimes syntax and semantics, which mark a speaker as belonging to one or more social groups. These variations in language behavior mark one as being a white, male, middle-class blue-collar worker from the northeast, or as a teen-aged black girl from Chicago, a young gay man from Texas, or a French-born elderly woman who learned English in high school.

These are all judgments and identifications that members of English-speaking American culture make about language users every day. Very often these judgments are not on the basis of language alone, but are aided by the visual cues of nonverbal communication and general appearance. Much of this social information, however, can be transmitted by voice and speech alone, as in telephone conversations. It is possible to judge by telephone whether callers are foreign, to determine their age, race, and sex, and possibly to guess at their educational level and socioeconomic status. And of course skilled mimics can fool the judge by altering their accents— their voices and their choices of language varieties. This means, in essence, that there is a lot of *who we are* encoded into *what we say*. It also follows that we present ourselves to others in the world when we use language, and we expect these others to be able to understand something very personal and important about us when we speak. We feel frustrated when our ideas or our projections of our selves are being misinterpreted.

It should not surprise those who have had extensive experience interacting with deaf people that the need for self-expression and social integration through language is just as important as the need for basic communication. Deaf people in the United States form a subculture bound together by common social, educational, and vocational experiences, but most important, they are socially unified by their use of a shared language, ASL. Like English or any other language, ASL can also vary vastly (or subtly) from region to region, from one social situation to another, or from one individual to another. While there are many people (especially beginning signers) who deplore the fact that there seem to be a great variety of signs for things like birthday, popcorn, tomato, etc., and that there are a number of ways of producing signs and making syntactic constructions in sign language, the fact is that this type of variation is quite natural to any linguistic system. This variety is part of the richness of any language, and it also serves social functions. Research on how deaf people use their language shows clearly that (1) there is a linguistic pattern to much of this variation—it is not random; and (2) there is a social pattern to this language variation, such that social, regional, and ethnic groups can be distinguished by the way they sign (Padden & Markowicz, 1975, Woodward & Erting, 1974). This is a necessary part of any stratified society, be it the hearing majority or the deaf minority. Demarcation of social groups through language use is relevant to both group identity and self-identity.

For example, English speakers from the Northeast and the South may regard each other's language with a mixture of amusement and scorn; younger speakers react with amused tolerance (at best) when their parents attempt to use youthful language or expressions (which are usually culled from reading, and thus are hopelessly out of date). Many similar situations can be found among deaf signers. There are signing styles used only with family, only with friends, only on the job, or only in a certain region. Signers can and do make judgments of others like ''She's obviously from New York,'' or, ''He must have gone to such-and-such a school,'' or ''He signs just like his father and his uncle.''

The easiest judgment to make, of course, is whether a person is a deaf signer or a hearing signer. Just as one can usually tell that a person is deaf because of the way he or she speaks or writes English, one can usually tell if a person is hearing by the way he or she signs. Hearing and deaf people sign quite differently; the differences are apparent to any moderately skilled signer, and the categorical judgment, hearing or deaf, is readily made. However, these basic differences are often obscure to an unskilled signer or to a signer skilled in a sign language other than ASL (Battison & Jordan, 1976).

This is not at all surprising. Someone with a high school course in French cannot discern the differences between the French language as spoken in Paris, in the provinces, or in Switzerland, and can't tell the difference between a native French speaker and an immigrant of 10-years' residence. These differences are nevertheless important to French speakers.

Similarly, within the deaf community, the identification of a person as either deaf or not can be complex. Some people regard themselves as ''more deaf'' than others. It is not a measure based on degree of hearing loss, but a sociologic measure of inclusion in the deaf community. One very common criterion is whether or not the person attended a state residential school for the deaf. If so, then it is reflected in the type of sign language used, it is perceived by other skilled signers, and the person is perceived as belonging to a distinct subgroup of deaf people, one that is ''more deaf'' than others by virtue of having had more interaction with deaf people while growing up. These issues of identification and consequent interaction have been explored by Padden and Markowicz (1975) and by Markowicz and Woodward (1975).

Of course, signing skill depends in general on signing experience and exposure to other signers, but most importantly, it depends on whether or not the signer learned sign language as a child from deaf parents or later in other circumstances. Only about 10 percent of deaf children are born to deaf parents, and in America most of these children will learn ASL as a first language, in very similar fashion to hearing children learning a spoken language. Deaf children of deaf parents learn the language and social interaction of their culture naturally, without technical instruction.

Conflicts of Code and Culture

All of these comments about language differences setting people apart are very important for another reason. When talking with someone who shares your language and your social identification with it, you not only feel that you can communicate effectively, but also that you have a good idea of who you are, of who the other person is, and of the nature of your relationship. For deaf people who have grown up with it, sign language and feelings about it work the same way.

Conversely, when languages and codes are not fully shared, communication and social interpretation of it become disordered. Foreigners are often excused when they make mistakes in telling or comprehending jokes, asking questions, or expressing judgments verbally, because they are not expected to know all the rules. But it is not so easy to accept such behavior from people who are regarded as members of one's own culture. They are expected to follow well-established patterns of language use and if they do not are judged negatively.

A person who does not respond to verbal commands or questions unless they are finally directed to his or her face arouses ill-feelings for not playing the communication game as hearing people do. In our society, the question "What's the matter, are you deaf?!" is an expression of frustration, accusation, and anger—not an inquiry into the processing capacity of the person's ears. Deaf or hearing, someone who is not perceived as using or understanding language appropriately creates a tension that inhibits smooth social interaction.

Since deaf people do not have a visible handicap, hearing people initially judge them as members of hearing culture by applying hearing norms for behavior. Since deaf people are not perceived as being "different" or "foreign," they are instead perceived to be people who know all the communication rules but do not follow them, and may be judged to be crazy, stupid, evil, etc. At the extremes, deaf people have been shot and killed, or have had narrow escapes because they did not respond properly to verbal commands put to them by gun-carrying citizens—in short, because they did not behave as hearing people would have in the same circumstances.

Much of the behavior that leads to conflicts between people with different standards of behavior is nonverbal behavior. While we can accept the fact that a foreigner uses a different language or uses our own imperfectly, we generally have a harder time accepting completely different approaches to conversations and verbal behavior. Recent anthropologic research has shown in detail how interaction can be inhibited by conflicts arising from nonverbal communication (Hall, 1974). Personal distance, head nodding, eye contact, voice inflections, body contact—even as innocent a thing as the time between the utterances of two speakers can vary from one culture to another. The people who normally allow a comfortable pause between speakers (for example, the "slow talkers" of the American South or Southwest) may think that it is rude or indicative of hostility not to allow these pauses. The people who alternate speakers without much blank transition time (for example, urban New Yorkers) may think that the other people are slow or slow-witted. Their differences thus lead to ill feelings.

We would claim that hearing and deaf people also differ in their communication on the linguistic level and on the nonverbal level, and that such code differences can result in misunderstandings, and in mutual judgments of "madness (craziness) or badness."

Actually, the signing of the deaf is itself a sensitive issue for many hearing people. Sign language still elicits stares on the street, slaps on the wrists in some schools for the deaf, and sometimes dismissal for teachers who use it to communicate with their students. Here, however, we wish to consider potential conflicts with hearing people, even those who know something about sign language. Some of what we say will be relevant to spoken communication, however.

We mentioned before that hearing people do not sign like deaf people; of course this varies with their experience in using sign language. Their signing does not flow together or follow a rhythm appropriate to skilled signers; it is often monotonous because the appropriate facial expressions, the "intonation" of signs, are not supplied, but rather are suppressed or performed incorrectly. All of these things can and do lead to misunderstanding, inattention, avoidance, and ill feeling.

To a hearing person, the face of a deaf signer often appears much too animated to be "normal," and the deaf person sometimes appears excited when he or she is not, or appears negative, disapproving, or angry when this is not the case. On several different occasions we have heard hearing people (some of them professionals working with deaf children or adults) react to the "animation" in signers' faces literally; the combination of "imperfect" speech, "excessive" gesturing, and "wild" facial expressions can lead to comments like, "They acted just like animals!" This is not a pleasant thought, but it is an attitude that must be dealt with in professional situations involving deaf and hearing people.

Neither deaf nor hearing people seem to realize that they have different codes for interpreting the facial expressions accompanying sentence production, and that these expressions are not random or meaningless disturbances of facial muscles. Sign-language textbooks commit the same error when stressing the importance of facial expression in signing but never specifying how to do it, as if it were both a natural and universal talent.

In informal experiments we have conducted, we have come across facial expressions made by signers that were interpreted as "emphatically negative" by hearing signers, and "emphatically positive" by deaf signers. This is clearly a code conflict. Actual misunderstandings based on this particular expression in conversation have been observed. We offer the following example.

A deaf woman who was fluent in both ASL and English was in a hearing friend's home looking at some art prints on the wall. They were speaking because the friend knew no signs:

Hostess (noticing the deaf woman looking at the prints): Oh, do you like Escher (the artist)?

Guest (makes the facial expression that means "emphatically positive"—"Oh, yes!"—in ASL)

Hostess (misinterpreting the facial expression): Oh, you *don't* like him then? (annoyed and disappointed)

Guest (confused and alarmed because her message got scrambled): Oh no—I *do* like him!

At this point both participants were confused by this breakdown in communication, and then someone else in the room (a bilingual) pointed out the misuse and the misinterpretation of that one facial expression.

Eye contact is another important aspect of nonverbal communication. In hearing people's conversations, eye contact, or a lack of it, is used to express respect, attentiveness, boredom, preoccupation, and various other states and affects. Since signers are visually dependent, lack of eye contact is naturally interpreted as something stronger than inattentiveness. If the receiver breaks eye contact, communication is broken.

More dramatically, eye contact plays a part in turn-taking and competition for the floor (i.e., the right to speak) in sign conversations. Two hearing people will compete by raising their voices gradually until one gives in and stops talking. The winner then lowers his voice to a normal level and continues speaking. As a direct analogue, you might expect two signers competing for the floor to sign larger and faster until one gives in—but they do not. Instead, with both signing at the same time, one signer will avert his eyes long enough to force the other person to stop signing. After all, if you lose your audience, you are in the silly position of signing to yourself. Beginning signers nearly always lose at this conversation regulating game, because they avert their eyes too soon, or not at all. It takes time to learn the complex rules of language use. Studies by Baker (1975, 1976) have focused on facial expressions and eye contact in sign conversations. Deaf signers also use eye contact and eye movements productively at other levels of the grammar—to mark boundaries between sign phrases and sentences, and some eye movements may be used in place of pronouns. Hearing signers are notorious for their incorrect (i.e., unregulated and ungrammatical) use of eye contact, and often appear shifty-eyed and evasive to deaf people.

Signers, who are visually dependent, will position themselves in a room very carefully with regard to room lighting and lines of sight between conversants. A hearing person in the same room will try to avoid sitting next to an air conditioner or a door opening onto a hallway, two very common sources of distracting noise. The logical position for the deaf person is not necessarily logical for the hearing person, nor are comfortable conversational distances necessarily the same.

In small gatherings involving mixed groups of hearing and deaf, hearing people who are sensitive to the visual dependence of deaf people will frequently wait until deaf people have rearranged chairs and bodies and are seated before finding a seat for themselves. To a hearing person who is not sensitive to this aspect of visual dependence, it must seem that deaf people do a lot of pointless (and annoying) shuffling of chairs and bodies. (An aspect of visual dependence and communication comfort that is applicable to the clinical setting is the seating arrangements of interviews between clinicians and clients. Very often seating arrangements in a small office are inflexible and are determined by the hearing clinician.)

At the production level, a skilled deaf signer may alternate signing with dominant and nondominant hands, may delete, contract, or assimilate signs or parts of signs according to regular linguistic rules, and will sometimes sign two separate things simultaneously (Battison, 1974, 1978). These skills are beyond average hearing signer's ability to produce, understand, or sometimes even to notice. A person who signs with one hand rather than two may do so because he or she is tired or is bored with the conversation. It may be a signal of dismissal or an expression of a wish to terminate the conversation. Other subtleties of style and affective state are communicated in the articulations of the signs themselves.

At the level of individual signs, the English-based signer may use some signs that were invented specifically for translating English words—the signs or the words themselves might not be in the deaf person's vocabulary. Also, the deaf ASL signer may use signs that can be interpreted correctly only with a knowledge of ASL lexical structure or syntax.

The Clinical Setting

With the various situations described above, it is a wonder that *any* communication takes place between deaf and hearing signers. Of course it does, but the point is that it is subtly limited by potential conflicts that arise from not sharing the same linguistic or nonverbal codes. There is far more to using a language correctly than simply knowing one or two thousand words.

By now it is apparent why we chose to focus on signing interaction between a hearing and deaf person. This most frequently characterizes the situation when a deaf person seeks counseling. A mental health specialist, generally hearing, has a client or patient who is deaf. Much of the conversation is signed directly or is interpreted. The clinician makes judgments about the client based on information received, and the client makes judgments about the clinician.

The client has come (or has been sent) for help and is trying to decide how much he or she can trust the clinician and how open to be in discussing problems. Deaf people are at a disadvantage because they are not in control of the situation; the clinician usually asks most of the questions. The clinician, on the other hand, is trying to assess the client's problems or provide therapy in a limited time. He or she is trying to make sense of what the client says, looking for indications of fears, confusion, excitability, etc and judging whether or not the client's communication is appropriate to the situation, and whether responses to questions are appropriate answers. Both are judging affective display and its congruence with what the other person is signing (does this person say one thing but mean something else . . . ?).

We have sketched the potential for culture and communication conflict between hearing and deaf people, even when the hearing people can sign and such conflicts arising from the transmission and reception difficulties are minimized. We feel that this has great relevance to mental health professionals because proper diagnosis and treatment both depend upon the correct interpretation of very subtle verbal and nonverbal interactions.

We believe it is inadvisable to assume, as many hearing people seem to do, that deaf people have the same standards for behavior or the same communication codes as hearing people. As recent sociologic and linguistic research shows, the deaf community constitutes a subculture with different cultural norms, institutions, beliefs, attitudes, and experiences. Thus, it is important for hearing people who do therapy with deaf people to appreciate these cultural differences, to gain a sensitivity about normal communicative and social behavior in the deaf community, and to apply this knowledge in their clinical practice.

As a practical measure for therapists, we suggest frequent consultation with deaf and hearing signers who have extensive knowledge of the deaf community and who also have a background in linguistics. If not actually part of the clinical staff, they can still expand staff sensitivity regarding deaf people and advise staff on communication with deaf people in clinical settings. We believe that very few hearing people are competent observers or judges of deaf social and communicative behavior; many more should be so trained.

We also advocate the training and placement of more deaf individuals in the mental health professions, as well as in the fields of social work and counseling. Deaf clients will always be served best by those who are able to fully communicate with them, and by those who are best able to understand the full meaning of their experiences.

Finally, we suggest that there is a need for collaborative research between linguists and clinicians on the topics we have raised: (1) normative deaf communicative and social behavior and its acquisition; (2) communication conflicts between deaf and hearing people; (3) educating (or re-educating) hearing people about deaf people; (4) deaf–hearing interaction in clinical settings; and (5) the role of the deaf professional in the delivery of social, clinical, and educational services.

CONCLUSION

We have taken an opposing viewpoint to the one that considers deafness as a pathologic condition afflicting people. We have discussed matters from a view in which the focus is not so much on deafness as it is on deaf *people* and their communicative and social behavior. It would help if mental health specialists could view the deaf person not as a hearing person with something lacking, but as a person who had learned different ways of receiving information about the world, different social survival skills, and different rules for personal interaction. The difference can be a crucial one in the testing, evaluation, diagnosis, and therapy associated with the delivery of mental health services to deaf people.

REFERENCES

Baker, C. *Regulators and turn-taking in American Sign Language.* Paper presented at the 50th Annual Meeting, Linguistics Society of America, San Francisco, December 1975.
Baker, C. *What's not on the other hand in American Sign Language.* Papers from the Twelfth Regional Meeting of the Chicago Linguistic Society, 1976.

Battison, R. M. Phonological deletion in American Sign Language. *Sign Language Studies,* 1974, *5,* 1–19.

Battison, R. M. *Lexical borrowing in American Sign Language.* Silver Spring, Maryland: Linstok Press, 1978.

Battison, R. M., & Jordan, I. K. Cross-cultural communication with foreign signers: Fact and fancy. *Sign Language Studies,* 1976, *10,* 53–68.

Brown, R. *A first language: The early stages.* Cambridge Mass.: Harvard University Press, 1973.

Goldin-Meadow, S. J., & Feldman, H. The creation of a communication system. *Sign Language Studies,* 1975, *8,* 225–234.

Goodenough, W. H. Componential analysis. *Science,* 1967, *156,* 1203–1209.

Hall, E. T. *Handbook for proxemic research.* Washington, D.C.: Society for the Anthropology of Visual Communication, 1974.

Kavanagh, J. F., & Cutting, J. E. (Eds). *The role of speech in language.* Cambridge, Mass.: Massachusetts Institute of Technology Press, 1975.

Krauss, R. M., & Glucksberg, S. The development of communication: Competence as a function of age. *Child Development,* 1969, *40,* 255–266.

Lane, H. *The wild boy of Aveyron.* Cambridge, Mass.: Harvard University Press, 1976.

Lewis, M. M. (Ed.). *The education of deaf children.* The British Ministry of Health, Her Majesty's Stationery Office, 1966.

Markowicz, H., & Woodward, J. C. *Language and the maintenance of ethnic boundaries in the deaf community.* Paper presented at the Conference on Culture and Communication, Temple University, Philadelphia, March 1975.

Padden, C. A., & H. Markowicz. Cultural conflicts between hearing and deaf communities. In Crammatte, Crammatte, & Markowicz, (Eds). *VII World Congress of the World Federation of the Deaf.* Silver Spring, Md.: National Association of the Deaf, 1976, pp. 407–413.

Sarles, H. *After metaphysics: Toward a grammar of interaction.* Lisse: Peter de Ridder Press, 1977.

Schlesinger, H. S., & Meadow, K. P. *Sound and sign: Childhood deafness and mental health.* Berkeley, Calif.: University of California Press, 1974.

Selby, H. A. *Zapotec deviance.* Austin, Tex.: University of Texas Press, 1974.

Spradley, J. P. (Ed.). *Culture and cognition: Rules, maps, and plans.* San Francisco: Chandler, 1972.

Tinbergen, N. Ethology and stress diseases. *Science,* 1974, *185,* 20–27.

Williams, J. S. Bilingual experiences of a deaf child. *Sign Language Studies,* 1976, *10,* 37–41.

Woodward, J. C., & Erting C. *Synchronic variation and historical change in American Sign Language.* Paper presented at Linguistic Society of America's annual conference, Amherst, Mass., 1974.

Sy Dubow, J.D.
Larry J. Goldberg, J.D.

13

Legal Strategies to Improve Mental Health Care for Deaf People

Despite some progressive reforms, mentally ill deaf people suffer neglect and abuse in many of our state mental health systems. These abuses can range from misdiagnosis and improper intake procedures, to inadequate treatment once hospitalized, to a lack of suitable aftercare. Initiating reform in major government agencies can be a frustrating and time-consuming procedural exercise. However, the courts and legislatures offer an alternative and, perhaps, a more direct approach to the problem. The purpose of this chapter is to provide professionals concerned with the plight of mentally ill deaf people an arsenal of legal weapons with which to begin to eliminate barriers to effective treatment and rehabilitation.

BACKGROUND

A survey of New York state psychiatric hospitals revealed that over one fourth of the deaf patients were initially diagnosed as mentally deficient as contrasted to only 3.7 percent of the hearing.[1] Vernon[2] noted that despite the fact that IQ is essentially normally distributed in the deaf population, gross errors have been made in the diagnosis of mental retardation. Too often, a patient's inability to communicate through speech is interpreted as a sign of mental retardation rather than a sign of deafness. Such a patient may remain in an institution for years before the mistake is discovered. An extreme example of this is the case of a deaf patient who, because of misdiagnosis, spent 35 years at a state hospital for the mentally retarded.[2] Deaf people have often been institutionalized because no suitable alternative, such as sheltered care facilities, exists. Instead of developing appropriate social and vocational rehabilitation facilities, state agencies have resorted to the expediency of placing the problem deaf person in an institutional or custodial setting.

Unless special facilities exist, deaf patients are often housed in a general ward, where they are unable to communicate with either staff or fellow patients. They may be denied treatment because they cannot participate in therapies that depend on the ability to hear. Unable to communicate other than through the cumbersome process of writing notes, they may languish on the wards without companionship or hope for treatment. Grinker[3] in a study of Illinois state mental hospitals, found that in only one of four facilities did the staff know which patients were deaf. One facility provided a list of 200 names of patients who were thought to be deaf out of an approximate population of 4000. Only 1 proved to be deaf. In contrast, 5 deaf patients, none of whom were on the list, were found in just one unit. Many thought they were the only deaf patients in the hospital. As Grinker[3] observed:

Obviously, if the deaf patients were not even identified as deaf, no real effort was made to treat them. No staff members or other patients could communicate with them in the language of signs. Thus, they were total isolates. In fact, in this sense, their hospitalization was actually anti-therapeutic (Grinker, [3] p. 24).

Even in those instances where intake is appropriate and diagnosis correct, the quality or even the existence of therapy appropriate for the deaf patient is questionable. In addition, the abuse sometimes inflicted upon deaf patients is a frightening problem. Unable to summon help or to readily identify attackers, deaf patients are easy targets for the more aggressive patients. They may have their food or personal property stolen, or they may be victims of outright assault. Even in the model institution where none of these abuses occur, the very process of institutionalization is fraught with pain to deaf individuals unless special programs and staff are available. Patients undergo loss of privacy and loss of dignity to which we all have a right. Their lives, more than that of hearing patients, are controlled and ordered through a process that they cannot hope to understand because they cannot be easily informed about what is happening to them. Frustration and bewilderment are natural results, often misdiagnosed as psychotic behavior leading to inappropriate treatment.

FUNDING SPECIAL PROGRAMS FOR MENTALLY ILL DEAF PERSONS

In several states, mental health services for the deaf are funded directly through the state's department of mental health. These programs are a legitimate and necessary component of the state mental health system and are allocated funds from the general budget. The state department of vocational rehabilitation is another source of funding. Several programs have successfully sought federal grants to provide services to the deaf; however, such funds are usually temporary and thus continuation funds constantly must be sought. Typically, programs designed to meet the special needs of deaf people were established through the efforts of a number of key citizens who became interested in the problem and pursued sources of funding within their state or community. This can be a frustrating experience, given most states' reticence or inability to commit funds for new programs. At this writing, failures have far exceeded successes, and alternative methods of initiating changes must be found.

In the following sections, we shall first take up how an unusual criminal case may affect the rights of deaf people to receive appropriate treatment. We shall then cite how litigation, both on an individual and class basis, and legislation can be used as means to initiate appropriate diagnostic and treatment programs.

CRIMINAL LAW

The case of Donald Lang is unique in criminal justice. Lang, who is deaf and cannot speak, lip-read, sign, read, or write, grew up in the streets of Chicago. He received minimal schooling because he was mistakenly judged retarded. Despite his handicap, he developed remarkable independence, including employment as a laborer. In 1966, Lang was charged with the murder of a prostitute. On the basis of testimony presented by experts who examined Lang, he was found mentally and physically incompetent to stand trial on the murder charge, was remanded to the Illinois Department of Mental Health, and placed in an institution for the mentally retarded. Lang remained there for 5 years while the courts wrestled with a situation that had no American legal precedent. Finally, the Illinois Supreme Court relied on an English case, *Regina v. Roberts,*[4] that dealt with a similar situation. The Illinois Supreme Court, in *People ex. rel. Meyers v. Briggs,*[5] held that Lang should be given a trial to determine whether or not he was guilty as charged or else be released. Due to the time that had elapsed, key witnesses had either died or could not be located and the case could not be prosecuted. Lang was released.

In 1972, shortly after being released from the state facility for the retarded, Lang was charged with a second murder similar in facts to the first. He went on trial under the previous Illinois Supreme Court decision, was found guilty and sentenced to 14–25 years in prison. Appeals were filed and in 1975, the Illinois Supreme Court reversed the earlier conviction on the grounds that the conviction was constitutionally impermissible without trial procedures to compensate for Lang's handicap. In other words, this ruling held that Lang's handicaps prevented him from communicating with his attorney and participating in his own defense. The case was again remanded to the Illinois Department of Mental Health for a hearing into Lang's need for hospitalization and treatment. In 1972, Lang was judged unfit to stand trial on the basis of tests and opinions that found him mentally retarded and dangerous to others. In a subsequent judicial action, Circuit Court Judge Joseph Schneider found that the tests employed with Lang were not proper for a deaf person and that the state's examiners were not skilled and experienced in working with deaf people. Judge Schneider gave greater weight to the testimony of examiners secured by the defendant's attorneys because they were more experienced in working with deaf people. Although Judge Schneider found that Lang was not in need of mental treatment and not mentally retarded, he ordered the state to retain custody of Lang during bail proceedings. He further requested the state and the defendant's attorneys to develop a plan to provide treatment or therapy that would make Lang fit for trial.[6] In the meantime, Lang's attorneys sought assistance for him by arranging voluntary admission to a state mental health facility where it was hoped that appropriate treatment or therapy could be initiated. During the year he spent in a mental health facility, Lang for the first time showed some capacity to learn sign language. There appeared to be a lessening of previous idiosyncratic gesturing and gutteral expressions and a beginning of what was felt to be a formalized language system.

In 1978, the Illinois Department of Mental Health appealed Judge Schneider's order to retain custody of Lang during bail proceedings on the ground that the court had no jurisdiction to order Lang into its custody. Subsequently, Lang was discharged and returned to the maximum-security section of the Cook County jail. In June, 1978, the Illinois Appellate Court ruled that the Illinois Department of Mental Health does not have to develop a training program to make Lang fit for trial because he is neither mentally ill nor retarded. At the same time, the court criticized the state's attorney's office, the mental health agency, and the legislature of Illinois, holding that Lang's case demonstrates the desperate need for substantial change in Illinois law. In Illinois, contrary to the laws of some other states, the courts do not have the power to commit defendants unfit to stand trial to mental health departments for proper treatment. Without such changes in Illinois, Lang cannot get treatment until he is exonerated, but he cannot be exonerated until he gets treatment.

A case similar to Donald Lang's was decided by the United States Supreme Court (*Jackson v. Indiana*[7]). Theon Jackson, an illiterate, mentally retarded deaf person, without basic communication skills, was accused of purse snatching. An Indiana court committed Jackson to a mental institution due to his inability to understand the nature of the charges against him. His commitment was to continue until his sanity could be certified to the court.

The Supreme Court reversed the state court decision, declaring that Jackson's constitutional rights were violated since he was condemned to permanent institutionalization without the necessary showing required for commitment under the state statute. If it could not justify continued confinement after 6 months, the state was ordered to proceed to trial or dismiss the case.

Both of these cases raise the issues of a deaf person's fitness to stand trial for a criminal offense and the applicable standard for commitment. Both Lang and Jackson were found incompetent to stand trial. The traditional test for competence is whether the defendant understands the proceedings and charges and whether he or she can consult with a lawyer and assist actively in the defense (*Dusky v. United States*[8]).

Lang and Jackson were found incompetent to stand trial, but this stemmed from an inability to communicate, not from mental illness. A finding of incompetence usually results in commitment to a mental health facility until such time as the individual becomes competent. Yet restoration of competence for Lang and Jackson was highly unlikely. In *Jackson v. Indiana*,[7] the Supreme Court realized that the result of this procedure—permanent institutionalization—violates the constitutional rights of the defendant.

To remedy this inequity, the Supreme Court held that any incompetency commitment must be temporary and reasonably likely to be effective in restoring the defendant to competency. If there is no substantial probability that the defendant's condition is treatable, commitment is either not allowed or must be terminated if it has already taken place.[7] The court thus attacked the rigid interpretation of competency and commitment standards applied by the state that resulted in the deprivation of Jackson's constitutional rights.

Presumably, the law that has developed as a result of these two cases would prevent deaf people accused of crimes from being institutionalized without proper treatment and without hope of being tried for the crime charged. Yet, practical problems remain in the implementation of these two judicial decisions. The Lang case demonstrates the problems in developing programs to train "incompetent" individuals to improve their communication skills and participate in their criminal defense. Who is responsible for developing these programs and what they will consist of remain unanswered questions. And although the court in *Jackson v. Indiana*[7] spoke of commitment for a reasonable time until competency is restored, no guidelines were provided as to how long a reasonable period of time is.

These practical problems seriously impair any protections guaranteed by the cases of Lang and Jackson. Until judicial decisions or legislation further clarify these issues and find solutions for these problems, deaf defendants, adjudged incompetent to stand trial, will continue to suffer the loss of their constitutional rights.

LITIGATION

The courts' evolving recognition of a mental patient's legal rights encourages legal action to improve mental health services for deaf patients. Litigation on both an individual and class basis, to establish new rights to adequate treatment for the mentally ill, can serve as models for the problems of deaf patients in mental hospitals.

Individual Rights of Action

Individual patients have sought relief through two methods. One method used is the civil damage suit against physicians who neglect their patients' care. A Florida man, in *Donaldson v. O'Connor*,[9] successfully sued two of his doctors for violating his constitutional rights under the Fourteenth Amendment. Although committed to a Florida state hospital for over 15 years, he had received no treatment.

The lower courts reasoned that the state may curtail one's liberty only for a permissible governmental goal, that of treatment of the person. Therefore, the person has a constitutional right to receive treatment when involuntarily committed. Without treatment, continued confinement is unconstitutional. The federal court jury awarded $38,000 in money damages against the doctors for their denial of the patient's constitutional rights.

Upon appeal, the Supreme Court of the United States, in *O'Connor v. Donaldson*,[10] upheld the outcome of the lower court's decision. The Supreme Court held that it is unconstitutional to involuntarily confine a nondangerous individual capable of living outside the institution, if he or she is not receiving treatment:

In short, a State cannot constitutionally confine without more [than custodial care], a nondangerous individual who is capable of surviving safely in freedom by himself or with the help of willing and responsible family members or friends (p. 576).

The court, however, sent the case back to the lower court for retrial to consider whether the defendant officials were immune from paying damages to Donaldson. In 1977, the case was settled out of court for $20,000, thereby leaving legally unresolved the question of the official immunity of the defendants in this case.

In order to obtain money damages, a patient must prove that doctors acted willfully and maliciously to deprive him or her of constitutional rights. To prove this contention, patients must show (1) that they clearly fit the description of being nondangerous and capable of surviving outside the institution; (2) that they received no treatment; and (3) that their physicians, although they knew or should have known the condition, still blocked release. Meeting these requirements may be difficult in court. Many individual patients have, therefore, tried a different legal approach. They have sought relief through a writ of habeas corpus.

Traditionally, habeas corpus has been a legal tool used to challenge the conditions of confinement, whether in jail or in other institutions. It has successfully been used in the District of Columbia to challenge placement of patients in excessively restrictive treatment settings. According to the District of Columbia statutes the purpose of involuntary commitment is treatment. Therefore, the District of Columbia courts have held that confinement must take away liberty only insofar as is necessary to treat the patient. A patient with a mild disorder, for example, cannot be locked in a maximum security ward used to house the criminally insane. Patients have a right to the least restrictive form of treatment consonant with their needs (*Covington v. Harris*[11]). Some courts have even held that the hospital has an obligation to explore alternative placements for the patient and to select that which is least restrictive (*In re Henry Jones*[12]).

For those patients who were misdiagnosed or committed because there were no alternatives available, the writ of habeas corpus may be the appropriate legal approach. It gives them the means to challenge their placement and the chance to seek release from overly restrictive conditions.

However, the problem with a habeas corpus proceeding is the standard that the court uses. This standard is not whether the hospital has made the best choice of treatments, but whether it made a permissible and reasonable choice in view of the relevant information the hospital possesses.[11] This relaxed standard makes it harder for the patient to prove that the hospital has acted unreasonably in choosing treatment. There are other problems with using a writ of habeas corpus. Success depends upon finding affected individuals and then individually litigating their cases. This process is both costly and time-consuming. An even greater problem is that the hospital may reassign the patient or change the terms of confinement while the legal case is pending in court. A court can then say there is no longer a need to decide the merits of the patient's claim of inadequate treatment, since the patient's status has changed.

Class Action

Because of the difficulty in bringing individual suits and the limitation of the remedy to only one particular patient, the class action has been utilized as a more effective means of institutional change. A class action is filed by a patient representative of all persons similarly situated. The case of *Wyatt v. Stickney*[13] is the leading precedent establishing a constitutional right to treatment. The court held that where patients are involuntarily committed through noncriminal procedures to a state mental hospital, they have a constitutional right to receive such *individual* treatment as will give them an opportunity to improve their mental condition or be cured. The court's decree on the minimum constitutional standards for adequate treatment emphasized that each patient shall have an individual treatment plan that included a statement of the least restrictive treatment conditions necessary to achieve the purposes of commitment. On the basis of this decree, an individualized treatment plan for a deaf patient would require a program such as a deaf ward where the patient could fully participate in his or her therapy.

A staff trained in sign language and the opportunity for a patient to interact with other deaf patients would be essential to achieve meaningful participation in the individual plan. Deaf patients who do not know sign language could be trained, if possible, to enable them to be involved in a deaf ward.

The *Wyatt v. Stickney*[13] decree also emphasized the right of patients to a humane psychological and physical environment. This includes the right to privacy and dignity and the right to be free from isolation. A human rights committee was established by the court to investigate violations of a patient's right and to oversee implementation of the plan. Protection of these rights will help alleviate the neglect and abuses a deaf patient endures. The court order also stresses minimum numbers of treatment personnel per 250 patients and standards to be followed to ensure more humane living conditions. To guarantee effective programs for the deaf patients, however, court orders should specify the special needs of deaf patients, such as deaf units in mental hospitals.

Another approach based upon constitutional law is the "protection from harm" theory. This theory embodies the concept that no person should suffer from a deteriorating condition caused by confinement by the state. This approach was successfully employed in correcting some of the overcrowded conditions in New York State institutions. In *New York State Association for Retarded Children (NYSARC), Inc. v. Rockefeller,*[14] the plaintiff challenged conditions at Willowbrook State School. The courts held that the patients of a state institution have a right to protection from inhumane treatment, which constituted cruel and unusual punishment under the Eighth Amendment. The *NYSARC* decision found that impermissible treatment existed not just when physical deterioration took place, but when conditions frustrated the full development of a person's capabilities.[15] The court ordered defendants to place plaintiffs in community residences and to hire and train direct-care staff. The court stated that financial or staff limitations imposed by the state could not deter defendants from complying with this deinstitutionalization process.

In *Michigan Association of Retarded Citizens v. Smith,*[16] a suit to prevent the physical, emotional, and sexual abuse of children in an institution for the mentally retarded, the court held that such treatment denied the children the right to a safe and humane environment. The court ordered an increased staff to monitor patient treatment, required that patients undergo annual physical exams to determine their health condition, and also increased parental participation in the investigation of abuses. Such decisions based on protection from harm can be helpful in attacking the present lack of individual treatment for deaf patients.

A third successful approach has been to rely on state law as a basis for suit. Many states now have statutes that guarantee the person a right to treatment in state institutions. This trend was begun by the highly influential decision of *Rouse v. Cameron.*[17] This case was a proceeding on a petition for habeas corpus. The patient relied upon the statutes of the District of Columbia to establish his right to treatment. This law states:

A person hospitalized in a public hospital for a mental illness shall, during his hospitalization, be entitled to medical and psychiatric care and treatment. The administrator of each public hospital shall keep records detailing all medical and psychiatric care and treatment received by a person hospitalized for a mental illness. . . .[18]

The court construed this statute to grant to each person a right to treatment. Other states have ruled similarly when interpreting their own state laws. One advantage to utilizing this approach is that state judges will probably be more inclined to enforce a state law than declare a constitutional right to treatment.

In the last two decades there has been a substantial movement away from large institutions and toward community-based care. The President's Commission on Mental Health found that "[i]n 1955 approximately seventy-five percent of people receiving care were treated as inpatients, primarily in large institutions. By 1975 approximately seventy-five percent were being seen as outpatients, primarily in community based settings."[19] The Preliminary Report found a variety of factors causing this shift. The Mental Retardation Facilities and Community Mental Health Centers Construction Act of 1963[20] and the subsequent Community Mental Health Centers Act[21] provided the federal legislative push toward the development of community-based care. Successful court challenges, coupled with state legislative reform of state commitment procedures and policies and recent court decisions setting minimum standards for patient care, have accelerated the movement toward providing mental health services in the community.[22]

This movement creates opportunities for deaf mentally ill patients to receive treatment in the least restrictive environment. While there have been several court cases requiring individualized treatment in the least restrictive alternative, and protection of patient's civil rights within institutions, there have been only a few law suits alleging that there is right to community placement.

In *Dixon v. Weinberger*,[23] a federal court held that under the Hospitalization of the Mentally Ill Act[24] patients in a federally administered mental institution in the District of Columbia have a right to treatment that includes placement in facilities outside the institution where the institution has determined that such treatment is appropriate. The court found that both the Federal Government and the District of Columbia violated the act by failing to place inpatients at St. Elizabeth's Hospital, who have been determined suitable for placement, in alternative less-restrictive facilities. Less-restrictive alternatives to the hospital include nursing homes, foster homes, personal care homes, and halfway houses.

A federal district court in Maine has approved the first consent decree that establishes detailed standards for the care and treatment of mentally retarded persons who are placed in community settings. Under the decree, persons released from institutions into the community will have the right to receive "habilitation," which includes suitable medical treatment, education, training, and care, regardless of their age, degree of retardation, or handicapping condition. Persons living in the community are to receive an individualized plan of care, education, and training including the services of physical therapists, psychologists, speech therapists, doctors, and dentists. A court-appointed master will monitor the implementation of the consent decree.[24a]

A federal court judge in *Halderman v. Pennhurst*[25] ruled that mentally retarded individuals institutionalized at Pennhurst State Hospital in Pennsylvania were deprived of opportunities for treatment, education, and training that are available in smaller, community-based facilities. This was held to be a violation of section 504, which requires services to be provided in an integrated setting on a community level where appropriate. Thus, defendants in this case were ordered to provide plaintiffs with suitable community living arrangements as well as such community services as were necessary to provide them with minimally adequate habilitation until such time as the plaintiffs were no longer in need of such living arrangements and/or community services. This case can be used by deaf people as well to attack the denial of appropriate mental health care on a community level.

Further judicial construction of a right to community-based treatment for the mentally ill could have a far-reaching impact on improving noninstitutional care for deaf people. Yet attitudinal and communication barriers prevent existing community facilities from adequately meeting their mental health needs. For deaf people to be released from institutions where they receive custodial care at most is no solution if all they have to look forward to is inaccessible community services. Once outside the institution and inside the community, deaf people need additional protections. Again, this consists of professionals trained in working and communicating with deaf people, interpreters, and specialized training and licensing programs to meet the demand for more professionals in the area. The creation of community centers that can provide specific services for deaf patients is a logical extension of the right to minimum treatment in the least restrictive setting.

LEGISLATION

Another tool to improve services for deaf people in mental hospitals is legislation. Meaningful legislation would guarantee to each patient the right to individualized treatment. Illinois, Massachusetts, Michigan, Pennsylvania, and Georgia have recently changed their mental health laws to require individualized treatment plans[26-32] A 1977 amendment to the Mental Health Code of Illinois[26] specifically provided for accessibility by deaf patients to individual treatment plans. The 1977 amendment mandated the use of sign language with any hearing-impaired patient for whom sign language is a primary mode of communication. That amendment stated:

Wherever this Act requires an oral explanation to be made to a patient, such explanation shall be given within 12 hours as provided for in Section 3–8 of this Act, in a language the patient understands, *or in sign language for any hearing-impaired individual for whom sign language is a primary mode of communication,* and a note of that explanation, and by whom made, shall be put into the patient's record.

Every patient shall be provided with adequate and humane care and treatment pursuant to an individual treatment plan. *Such care and treatment shall include the regular, daily use of sign language for any hearing-impaired individual for whom sign language is a primary mode of communication* (emphasis added).[26]

Due to an administrative error, this 1977 Amendment to the Mental Health Code of Illinois was excluded from a comprehensive reform of its mental health laws in 1978.[27] However, this provision to ensure accurate communication can be used as a model in any state mental health law guaranteeing accessibility of mental health services to deaf people.

Pennsylvania's Mental Health Procedures Act of 1976 requires the development of an individualized treatment plan appropriate to the patient's specific needs in the least restrictive setting.[28,29] Treatment may include inpatient treatment, partial hospitalization, or outpatient treatment.

The Massachusetts Mental Health Code[30] provides that institutionalized patients must be subject to periodic administrative review. The institution must consider all possible alternatives to continued hospitalization or residential care, including a determination of the person's relationship to the community and to the family, employment possibilities, and the availability of community resources.

The Georgia legislature amended its mental health law to extend the rights of patients in mental health facilities.[31] Such rights include the right to refuse treatment, the right to the least restrictive alternative for every patient, placement in noninstitutional community facilities and programs, and an established complaint procedure.

The Massachusetts, Pennsylvania, and Georgia laws[28-31] provide good models for requiring individualized treatment for mental patients in the least restrictive environment. Alternative facilities for deaf patients should include but not be limited to community mental health centers, nursing homes, personal care homes, foster homes, and halfway houses. The Michigan Mental Health Law[32] provides for individualized plans and the establishment of a violations office within the Department of Mental Health to investigate apparent violations of patients' rights and act on behalf of patients to obtain a remedy for any apparent violations.

It is most important, however, for state laws to include independent advocacy agencies to protect the rights of mental patients. Section 113 of the Developmentally Disabled Assistance and Bill of Rights Act[11] requires that each state receiving formula grants for developmental disabilities services have in effect by October 1, 1977, an independent system for protection and advocacy of the rights of persons receiving such service with "the authority to pursue legal, administrative, and other appropriate remedies." The protection and advocacy agency must be independent of any state agency that provides treatment, services, or habilitation to persons with developmental disabilities.

FEDERAL REGULATIONS

The Regulations to Section 504 of the Rehabilitation Act of 1973[33] offer another avenue for deaf people to challenge inaccessible mental health services. The Regulation requires mental health facilities receiving HEW funding to provide effective benefits or services, and a recipient may not provide benefits and services in a manner that limits or has the effect of limiting the participation of qualified handicapped persons. A mental health funding recipient

that employs fifteen or more persons shall provide appropriate auxiliary aids to persons with impaired sensory, manual, or speaking skills, where necessary to afford such persons an equal opportunity to benefit from the service in question. [For the purpose of this paragraph,] *auxiliary aids may include* brailled and taped material, *interpreters,* and other aids *for persons with impaired hearing* or vision (emphasis added).[33]

This regulation thus places the responsibility on mental health services to provide interpreters for deaf patients to enable them to participate in treatment programs. If facilities refuse to provide interpreters, they face the possibility of the withholding of and/or cutting off of HEW funds or a private law suit against the mental health services. Several successful suits have been brought against universities, social service agencies, and hospitals to require them to pay for interpreter services.[34-38]

CONCLUSION

This chapter has provided an overview of litigative and legislative strategies adaptable to the deaf patients in mental hospitals.

Some of the established methods mentioned are the individual civil suit, habeas corpus, the class action, and legislative reform. Although these legal precedents have applied to mental health patients in general, they can and should be used to challenge the present plight of the deaf patients in mental hospitals and outpatient programs.

In determining whether to pursue a litigation, administrative, or legislative approach in obtaining effective mental health services for deaf people, it is important to evaluate, along with other factors, the possible remedy under each approach.

To be afforded the right to treatment and equal services required by state statutes and Section 504, deaf people need comprehensive mental health services, including a professional staff trained in the psychology of deafness and in sign language, as well as specialized inpatient and outpatient treatment facilities. Yet such a comprehensive program would not clearly be ordered by a court or administrative agency interpreting the above statutes. All that might be required is interpreters.

For example, as previously mentioned, the Regulation to Section 504[33] generally requires equal benefits and services for handicapped individuals. The only section of this regulation that specifically deals with deaf and hearing-impaired individuals requires recipients to provide interpreters to deaf people in health services settings.

Under the general nondiscrimination provisions of the regulation, the provision of an interpreter is probably the most expedient remedy.[33] Only by proving that the mental health services provided to deaf people are not as effective as provided to those who can hear[33] could it be argued that comprehensive services are the required remedy. To prove this, one would have to show that most deaf people in need of mental health services could be effectively served only by specially trained personnel and by facilities reserved solely for deaf people. If this could not be shown, a Section 504 recipient would be precluded from setting up separate facilities and services.[33] Even if an individual was successful in proving this factor, it is not certain that more than an interpreter would be the ordered remedy.

This problem raises the issue of the sufficiency of an interpreter in making mental health services accessible to deaf people. Most professionals providing mental health care to deaf people agree that the provision of an interpreter alone is not sufficient. What is needed is a professional staff trained in communicating with deaf people. Important in psychiatric or psychological counseling is the one-to-one relationship between the counselor and the patient. The addition of a third person—an interpreter—could adversely affect this relationship and any possible benefits the deaf person might receive.

Because existing laws do not ensure that a deaf person will receive more services than an interpreter, there is a need for laws more comprehensive and specific than Section 504 and present state mental health statutes. Thus, improved legislation is necessary to truly meet the mental health needs of deaf people. Comprehensive legislation, with appropriate fiscal planning consistent with these needs is the alternative that might guarantee the provision of specialized services for deaf people. With an increased opportunity for direct involvement through drafting bills, lobbying, and testifying before legislators, deaf people could advocate specific services not available under existing statutes and regulations. In addition, the time and expense involved in the legislative process usually requires less than that entailed in litigation.

One of the first legislative efforts to establish a comprehensive outpatient program for deaf people was started in Maryland.[39] While this bill failed to pass the legislature in 1979, that legislative experience provided some helpful lessons on how to pass such a bill in the future. The bill overwhelmingly passed the house after a well-received committee hearing. In the senate, however, some parents of children brought up in the oral method of communication raised questions whether the definition of deafness would include their children. This issue was raised during the closing days of the legislative session and created confusion for the Chairman of the Senate Committee considering the bill. A last-minute amendment was made on the definition to remove any doubt that all deaf people were covered regardless of their method of communication. This amendment necessitates house approval but there was not sufficient time in the session to act on the bill, and it therefore was not passed. An agreement on the bill's provisions by all interested deaf organizations prior to its filing in the legislature will show the legislators that all representatives of their deaf constituency support the bill. Any disagreements on a bill voiced by organizations of and for deaf people will ensure its defeat.

Thus, before efforts are made to make legislators aware of the dearth of appropriate mental health care for deaf people in their state and the need for comprehensive, specialized services, deaf groups must organize and advocate a united position. Only then can the legislative process work to the advantage of deaf people.

In 1980, a united effort by Maryland groups resulted in the State General Assembly passing H.B. 196,[40] which establishes an outpatient program for hearing-impaired people. The governor then recommended $110,000 in his supplemental budget to begin the program.

The difficulties in effecting change through the law cannot be ignored. But active involvement of interested persons in the problems of deaf people can help assure that they will receive appropriate mental health care.

REFERENCES*

1. Rainer, J.D., Actshuler, K.A., Kallman, F.J., et al. *Family and mental health problems in a deaf population.* New York: New York State Psychiatric Institute, 1963.

2. Vernon, M. Techniques of screening for mental illness among deaf clients. *Journal of Rehabilitation of the Deaf,* 1969, *2,* 24–25.

3. Grinker, R. R. *Psychiatric diagnosis, therapy, and research on the psychotic deaf.* Washington, D.C.: U.S. Department of Health, Education and Welfare Social and Rehabilitation Service, 1969.

4. *Regina v. Roberts,* [1953] All England Law Report 340.

5. *People ex. rel Meyers v. Briggs,* 46 Ill. 2d 281, 263 N.E. 2d 109 (1970).

6. *In the Matter of Donald Lang,* 76 Crmmt 064 (Cir. Ct. Cook County, Ill., Dec. 8, 1976); Reversed *People of the State of Illinois v. Donald Lang,* No. 77–1541, No. 78–250. (consolidated) Second Division, Illinois Court of Appeals (June 20, 1978).

7. *Jackson v. Indiana,* 406 U.S. 715 (1972).

8. *Dusky v. United States,* 362 U.S. 402 (1960).

9. *Donaldson v. O'Connor,* 493 F. 2d 507 (5th Cir. 1974).

10. *O'Connor v. Donaldson,* 422 U.S. 563 (1975).

11. *Covington v. Harris,* 419 F. 2d 617, 623 (D.C. Cir. 1969). Developmentally Disabled Assistance and Bill of Rights Act, 42 U.S.C. §6001 *et seq.* at §6012.

12. *In re Henry Jones,* 338 F. Supp. 428, 429 (D.D.C. 1972).

13. *Wyatt v. Stickney,* 344 F. Supp. 373 (M.D. Ala. 1972); aff'd sub. nom. *Wyatt v. Aderholt,* 503 F. 2d 1305 (5th Cir. 1974).

14. *New York State Association for Retarded Children, Inc. v. Rockefeller,* 357 F. Supp. 752 (E.D. N.Y. 1973), enforced sub. nom. *N.Y.S.A.R.C. v. Carey,* No. 72–C–356/ 357 (E.D. N.Y. Sept. 29, 1978).

15. *New York State Association for Retarded Children, Inc. v. Carey,* 393 F. Supp. 715, 718 (E.D. N.Y. 1975).

16. *Michigan Association of Retarded Citizens v. Smith,* C.A. No. 8–70384 (E.D. Mich. March 3, 1978).

17. *Rouse v. Cameron,* 373 F. 2d 451 (D.C. Cir. 1967).

18. D.C. Code §21–562 (Supp. V. 1966).

19. President's Commission on Mental Health, p. 8–10 (September 1, 1977).

20. Mental Retardation Facilities and Community Mental Health Centers Construction Act of 1963, 42 U.S.C. §2681.

21. Community Mental Health Centers Act, 42 U.S.C. §2689.

22. President's Commission on Mental Health pp. 9–10 (September 1, 1977).

23. *Dixon v. Weinberger,* 405 F. Supp. 974 (D.D.C. 1975).

24. D.C. Code §21–501 *et seq.* (Supp. V. 1966).

24a. *Wouri v. Zitnay,* No. 75–80–SD (S.D. Maine, July 14, 1978).

25. *Halderman v. Pennhurst,* 446 F. Supp. 1295 (1977), aff. in part, rev. in part, 612 F. 2d 84 (3rd Cir. 1979).

26. Illinois H.B. 1612. The 1977 Amendment passed the Illinois legislature as H.B. 1612,

---

*Legal citations used herein conform to legal format and can be found in a law library according to information given.

September 21, 1977. A copy of this bill can be obtained from the Illinois legislature in Springfield, Ill.

27. Mental Health and Developmental Disabilities Code, Smith-Hurd Annotated, Ch. 91–1/2 (1978).

28. Mental Health Procedures Act of 1976, Pa. Stat. Ann. Tit. 50 §7107 (1976).

29. Mental Health Procedures Act of 1976, Pa. Stat. Ann. Tit. 50 §7104 (1976).

30. Mental Health Code, Mass. Gen. Laws Ann. Ch. 123 §4 (1974).

31. Code of Georgia Ann. §§88–502 (1978).

32. Mental Health Law, Mich. Stat. Ann. §§330.1712 and 330.1754 (1974).

33. Regulations to Sec. 504 of the Rehabilitation Act of 1973, 45 C.F.R. §84.52(a) (1), (2), (3), (4), and (5), *text below;* and 45 C.F.R. §84.52(d).

§84.52(a) *General.* In providing health, welfare or other social services or benefits a recipient may not, on the basis of handicap:

(1) Deny a qualified handicapped person these benefits or services;

(2) Afford a qualified handicapped person an opportunity to receive benefits or services that is not equal to that offered nonhandicapped persons;

(3) Provide a qualified handicapped person with benefits or services that are not as effective (as defined in §84.4(b)) as the benefits or services provided to others;

(4) Provide benefits or services in a manner that limits or has the effect of limiting the participation of qualified handicapped persons; or

(5) Provide different or separate benefits or services to handicapped persons except where necessary to provide qualified handicapped persons with benefits and services that are as effective as those provided to others.

34. *Camenisch v. University of Texas,* 616 F. 2d 127 (5th Cir. 1980)

35. *Crawford v. Univ. of North Carolina,* 440 F. Supp. 1047 (M.D. N.C. 1977);

36. *Herbold v. The Trustees of California State Univ. & Colleges,* C–78–1358 RHS (N.D. Cal. 1978);

37. *Riker v. Holy Cross Hospital,* 78–1437 (D. Md. 1978);

38. *Williams v. Quern,* 78–C–656 (N.D. Ill. 1978).

39. Maryland H.B. 269, introduced by Delegate Beck on January 22, 1979, to add to Article 59—Mental Hygiene an Act under the new subtitle "Mental Hygiene Services for the Hearing Impaired," Annotated Code of Maryland (1978 Supplement).

40. Maryland H.B. 196, Article 59, §70 *et seq* of Annotated Code of Maryland.

McCay Vernon, Ph.D.

14

Employment, Deafness, and Mental Health

"I think most of us are looking for a calling, not a job. Most of us, like the assembly line worker, have jobs that are too small for our spirits. *Jobs are not big enough for people.*"

Nora Watson in *Working**

An understanding of both the psychology of deafness and the mental health of deaf people must include the influence of vocation. Seldom do we see work as an integral part of human psychology. But the average person spends more waking hours on a job than in any other type of activity. If to those hours is added the time used in commuting, studying for job advancement, and, for many people, the hours spent on a second job, one fact becomes clear. Quantitatively at least, work is human's primary activity in life.

Work is even more significant in deaf people's lives for several reasons. For one, when on the job they tend to be more totally involved in it than hearing people. They cannot socialize as much, due to communication problems. Other diversions are denied, such as the radio or background music. Deaf workers are left primarily with the stimulation, or stultification, of the job itself. For example, the deaf hair stylist's day is spent almost exclusively in cutting and styling hair or else in fantasy. By contrast, for the hearing hair stylist, social interaction, radio, and television are often the major pleasures of the job, not the work itself.

The point, in terms of mental health, is that work is more important for the deaf person than for the hearing person. Paradoxically, deaf people as a group tend to be relegated to the more mundane uninteresting types of jobs (Schein & Delk, 1975, pp. 73–98).

In our desperation to escape the frustration and monotony of our jobs, we often make the assumption that work and the rest of life can be divorced from one

*From *Working: People talk about what they do all day and how they feel about what they do,* by Studs Terkel. Copyright © 1974, by Studs Terkel. Reprinted by permission of Pantheon Books, a Division of Random House, Inc.

another, that despite what we may do for a living, once we leave the job we are transformed. The naiveness of this view is best expressed by Roberta Victor.

"You become your job. I became cold, I became hard, I became turned off, I became numb. I don't think it is terribly different from somebody who works on the assembly line forty hours a week and comes home cut off, numb, dehumanized. People aren't built to switch on and off like water faucets."

Roberta Victor in *Working**

With this cursory overview of the relationship of work to mental health, let's examine some of the major variables affecting deaf people and work.

STATE OF THE ECONOMY

The primary consideration relevant to deaf workers in the current economy is unemployment. Presently, the national rate for hearing people is up over 7 percent, with no substantial evidence that in the foreseeable future this figure will decline to the rates of the previous several decades, which generally were below 5 percent (Levine, 1978). While the overall unemployment rate is above 7 percent, in manufacturing and goods producing industries (automobile production for example), the unemployment rates are much higher. This is important to deaf people because it is in these fields that a disproportionate percent of them work. For example, 3 out of 10 deaf people are employed in the manufacture of nondurable goods (Schein & Delk, 1975, p. 79).

The high rate of unemployment has another negative effect on deaf people, one which has long-range implications. The money that formerly went into job training centers and the Division of Vocational Rehabilitation is now being diverted to public service "make-work" type jobs (Mossberg, 1975). Traditionally, over half of all deaf workers use the states' Divisions of Vocational Rehabilitation for training and job placement, and many are given vocational-technical training in job training centers (Schein & Delk, 1975, pp. 85–87). Thus, money diverted from these agencies into public service jobs tends to hurt deaf peoples' chances for work both on a short-term and long-term basis. The significance of this must not be overlooked.

VOCATIONAL REHABILITATION ACT OF 1973

The Vocational Rehabilitation Act of 1973 had many positive implications for deaf people. Section 503 is probably the most important part of the act because it says that every federal agency contract of more than 2500 dollars must have an affirmative action clause for the employment of handicapped people (Krents, 1975).

---

*From Terkel, S. (1974). Reprinted with permission.

This law affects over 50 percent of the nation's corporations (Krents, 1975). It calls for these businesses to submit plans describing the specific actions they are taking to employ handicapped people, including the deaf. In essence, this means that deaf people will be accorded the same legal protection from discrimination that has been of such great advantage to blacks and other ethnic minorities in their efforts to gain equal job rights. For the black deaf person, who has the most severe unemployment problem within the deaf population, Section 503 could prove a double blessing. By hiring a black deaf worker, the employer will have fulfilled two major requirements of the affirmative action law. If the worker is also female, the benefits to the corporation in complying with the law are threefold.

The problem with Section 503 is that the federal government has not yet hired the people to staff the office that will enforce the law. Administrative resistance to advocacy legislation and bureaucratic red tape are the reasons for the delay. However, some money has been appropriated, and it is not unrealistic to assume that eventually the staff positions will be filled and the called for actions implemented. The little implementation that has occurred resulted from class action suits brought by the handicapped themselves.

One reason Section 503 has special value to deaf people is that deaf people are seen by employers as a preferred group of the handicapped (Tringo, 1971). Thus, when faced with a mandate to hire a certain percentage of handicapped workers, it is probable that employers will turn to deaf applicants first, rather than to the mentally ill, the epileptic, the mentally retarded, or others classified as handicapped.

Deaf people themselves and their advocates such as vocational rehabilitation counselors, rehabilitation center staff, and placement officers have the most important responsibility of all. They must demand implementation of the law. At present, fewer than 1 percent of them even know of the law and not one case has yet been reported of any effort by these professionals to force implementation of Section 503.

INDUSTRIAL NOISE AND DEAF EMPLOYEES

The high cost to industry of reducing noise to levels acceptable to the Environmental Protection Agency is estimated between 11.7 and 31.6 billion dollars over the next 10 years (Fankhauser & Katsarkas, 1975; Ross, 1975). These costs may threaten economic growth, and represent a huge expense to many major industries such as steel and textile manufacturing and newspaper printing.

One way industry can partially circumvent such expenses is to hire deaf workers since they are less susceptible to the destruction of their hearing by excessive noise levels. The Samsonite Luggage Factory has deaf operators on certain very noisy stamp presses. *The Washington Post* faced a strike by printers if the noise level of certain presses was not reduced. The cost to the paper would have been exorbitant, yet there were enough deaf printers at the *Post* to have completely staffed these presses and the work areas in which they were located. Throughout the printing industry, noise pollution control represents an awesome expense. Many deaf persons are trained for work in printing. They could be hired to work around the noisy machinery at a tremendous savings to the publishing business.

The generality that derives from these specific cases is that the hiring of deaf workers in certain jobs involving exposure to excessive noise could be attractive alternatives to employers who otherwise face tremendously expensive machine and plant renovation. Unfortunately, no effort has been made to capitalize on this opportunity. No research has been done on the types of jobs or the kinds of training that are involved in noise-related employment. This lack of research data is a gross deficiency because the employer who, by hiring deaf people, could save thousands of dollars of industrial noise-reduction costs, while simultaneously meeting affirmative action demands, would have every reason to be receptive to deaf applicants.

THE CURRENT PICTURE—PERSONAL OBSERVATIONS

Up-to-date, meaningful, specific information about what is happening in the world of work is impossible to obtain. The Bureau of Labor Statistics and other government agencies provide some broad general statements and figures. However, their projections are notoriously inaccurate (Schein & Delk, 1975, p. 98). They are also subject to considerable political manipulation, especially around election time. In view of the problem of obtaining scientifically sound data, especially on deaf workers, some personal observations are permissible. These observations are based on close contact and work over the last decade with vocational rehabilitation counselors and their deaf clients.

First of all, the repeated failure of congress and the President to appropriate funds for rehabilitation in time for the fiscal year for which they are intended has left rehabilitation agencies in the untenable position of not knowing how much money they are to have or when they are to receive it. The result is poor use of money and fragmented inadequate services. The freezing of funds that results, and the requirement that agencies run on "continuing funds" that make no adjustment for inflation, has left many rehabilitation counselors without adequate client services money. At the same time funds have been reduced, case loads have been increased by legislation transferring more clients to rehabilitation roles from other agencies such as welfare.

The result has been that for the last several years, fewer deaf clients are getting technical vocational training. Consequently, their potential for high-level employment has been reduced. Concurrent with this problem has been a sharp decrease in the number of available jobs and of some programs such as Social Security Income (SSI) and Social Security Disability Income (SSDI), which make "welfare"-type money available to deaf people. Until recently, relatively few deaf persons had turned to welfare (Schein & Delk, 1975, p. 103). Currently it is becoming a more common practice.

The psychological effects of welfare and unemployment, while not adequately understood, are generally agreed to be highly negative. In the Baltimore–Washington area alone, an increasing number of deaf individuals, especially youths, are turning to the various forms of government assistance such as SSI and welfare. This is especially significant as these two cities have been spared the high unemployment of much of the United States. In other areas, the trend must be even more pronounced. Some of this increased tendency to ask for welfare or other assistance has to be seen as a function of reductions in Division of Vocational Rehabilitation (DVR) client services funds as well as a consequence of the overall slump in the economy.

In addition to negative effects on deaf clients, the current situation with DVR is lowering rehabilitation counselors' morale. Often these individuals feel powerless to do anything for their deaf clients. More and more of their time is spent in placement, a function that most dislike and for which few are trained.

AUTOMATION

Before moving on to data from the Bureau of Labor Statistics, it is of value to relate the general concept of automation and its implications for deaf people in a specific industry, printing. Then and only then does the full impact of automation become apparent.

Formerly, some 14 percent of deaf people were printers (Lunde & Bigman, 1959). Printing was one of the highest paid of all crafts, and working conditions were among the best. There were advancement possibilities in the sense that deaf printers often owned their own businesses or were able to edit small weekly newspapers or manage printing businesses.

Residential schools for the deaf could train deaf students sufficiently for them to be employed as printers when they graduated. The cost of equiping a school shop was relatively low. It included the purchase of a few linotype machines, small presses, and some other machinery. None of it was especially costly nor did it become obsolete overnight.

By contrast, printing today offers little opportunity for deaf youth. Linotypes are becoming anachronisms. There are 20–30 applicants for every position as a linotype operator. Cold-type processes are taking over. The result is a massive reduction in the number of printers needed. In place of the highly paid and respected linotype operator, there is the new phototypesetter who can produce far greater volume than the linotyper, and who gets paid far less. New computers that can set type each take the place of 25 men. Large companies that formerly farmed out their printing to huge printing facilities that were almost all unionized now do the work themselves, usually on a nonunion basis.

Of equal importance, the machinery for cold-type printing is exorbitantly expensive and must be continually updated. Hence, few if any residential schools can afford to purchase it. This means that the schools either have given up teaching printing or else teach on antiquated obsolete machines that leave their graduates unqualified for jobs. In other words, automation has taken a highly desirable lucrative trade that once employed 14 percent of deaf people and transformed it into a vocation relatively closed to entering deaf workers.

CURRENT TRENDS IN WORK AND THEIR EFFECTS ON DEAF PEOPLE

The major source of data on occupational trends is the Bureau of Labor Statistics. It divides the national industries into major categories and projects occupational outlooks within these broad fields. What follows is a reporting of some of this information and an interpretation of its impact on deaf people (*Occupational Outlook Handbook,* 1974–1975, pp. 16–22, 25, 85, 153, 203, 218, 245, 285, 329, 403, 463, 529, 543, 575, 619, 629, 641, & 787).

The area of most rapid growth will be service-producing industries. Here the major demand will be for the technical and professional occupations. Deaf people tend to be underrepresented in these fields (Schein & Delk, 1975, p. 95). Clerical and sales work will also increase at high rates, but here again deaf people are not well represented (Schein & Delk, 1975, p. 95). Areas such as semiskilled work and trades will either decline or grow less rapidly than the general economy. It is these types of jobs in which the deaf worker is generally found (Schein & Delk, 1975, p. 95). The projected slump in farm workers does not hurt deaf people as few of them are in agriculture.

The decline in manufacturing poses a serious threat to deaf workers. About half of them are in this field, yet in the 1980s only one fourth of available jobs will exist in manufacturing. In other words, the type of work over half of the deaf working population now does is diminishing (Schein & Delk, 1975, pp. 80, 95).

The overall picture yielded by combining the Bureau of Labor Statistics economic forecasts with the knowledge we have of the kind of work deaf people do is not encouraging. It indicates that the type of jobs deaf people have typically held are either going to decrease in number or else their growth will be less than that of the general economy. Some of the occupations that will be growing the fastest, such as sales and management, are not open to most deaf people.

Occupational areas that are expected to grow and in which deaf people could do well are health and business services. For example, medical technicians are needed, and the work requires little oral communication.

A field of work of particular interest to deaf people is computer science and its related occupations. The deaf community has seen the computer field as having the promise for them that printing had had until recently. For the college or technically educated deaf person, the computer field has proven an excellent source of employment and a continued demand is projected. However, at lower levels, such as in keypunching, automation will be eliminating many jobs. Thus, the employment picture for computer-related work is optimistic only for educated deaf persons. This is still only a minority of the deaf population. It does not continue to hold the promise for deaf semiskilled clerical workers it had in the past.

Another area of work of potential importance to deaf people is government service. Projections call for continued growth in this sector, and deaf people need to be assured of their share of government jobs. The major problem posed is that many of the jobs require written civil service examinations. These tests deny deaf people jobs that they are fully capable of doing. Some progress is being made in breaking down this barrier. For example, the Post Office has given job performance trials rather than written tests as a requirement for hiring in certain positions. The Civil Service Commission is trying to use more nonverbal tests in some of their examinations. It is essential that the barrier posed by written examinations for government jobs be reduced or many deaf people will miss out on job opportunities.

POSTSECONDARY EDUCATION

The need for more and better education for deaf persons is urgent if they are to compete in today and tomorrow's job market. Fortunately, many new postsecondary programs providing supporting services for deaf students have been developed (Merrill, 1972; Vernon & Harkins, 1978). A number of these emphasize technical–vocational education.

Adult education (also called continuing education and community education) is now being made available nationally to deaf adults through efforts growing out of Gallaudet College and California State University at Northridge. With the average worker, hearing or deaf, switching careers 4–6 times during a lifetime, opportunities for re-education must remain open to deaf people of all ages if they are to compete.

The educational vacuum is in the lack of facilities to serve post-school-age deaf people whose educational achievement is below fifth grade. This constitutes one-half or more of the deaf population (Vernon, 1975). These are the people for whom current trends in occupational outlook pose the greatest threat, as they who face the greatest danger of unemployment. Yet for them there is almost no vocational training available. Unless the gap in post-school services is filled quickly, this large segment of deaf people, many of whom are already out of work, will soon face a long-term bleak employment outlook.

DISCUSSION

America has been built on a work ethic. Other societies have advocated this ethic for the masses and leisure for the elite. Our society is one in which a human being's value, income, opportunities, and life during most waking hours depends in large part on his or her job. Thus, mental health is in many respects determined by (and determines) employment.

Having created a work-oriented society, our country now faces the reality of up to 10 percent of its work force being without jobs. These unemployed individuals are often seen by the majority as parasites and are devalued as human beings.

Alcoholism, drug addiction, and crime are among the psychological and sociologic problems associated with unemployment in a culture that holds a deep respect and reward for work but is unable to provide a sufficient number of jobs.

As is so often the case, the deaf population represents a microcosm of the problems and reactions of the total society. Thus, without reasonably rewarding work, deaf people will increasingly have the aforementioned psychological illnesses that characterize the unemployed and the devalued members of a work-oriented society. Given the present and projected state of the economy, there is a high probability of at least a 20-percent unemployment rate among deaf people and along with it inevitable mental health problems. Only through the support of job training programs, vocational rehabilitation, affirmative action, continuing postsecondary education, and career guidance geared to the needs of deaf people can the deaf population hope to hold its own in the world of work.

REFERENCES

Fankhauser, C., & Katsarkas, A. Industrial hearing conservation. *Hearing and Speech Action,* 1975, *43,* 20–22.
Krents, H.E. Section 503 of the Rehabilitation Act of 1973. *Hearing and Speech Action,* 1975, *43,* 12.
Levine, R.J. Tighter reins? *Wall Street Journal,* 1978, *188,* 1.
Lunde, A.S., & Bigman, S.G. *Occupational conditions among the deaf.* Washington, D.C.: Gallaudet Press, 1959.
Merrill, E.C. A perspective on higher education for the deaf. *American Annals of the Deaf,* 1972, *117,* 597–605.
Mossberg, W.S. Jobless tech: Skill training centers say recession causes cutbacks in programs. *Wall Street Journal,* 1975, *185,* 1, 23.
Occupational Outlook Handbook. Washington, D.C.: U.S. Department of Labor, 1974–1975.
Ross, N.R. Cost to cut job noise drops. *Washington Post,* 1975, *98,* F-1, F-10.
Schein, J.D., & Delk, M.T., Jr. *The deaf population of the United States.* Silver Spring, MD.: National Association of the Deaf, 1975.
Terkel, S. *Working: People talk about what they do all day and how they feel about what they do.* New York: Pantheon Books, a Division of Random House, Inc., 1974.
Tringo, J.L. The hierarchy of preference toward disability groups. *Journal of Special Education,* 1971, *4,* 295–306.
Vernon, M. Major current trends in the rehabilitation and education of the deaf and hard of hearing. *Rehabilitation Literature,* 1975, *36,* 102–107.

Robert I. Harris, Ph.D.

15

Mental Health Needs and Priorities in Deaf Children and Adults: A Deaf Professional's Perspective for the 1980s

This chapter reflects my conviction that traditional mental health services are not capable of sufficiently reducing emotional/behavioral disorders in deaf children and adults. Innovative planning at the community level is needed. We must create long-term strategies designed to reduce or prevent these disorders in this special population by fostering healthy family and school atmospheres and enhancing the visibility of deaf adults as healthy and proud citizens. Achieving these goals will require the talents of many creative people—people with both intelligence and lively imaginations.

In my clinical work, I have been frustrated by limited ability to stretch my schedule sufficiently to help the many deaf people who have emotional and/or behavioral problems. I have become increasingly aware that I can make a greater contribution by sharing with others what I see to be the mental health needs and priorities of deaf individuals and their significant others. Four major issues will be covered in this chapter: (1) overview of mental health problems in deaf children and adults, (2) preventive mental health school programs as one among several approaches in minimizing these mental health problems, (3) innovative uses of paraprofessionals in expanding mental health services to this special population, and (4) the need for political action from deaf leaders to enhance quality of life for deaf individuals of all ages.

Supported in part by St. Paul-Ramsey Medical Education and Research Foundation (Grant No. 801D147), the Bush Leadership Fellows Program, and the Phillips Foundation.

219

MENTAL HEALTH PROBLEMS IN DEAF CHILDREN
AND ADULTS

Articles and books on the mental health problems of the deaf abound (e.g., Altshuler, 1964, 1971, 1974; Grinker, 1969; Mindel & Vernon, 1971; Rainer et al., 1963; Rainer & Altshuler, 1966; Robinson, 1978; Schlesinger & Meadow, 1972; Shapiro & Harris, 1976). The pertinent literature indicates that the developmental handicaps and personality characteristics accompanying deafness reduce the effectiveness of traditional modes of psychotherapy for many deaf people. These deaf people are often educationally deprived; they have frequently experienced a prolonged period of dependence on family, educators, and rehabilitation specialists. As a result of these and other factors, they often appear emotionally immature, insensitive to others, and highly rigid and demanding. These problems compound the difficulties of the psychotherapist.

Overview of Mental Health Problems—
A Family Perspective

The emotional problems of many deaf adults are rooted in the responses of their families to them as children. Families of deaf children are frequently unable to come to terms with the guilt, sorrow, hostility, and resentment they feel as a result of having a child with a disability. Compounding the situation is the breakdown in communication that often develops between the deaf child and his or her family. For this reason, a preventive mental health model should include parent counseling as the first step in helping the parents accept their child's deafness. Parent education should follow as soon as the parents' acute feelings are resolved. An example of parents' limited capacity in coping with the child's deafness is presented below to illustrate some of the typical problems that develop in families of deaf children.

Unless a relative insists that the deaf child is not responding to verbal communication, the immediate family will often deny the child's deafness until the child is 2- or more years-old. This recourse to denial and the accompanying rationalization have been described by other authors (Harris, in preparation; Mindel & Vernon, 1971; Schlesinger & Meadow, 1972; Shapiro & Harris, 1976). When the child's deafness can no longer be denied, the parents' initial feelings of sorrow for their deaf child are followed by anger. The anger generates guilt. From this point on, as Vernon (1969) noted, rage and depression pervade the relationships within the family.

The presence of a deaf child can also indirectly precipitate family problems or even crises. For example, because deaf children rely much more on nonverbal communication than do their siblings, they develop extreme dependence on a parent, usually the mother. Even as children grow older, there are very few people with whom they can communicate effectively; this leads to more than a normal dependence on the mother. The dependent dyad of deaf child and mother has adverse effects on the mother's relationships with other members of the family.

Conflicts, often between the parents, result. It is not surprising, therefore, that a high divorce rate occurs among parents of deaf children (Hoffmeyer, 1976; Mindel & Vernon, 1971).

My own background is typical. My parents were divorced when I was 18-years-old. Later, while a graduate student in clinical psychology, I told my mother about my training in family therapy. She then read *They Grow in Silence* by Mindel & Vernon (1971). Later, when my mother and I talked about our past family problems she said that she thought that if she and my father had gotten family counseling or psychotherapy immediately after they knew I was deaf, they might have had a better chance of working out their problems and saving their marriage. Her remarks further brought home to me the importance of family therapy or counseling for the parents of deaf children.

Communication problems impede the development of healthy relationships between the deaf child and other family members. Very few hearing parents learn sign language or finger spelling to facilitate communication with their deaf child (Harris, 1978). This may be due to the belief that oral speech and lip reading should be forced on the deaf child (Mindel & Vernon, 1971), but it may also reflect the unwillingness of parents to come to terms with their child's deafness. The communication barriers between other family members and the deaf child create further complications that negatively affect family relationships. For example, parents typically have unrealistic expectations of their deaf child's potential to learn (Vernon, 1969) because impoverished communications never lead to an adequate understanding of the child's abilities to assume a more responsible role in the family. When parents have a mistaken sense of their deaf child's potential for leading an independent life, friction between the deaf child and the family results.

A discussion of one of my patients will illustrate how parents' misjudgments of their deaf child's potential can lead to behavioral problems.

Susan, a profoundly deaf 18-year-old, was referred to me because she screamed at her parents, threw objects in the house, and refused to attend school. Susan had not been encouraged to learn manual communication because her parents believed that reliance upon manual communication would inhibit her learning to speak and lip-read. Unable to communicate with her manually, they had no accurate sense of her present capacity or future potential. They became overprotective; they refused to allow her to take driver's education although a younger hearing cousin had a driver's license; they refused Susan's request to stay overnight with girlfriends at a nearby college for the deaf because they were afraid Susan, out of ignorance, would allow herself to become pregnant. Susan's resentment and violent behavior followed.

A second aspect of Susan's problems provides an illustration of the way in which the deaf child can become the focus of a family conflict (Mindel, 1969). In the language of family theory, the deaf child becomes a *scapegoat,* a displacement target for frustrations not the direct result of the presence of the deaf child in the family. The scapegoat role may be attractive to the deaf child because it satisfies needs for attention. Susan, for example, was frequently the target of the frustration her parents felt toward each other. Susan's father was an alcoholic who took out his anger at his wife's criticism of him on Susan. When, in response to her father's unjustified impatience with her, Susan screamed, her mother scolded her. Susan also became a scapegoat for frustrations that other members of the family experienced. Susan's younger sister expressed her anger at her parents' refusal to let her go out at night with friends by wearing some of Susan's clothes to school the next day, an action she knew would upset Susan.

It is not surprising that the experts who have studied families that include a deaf child make a number of suggestions in common (Altshuler, 1974; Harris, in press; Mindel & Vernon, 1971; Schlesinger & Meadow, 1972). The suggestions are crisis intervention for parents following their discovery that their child is deaf, parent counseling, parent education, and intensive instruction in sign language and exposure to the deaf community for the entire family.

Prevalence of Emotional/Behavioral Problems in Deaf Children

Investigators report that deaf children have emotional or behavioral problems or both in significantly higher percentages than do their hearing peers. Schlesinger and Meadow (1972) found emotional disturbance among deaf children at one residential school to be three times more prevalent than it was among a comparable group of hearing students at a public school. Jensema and Trybus (1975) reported that nearly 10 percent of the 44,000 hearing-impaired children they studied had "educationally significant emotional behavior problems." Meadow and Trybus (1979), having reviewed a number of studies, concluded that the prevalence of emotional or behavior problems is at least three to six times as high among deaf children as among hearing children. Any handicap a child has in addition to deafness increases the likelihood of having educationally significant emotional problems (Jensema & Trybus, 1975) and, according to Gentile and McCarthy (1973), one fourth to one third of all hearing-impaired children have one or more handicaps in addition to hearing loss.

Mental Health Personnel

Despite the high percentage of emotionally disturbed deaf children, there are few professionals trained specifically to help them. Most teachers of the deaf are not adequately trained to work with emotionally disturbed deaf children. Also, few mental health personnel have the skills to communicate with deaf children (Harris, 1976; Meadow & Trybus, 1979; Rainer & Altshuler, 1973; Sachs, 1978). Furthermore, there has been a lack of research in the early detection and amelioration of emotional disturbance in deaf children.

Mental Health Service Delivery Systems

Parents, teachers, administrators, and other concerned specialists must meet and decide how to use what available resources there are. Traditionally, a deaf child with emotional and behavioral problems has received clinical attention only after problems have become so severe and overt that parents and educators can no longer ignore or wish it away. Obviously, emotional/behavioral (EB) problems that reach this stage are difficult to overcome. A revolutionary approach is necessary if one is to increase the ability of mental health services to reach deaf children before their problems seriously impede their academic progress.

The need to prevent deaf children from developing severe psychological problems and the relationship of these problems to learning difficulties have prompted many to recommend the development of preventive mental health school programs (Chough, 1976; Harris, 1976; Harris, in press; Rainer & Altshuler, 1973; Schlesinger & Meadow, 1972). This recommendation rests squarely on the assumption that an "ounce of prevention is worth a pound of cure." Once educational failure sets in, negative consequences such as shame, ridicule by others, and anxiety follow, compounding the deaf child's emotional difficulties. The harmonious development of cognitive and affective faculties is, therefore, essential to the healthy development of the deaf child during school years. Put another way, one should not debate the relative importance of learning versus psychological development in deaf children; rather one should emphasize their reciprocity. Such a school program would enable us to prevent mental health problems from developing or worsening. It should be our first priority.

A PREVENTIVE SCHOOL MENTAL HEALTH PROGRAM:
A MODEL FOR DEAF CHILDREN

School programs designed to prevent mental health problems from developing in the deaf population should be capable of early diagnosis of emotional difficulties in deaf children and should provide a therapeutic milieu for early intervention. The rationale for developing these preventive school programs is based on the following: first, early detection is essential, since the reactions of peers and teachers to a deaf child's behavior is the most consistent predictor of later psychopathology (Bower, 1960; Zax & Cowen, 1972); second, schools can offer more hours of a therapeutic environment to more deaf children than a mental health clinic can; third, separating emotionally disturbed deaf children from normally adjusted deaf children deprives them of invaluable "learning" time as well as social experiences. These points are crucial, since, according to Albee's (1967) theory, most emotional disorders are defects in social participation. Albee maintained that socially deprived children or children with deviant parental models can benefit from "enrichment environments" and more adequate models of social behavior. While it is the intention of most federally funded programs to provide such environments, most schools fall far short of the ideal, due to the inadequate funding of programs for deaf children and the many other special needs of deaf children.

The present situation is even worse for the deaf child with well-entrenched behavior disorders. Often individual needs are too great or behavior too disruptive to be tolerated by the already overworked staff. Therefore, the emotionally disturbed deaf child who could benefit most from an "enriched environment" is often expelled from existing schools.

An ideal preventive school program would have (1) the means to identify the psychological and emotional problems of individual students; (2) a staff of sufficient number, commitment, and training to provide the needed therapy; (3) the expertise provided by mental health professionals and facilities within its reach; and (4) structures that ensure the input of the deaf consumers and parents to the governing body of the school. Toward the first goal, screening instruments are needed. Toward the second, if deaf students (high school or college) and other deaf adults were trained as teachers' aides, the number of potential staff interested in the problems of deaf children would increase dramatically, while an initial training program followed by in-house seminars could assure that these highly committed people were also adequately trained. Toward the third goal, the school should collaborate with a mental health facility, hiring mental health professionals as part of its staff or as consultants. Toward the fourth goal, the advisory committee should include deaf persons and the parents of deaf children. I also recommend that the school register all deaf children as "high-risk" subjects. These topics will now be considered individually.

Screening Instruments

A battery of tests for early detection of emotional and behavioral problems would enable us to identify deaf children who have emotional or behavioral problems that are not yet fully manifest. It would also enable teachers without training in mental health disorders to determine which children are likely to have emotional or learning problems without consulting mental health personnel, who would then be more free to work with deaf children who need immediate help, to consult with teachers, administrators, counselors, and parents, and to train paraprofessionals.

Some teachers may raise the questions: "Can we really identify high-risk deaf children?" and "Does a preventive approach help?" A review of literature on preventive programs for hearing children indicates two important facts. First, hearing children with a high risk for school failure can be identified in the first 3 years of school (Bower, 1960; Cowen et al., 1975; Zax & Cowen, 1972). Moreover, if nothing is done to help these high-risk children, they are likely to follow a downward spiral. In addition to the personal tragedies, the problems of delinquency, drug addiction, etc., which result ultimately involve major expenditures of public monies. Second, there are definite positive outcomes of the preventive programs, such as better school attendance, more consistent academic performance, better school grades, less disruptive behavior in the classroom, better relations with peers, and less manifestation of EB problems (Cowen et al., 1972; Newton & Brown, 1967; Zax et al., 1968).

A few studies have already been conducted in which behavior-checking lists were used to identify EB problems in deaf children (Goulder & Trybus, 1977; Jensema & Trybus, 1975; Schlesinger & Meadow, 1972). Meadow (1980) recently completed the development of a standardized behavior rating scale for deaf children. The author currently is conducting a study to explore which school behavior ratings are found to be most reliable in identifying deaf children who have EB problems.

Training Deaf People as Paraprofessionals

Training deaf people, especially deaf high school and college students, as aides would offer a cost-effective way of expanding services to the deaf people who have emotional or behavioral problems. The idea parallels programs already in existence for the hearing people who suffer from emotional disturbance (Cowen, 1968; Cowen, Chinsky, & Rappaport, 1970; Cowen et al., 1975; Cowen, Zax, & Laird, 1966; Goodman, 1967; Mitchell, 1966b). To identify and treat potentially severe maladaption problems, Cowen and his colleagues established the Primary Mental Health Project (PMHP). To overcome the shortage of mental health personnel, the PMHP associates sought committed and enthusiastic people, especially homemakers, and trained them as paraprofessionals. Selected on this basis and working under the supervision of school mental health personnel, these people have been judged remarkably effective by the hearing children they worked with, the school personnel, mental health workers, and parents (Cowen et al., 1975).

Can the training of paraprofessionals, such as high school deaf students, college deaf students, and/or deaf adults to work with young deaf children who have emotional disorders yield results similar to those reported in Cowen's PMHP? There are persuasive reasons to think that it would. In addition to expanding the numbers of staff, having experienced the problems of deafness would make the deaf paraprofessional uniquely qualified. Furthermore, using deaf college or high school students as aides to work with deaf children would be cost-effective, since students could be rewarded with academic credit. If the need to train deaf adults who were not students arose, their modest salaries could be easily assumed in the school budget. Suggestions as to what type of paraprofessional programs to train teachers' aides (among others) should be offered will be taken up later in this paper. For now I add only that after the initial training period, teacher aides, dorm counselors, and other personnel could attend supplemental weekly seminars on mental health. Such seminars have been tried on a pilot basis in a few schools for the deaf (Naiman, 1972; Rainer & Altshuler, 1970; Schlesinger & Meadow, 1972).

The Mental Health Consultant

A utopian mental health preventive program in a school for the deaf would establish a new division of mental health services in the school. Two reasons why school administrators are unable to reach this ideal are its cost and the limited number of people trained as mental health specialists who are able and willing to work with deaf children. A viable alternative to the hiring of full-time professionals is the hiring of a consultant.

RECRUITING, HIRING, AND TRAINING

A specialist in the mental health problems of the deaf population may not, however, be available, even as a consultant. Very few mental health personnel have the knowledge and skills in working with deaf people (Sachs, 1978). If no one is available, the school might hire a mental health specialist who lacks background in working with deaf children or adults. The person sought should be interested in deaf people, warm and sincere, should have a good reputation as both an educator and a clinician, and should have a faculty appointment at a nearby university or clinic for consultative and referral purposes.

In approaching the mental health professional, the school official is forewarned that the professional inexperienced in working with deaf individuals may well be nervous at the prospect of facing a new and complex problem. The school official should make the mental health professional aware that he or she is needed and that help and training will be available.

Once the consultant is hired, an in-service training program should be set up. The components of the program should be conducted in the following order:

1. The consultant should be given an orientation on the ramifications of hearing loss, brief literature review materials on mental health problems of deaf children and adults, and utilization of interpreting services;
2. The consultant should then participate in school staffing conferences, classroom observation meetings, and informal school faculty meetings to "get his or her feet wet";
3. As soon as the consultant's anxieties are reduced, the school official should arrange for him or her to interview a number of deaf children with the assistance of an interpreter;
4. The consultant, the interpreter, and the school official should have a supervision meeting to exchange clinical impressions with each other. The consultant, for example, may need to be reminded about the limitations of traditional modes of therapy with deaf children due to language problems, developmental immaturity, and/or poor communication skills. Likewise, the consultant may advise the school official about the role as a counselor; and
5. As soon as the consultant gains confidence in his or her ability to apply knowledge on the psychopathology of deaf children and their parents, he or she should be encouraged to take sign language classes.

This model was used at the Rochester School for the Deaf in cooperation with the University of Rochester Medical Center. A child psychiatrist was hired to spend a certain number of hours weekly at the school. The experiences have been very rewarding and profitable for both the psychiatrist and the school personnel.

ROLE OF A CONSULTANT

With time and an increase in confidence, the consultant could be asked to perform some of the following functions:

- Offer a weekly seminar on parent effectiveness training (PET), child development, psychopathology, parent counseling, behavior modification, or other related courses.
- Arrange a lecture series in which a number of mental health specialists from the university or clinic are invited to present a lecture on the areas of special interest to the school faculty or parents or both.
- Direct a school preventive program.
- Consult with teachers and dorm counselors on managing behavior.
- Train and supervise paraprofessionals.
- Arrange for one or more staff persons to obtain orientation or practicum seminars on various modes of treatment at the university or clinic.
- Interview parents on a crisis intervention basis if necessary.
- Interview and/or observe deaf children.
- Help others on the staff to gain confidence and take active roles by leading groups of deaf teenagers (with the aid of an interpreter) in the presence of cotherapists from the school staff.
- Participate in staffing and case conferences.
- Refer deaf children or their parents to appropriate specialists for evaluations and/or treatment not available at the school.
- Advise the school personnel about effective ways to establish a school register of all deaf children for early detection and immediate amelioration of their school adjustment problems.

The following narrative example is an illustration of the type of contribution a consultant can and should make.

Dick, a 5-year-old, was referred to me for a psychological evaluation. Having withdrawn from his peers and entered his own world of daydreams, he was reportedly behaving like a dog—barking and crawling. There were family problems: his parents were separated, his teenage brothers were hostile and rebellious, and family income was limited. Until his parents' separation, Dick was doing well academically. When his mother was taken to the hospital for surgery, Dick began to daydream. A visit to a farm removed him from his special education classes for 4 months. When he returned, school personnel observed his daydreaming, his withdrawal, and his adopting the behavior of a dog.

Confronting Dick's insecurity, fear, and low self-esteem, I asked myself whether it would be more productive to try to help Dick directly with weekly 1-hour play therapy sessions or whether it would be more productive to counsel his teachers and his mother on how to help Dick. I chose the latter.

I asked the teacher to describe Dick's animal-like behavior. She explained that Dick told her that he is a dog. The teacher responded, "No, you are not a dog." I suggested a different response: "Oh, you mean you are a dog; what does a dog do; does a dog brush his teeth or play baseball?" Through these questions, the teacher learns the extent to which Dick can tell the difference between reality and daydreaming. Should he recognize the differences and respond with a smile, he is coping with his anxieties; the daydream is less likely to be a sign of psychosis. The daydreaming helps him to regress and to feel more comfortable and secure. As soon as he feels more comfortable, he may return to previous level of functioning.

I gave the teacher a brief introduction to the therapeutic conditions that promote a child's sense of self-actualization. Such conditions are unconditional respect, recognition, and reflection of his feelings; communication with him at his own level; warmth; and a sincere interest in his welfare and health.

RATIONALE FOR HIRING A CONSULTANT

Generally, I believe it is more effective to offer a teacher 1 hour a week of consultation than to spend 1 hour a week with the child in play therapy, as the teacher has 30 hours each week to spend with the child. Furthermore, such an approach would indirectly help teachers become more effective in working with other deaf children.

To help defray the costs of consultants, school administrators and directors of special education should be made aware that all community mental health centers originally supported by federal funds have an obligation to serve the consumers from the neighborhood (Goldston, 1968, 1977). Among several functions a community mental health center must implement to meet federal regulations, one is to offer consultation and education services. Should a school for the deaf be located near a community mental health center, school administrators should initiate negotiations with that center to request the services of a mental health consultant and/or educator for the school for the deaf. In many places, the charge for consultation is very low or even free.

Establishing a collaborative relationship with a nearby medical or mental health center has many advantages for the school and its students. First, after school officials have trained some of the medical personnel from the facility to deal with deaf children, the school could refer deaf children to the medical facility. Second, the medical center should offer a tour of the facility to the students. Third, the school could invite medical personnel to present courses for the deaf students, their parents, or teachers on various subjects, such as sex, the use and abuse of drugs and alcohol, preventive health-care, child-raising and nutrition. Moreover, the collaboration can be mutually beneficial: the school can offer an elective course, including visits to the school for case conferences, panel discussion with deaf participants and other practicum experiences for interested medical personnel.

The collaborative relationship with the medical center serves four important functions: (1) it increases the visibility of deafness; (2) it makes medical and mental health services to deaf children and parents more available; (3) it increases the number of specialists who could be called upon to consult with school teachers and officials on an emergency basis; and (4) it expands the curriculum of deaf students to include medical and mental health education.

The following vignettes demonstrate the importance of establishing a collaborative relationship with a medical center.

Sharon, a 10-year-old profoundly deaf girl, was rushed from a nearby school to the University of Rochester Medical Center for heart surgery. Thanks to the orientation programs on deafness offered by the school, the medical specialist recognized Sharon's special needs immediately. An interpreter from the school was assigned to her at nearly all times, providing a way to comfort Sharon and a way to consult with her parents. Sharon was able to know what was going on around her prior to and following surgery. The surgery was successful, and Sharon had an easier time adjusting to the hospital environment. The hospital staff were very pleased with their ability to accommodate Sharon's needs prior to the surgery.

A second example involves Wendy, a deaf 19-year-old student at the National Technical Institute for the Deaf (NTID).

One day Wendy was acting suicidal. Since a collaborative relationship existed between NTID and the University of Rochester Medical Center, the counselor from NTID, without hesitation, arranged to have Wendy taken to the Medical Center. The school arranged for interpreting services and had the staff at Rochester Medical page me for consultation and evaluation. An in-patient hospitalization was recommended. The awareness of the hospital staff of Wendy's special needs facilitated her adjustment to the hospital environment. She was discharged after 3 days.

The third example illustrates how the school can benefit from collaborating with the hospital.

The Minnesota School for the Deaf in Faribault set up a collaborative relationship with the Mental Health and Hearing Impaired (MHHI) Program at St. Paul-Ramsey Medical Center. We were able to enroll two emotionally disturbed deaf boys who were being treated at Ramsey in their school program. Furthermore, the hospital staff developed a program that included instruction in behavior management in the classroom through discussion with dorm counselors, teachers, and parents; collaboration with medical specialists for neurologic and pediatric evaluations; setting up a behavior-modification program; and several staffing conferences. Lastly, the MHHI staff assisted the school in requesting with success (3) new civil service positions from the Minnesota Department of Education for a psychologist, a social worker, and a counselor.

Consumer and Parent Involvement in Governing the School

PARENT ADVISORY COMMITTEE

The school preventive mental health model should establish a parent advisory committee. Since many deaf children are sent away to residential schools for the deaf, there has been little parent involvement in the deaf child's educational program. This is detrimental to the child's education and adjustment, since many mental health problems in the deaf population are related to family problems and family communication breakdowns. The parent advisory committee would include hearing and deaf parents of deaf children, medical and mental health advocates from nearby medical centers, and school personnel. The goal of the committee should be to develop guidelines for parental counseling and parental education programs, establish ways to notify parents in emergencies, secure cooperation from parents and inform parents of different services and organizations that may offer assistance to deaf children and adults or their parents.

DEAF PERSONS AND THE SCHOOL ADVISORY BOARD

Appointment of deaf persons to the school advisory board is an indispensable part of the school preventive mental health model. It will help assure that the interests of deaf children and their parents are protected. Vernon and colleagues reported that children of minorities perform well academically, and socially, when their parents are involved in making decisions on guidelines for developing and implementing educational and social programs for their own children (Vernon & Estes, 1975; Vernon & Makowsky, 1969).

It is important to note that the advisory boards at National Technical Institute for the Deaf (NTID) and Gallaudet College include deaf people. Their participation has had a major impact on the college administrators' decisions, which greatly facilitates deaf college students' personal and academic success. NTID and Gallaudet College and their alumni should pressure school superintendents and directors of special education to appoint deaf persons to school boards. Such political pressure could be manifest by requesting public hearings by the state legislative bodies so that deaf citizens and their friends have an opportunity to testify that decision-making involvement of deaf individuals is essential in maintaining the best interests of deaf children.

It is important to keep in mind that deaf children of deaf parents generally do better in school work than deaf children of hearing parents. Deaf parents, however, are rarely consulted for their opinions on effective approaches in raising deaf children. Elsewhere, I have urged professionals working with deaf children and adults to use the findings in the studies showing the greater educational achievement of the deaf children of deaf parents to call for more participation of the deaf people in programs affecting them:

Educators, mental health specialists, and research investigators should be aware that studies of deaf children and their deaf parents would indicate better ways to educate a deaf child who has hearing parents.

Past, present and future findings on the relationship of parent hearing status to impulse control and language development in deaf children should be given serious consideration when drawing up guidelines for parent education and preschool programs for deaf children. For example, the findings in this study suggest that more deaf persons should be hired as teachers for pre-school deaf children, instructors of sign language for hearing parents and teachers, professors at teacher-training programs, and for positions that involve policy-making decisions that affect deaf children (Harris, 1977, p. 97).*

Appointment of deaf persons to the school boards would result in decisions that would better meet the needs of deaf children, foster a more healthy school atmosphere for deaf children, and maintain a two-way communication between deaf children and school teachers and/or school personnel. Some progress has

---

*Reprinted with permission from Harris, R.I. The relation of impulse control to parent hearing status, manual communication, and academic achievement in deaf children. In *Dissertation Abstracts International,* 1977, *37*, 4682B.

already been made in Minnesota. First, two deaf representatives from Minnesota Association of Deaf Citizens* recently were appointed by Assistant Commissioner, Department of Education to serve on the Advisory Council for the Minnesota School for the Deaf. Second, one deaf citizen was appointed by the Governor to serve on the Minnesota State Council for the Handicapped. Third, a number of deaf parents of deaf children participated as decision-makers in a two-week sign language workshop in a day program for hearing-impaired children. The workshop objective was to write a position paper regarding the philosophy of total communication and to standardize signs for instructional purposes. Fourth, a deaf consumer was elected as a chairperson of the Legislative Committee on the Hearing-Impaired. Through his leadership role in mobilizing lobbying efforts among deaf fellows, parents of deaf children, and professionals working with deaf people, a new state legislation bill—the Hearing-Impaired Service Act—was passed in 1980. Among several objectives of this act, one is to improve the coordination of services between home and school/community settings.

"HIGH-RISK" CHILDREN AND ESTABLISHMENT OF A SCHOOL REGISTER

Another equally important part of the preventive school program is its acknowledgement that all deaf children are "high-risk" and that the preventive model should include the establishment of a school register. The term high-risk reflects our concern that deafness has a profound impact upon a child's language, emotional, and communicative development—so profound that special therapeutic and educational correctives must be offered to parents of deaf children on a consistent ongoing basis from the time their child's hearing loss is detected. In order to deliver effective preventive services to deaf children and their parents, it is necessary for all medical, neurologic, pediatric, audiologic, psychological, and psychiatric impressions to be recorded as part of the school register. Such a record-keeping system is an invaluable resource in researching the incidence of emotional disturbance in deaf children, in delineating specific factors that account for emotional disturbance, comparing deaf children's behavior in later school years with that of earlier years, and making the prognosis of deaf children for treatment purposes. To illustrate the importance of a high-risk register, 45 percent of deaf mental inpatients at St. Paul–Ramsey Medical Center were found to have outstanding long-term medical complications that were not previously diagnosed by other physicians (Reisman, Scanlan, & Kemp, 1977). Such a register has been successfully implemented for hearing children with schizophrenic parents, antisocial parents, birth defects from prematurity, or impoverished social and economic backgrounds (Garmezy, 1971, 1975; Rolf & Harig, 1974; Sameroff & Chandler, 1974).

---

*At the state convention in Pengilly, Minnesota, July 16, 1977, the deaf members voted to change the old name from Minnesota Association of the Deaf to Minnesota Association of Deaf Citizens.

Summary: A Preventive School Program

A preventive school program should be implemented on a pilot basis. Evaluation of the pilot study would help us determine the degree to which we should direct our mental health effort to the young deaf children and to the schools that shape their development. It is suggested that we shift our emphasis to school mental health programs that help the many to adapt effectively rather than on programs that react to marked adaptive failure in the few. Also, it is suggested that we focus our efforts on detecting and preventing dysfunctions in deaf children rather than treating only a few deaf children whose problems are severe and difficult to reverse. The older, more entrenched the maladaptation, the more difficult and costly it is to treat and the greater the danger of irreparable personal consequences.

The pilot program would also shed light on which types of treatment modalities are most effective for the amelioration of emotional/behavior problems in deaf children. It would help determine the relative role of the following as a part of the preventive mental health model for deaf children: (1) early screening techniques for detection of emotional/behavior problems; (2) deaf paraprofessionals selected for their warmth, facility in interpersonal relations, and interest in children, to bring immediate assistance to children identified as functioning ineffectively; (3) mental health specialists used as consultants, training others but treating only the severely malfunctioning few; and (4) consumer and parent involvement in governing the school.

An additional potential of the proposed preventive model is that if it should prove to be successful in training deaf paraprofessionals to be capable of offering assistance to maladjusated deaf children, it would have far-reaching implications for parent education; that is, guidelines from the proposed model could be used to train deaf paraprofessionals to work with hearing parents of young deaf children. The benefits would be multiplied since deaf children would then receive helping services both from the deaf professionals at the school settings and from the ''trained'' hearing parents at home.

MENTAL HEALTH WORKERS WITH DEAF CHILDREN AND ADULTS

Increasing the reach of mental health services for deaf people will require finding and utilizing new manpower resources. We will need to develop innovative programs designed to train both professionals and nonprofessionals to deliver mental health care to deaf people. We will need to recruit and train deaf people as well as hearing people to serve in a variety of roles.

Deaf Paraprofessionals

One among several ways to increase the mental health manpower for deaf children and adults is to recruit and train deaf persons as paraprofessionals. Deaf paraprofessionals could help other deaf people who, while not in need of hospitalization, nevertheless have problems requiring attention. I am thinking, for example, of the deaf child painfully struggling in the attempt to communicate needs to hearing parents and siblings; a deaf adolescent who feels unbearably embarrassed about his or her ignorance of the moral and social aspects of sexuality; of a young deaf college student experiencing an acute developmental crisis; of a deaf young couple undergoing a marital crisis due to unrealistic expectations about each other's roles as spouses; of a deaf adult feeling uneasy in communicating unsatisfactory sexual experiences to his or her partner for fear of hurting feelings; of deaf parents feeling inadequate to raise their child.

When I refer to deaf people serving as mental health aides, I have especially in mind deaf college and high school students who are motivated, curious, and have other ego assets that would make them effective in helping deaf children and adults who have adjustment problems. I am also thinking about well-adjusted deaf parents who could offer young, shy, and withdrawn deaf children living in a residential facility the warmth and affection they desperately need, or who could be trained as aides to work with vocational rehabilitation clients with a long history of overly aggressive behavior, delinquency, and/or acting-out problems, to help these clients recognize the importance to their well-being of getting and maintaining a job.

Training deaf persons as paraprofessionals has many advantages for deaf persons with emotional problems. By increasing the number of trained, committed people, we would be able to increase the reach of mental health services for deaf children and adults. The deaf paraprofessionals would also provide deaf children with the models the children need to be able to accept their deafness and acquire confidence and motivation. In addition to the advantages to those served, the program would offer advantages to all deaf persons. Offering employment as paraprofessionals would introduce new job opportunities for qualified deaf persons. As a group, deaf people suffer relatively high levels of unemployment and underemployment. And the employment picture for deaf people is likely to grow worse. Automation is eliminating many of the unskilled and semiskilled jobs that deaf people have traditionally held (Tully & Vernon, 1965). The areas where new opportunities seem likely to develop (technical areas, service industries, and management) are areas in which currently, at least, deaf people are neither well-represented nor prepared to enter (Lowell, 1965). The opportunity to become mental health paraprofessionals will offer to qualified deaf people the satisfying, challenging jobs they are capable of performing. The following models are provided to help those interested in developing paraprofessional training programs for deaf people.

DEAF COLLEGE STUDENTS AS PARAPROFESSIONALS

Programs for deaf paraprofessional college students might parallel those already in existence for hearing paraprofessional college students. There are many studies describing these programs and those interested in establishing similar programs for deaf college students may want to consult them. Hearing students have, for example, been trained to work with the chronically ill (Scheibe, 1965; Umbarger et al., 1962); with children in hospitals (Kreitzer, 1969; Reinherz, 1963), in outpatient and clinical settings (Brennan, 1967; Davidson, 1965), and with children through play therapy (Linden & Stollak, 1969). Hearing students have also worked with children who were experiencing difficulty adapting to school (Cowen, 1968; Cowen, Carlisle, & Kaufman, 1969; Cowen, Zax, & Laird, 1966), sometimes in remote geographical areas beyond the reach of professional services (Mitchell, 1966a, 1966b), with emotionally-disturbed grade schoolers (Goodman, 1967, 1972a, 1972b), with institutionalized delinquents (Gorlich, 1967) and with other college students (Zunker & Brown, 1966). Deaf paraprofessionals might serve similar groups of deaf people.

Programs approximating the paraprofessional training I have in mind are in existence .at Gallaudet College, NTID, and California State University at Northridge. But the programs at these schools are not a part of the students' degree requirements. I believe that education in health and mental health care should be a part of every deaf college student's curriculum.

The education a deaf college student receives in health and mental health care should include a professional experience program, one that affords the opportunity to work in the community with deaf children or adults. These programs would extend the reach of helping services to more deaf children and adults, as well as provide invaluable experience for the students. Vocational rehabilitation agencies and other organizations should create supervised job opportunities for deaf college students to share on a rotational basis every semester. The students would discuss their experiences at their home college in subsequent semesters.

Deaf and hearing mental health personnel who work with deaf patients should be invited as guest faculty to colleges with paraprofessional programs. A short-term institute, which would include in-service training, panel discussions and seminars on helping services, and career education could be established. I can attest to how helpful and inspiring support and guidance from a professional in the field can be to a college student. While a sophomore at Lake Forest College, I met Drs. McCay Vernon and Eugene Mindel at Michael Reese Hospital in Chicago. They were working in a federally funded research program on emotionally disturbed deaf children and adults and their families (Grinker, 1969). They sensed my enthusiasm for their work. They helped me immensely—recommending books and articles on the mental health problems of deaf people, helping me clarify my career goals, and increasing my confidence in my ability to pursue an advanced degree. Furthermore, they encouraged me to meet deaf mental health professionals so that I could talk with and learn about their career experiences. Since that time, in meeting other deaf college students I have realized that my confusion and lack of confidence were typical. Many deaf college students have the ability to be helping agents. It would be a tragic loss if this resource were not tapped.

Still another way to establish opportunities for college student paraprofessionals to receive supervised training while providing needed service to the deaf community would be for the college to establish a crisis center. This center, staffed at least in part by the paraprofessional students, could set up programs and offer counseling on sex, alcohol, and drug education; dispense information on job opportunities; disseminate literature on organizations for the deaf (e.g., National Association of the Deaf, Alexander Graham Bell Association of the Deaf, etc.); and promote studies of deaf heritage.

DEAF HIGH SCHOOL STUDENTS AS PARAPROFESSIONALS

Programs using deaf high school students as paraprofessionals could be modeled on similar programs for hearing high school students. These programs have brought high school students to work with a number of groups, including preadolescent hospitalized youngsters (Walker, et al., 1967), mildly disturbed children (Perlmutter & Durham, 1965), grade schoolers experiencing adjustment problems (McWilliams & Finkel, 1973), and disadvantaged youngsters (Neale & Mussel, 1968). In addition to helping other people, these programs are beneficial to the helpers also. High school students learn best as teachers, and helping others promotes maturity as well as being rewarding in itself. Several schools currently require students to serve as teachers before they can graduate (Cowen, 1973).

DEAF HOMEMAKERS AS PARAPROFESSIONALS

To meet the severe shortage of therapists for emotionally disturbed hearing patients, Rioch and his colleagues (1963, 1967) trained hearing mothers as therapists to serve in schools, hospitals, and clinics. The women chosen were from the upper middle class, had excellent academic credentials, and were warm, empathic, and sincere. The results were encouraging, as were the results of studies that used mothers from different socioeconomic backgrounds and with less formal schooling to serve as counselors in prenatal and infant clinics (Rioch, 1967), to work with students having adjustment problems (Cowen, 1968, 1969; Zax & Cowen, 1967; Zax et al., 1966), and to work in telephone crisis and suicide prevention centers (Heiling et al., 1968). Still other studies have utilized homemakers as helping agents ministering to hospitalized mental patients (Cain & Epstein, 1967; Katkin et al., 1971).

Deaf mothers could play similar roles in working with other deaf people. They could work with hearing parents of young deaf children, with emotionally disturbed or multihandicapped deaf children in residential or day programs; with deaf clients in rehabilitation and sheltered workshops; with deaf clubs as mental health referral agents; and with the deaf community as mental health advocates or educators. Under my supervision, for example, a married deaf woman with a masters degree in preschool education is learning to do play therapy with young deaf children having school adjustment problems. Another deaf woman has learned to administer intelligence and drawing tests to deaf inpatients. Three deaf mothers were trained as research assistants in my research study on emotional disturbance in deaf children. As I write this, a screening program for selecting and training deaf mothers

as voluntary aides for a variety of roles is being explored as part of our mental
health and hearing-impaired program.

INNER-CITY DEAF PEOPLE AS PARAPROFESSIONALS

My experience indicates that deaf people from the inner city or the ghetto
rarely receive the mental health services they need. They are neglected because
they are hard to reach and because mental health personnel feel unequal to the task
of helping these people who often suffer from drug addiction, delinquency, and
the host of nutritional and medical problems that accompany poverty. To reach
these people, leaders from their community should be trained as paraprofessionals.
Here, again, the experience in the recruitment and training of hearing paraprofessionals is instructive to those interested in recruiting and training deaf paraprofessionals. Hearing native Puerto Ricans have been recruited and trained as bilingual
interpreters for patients and medical personnel. They have also worked in identifying problems in their communities and have worked with professionals to resolve
them. Indigenous paraprofessionals have also functioned successfully in areas such
as child care, housing, recreation, education, homemaking, health care, and cor-
rections (Cowen, 1973). Deaf paraprofessionals could serve their communities in
similar programs.

Associate Degree Programs

In addition to training paraprofessionals to staff special programs, another way
to increase the reach of mental health services to deaf people is by recruiting deaf
high school students and adults into associate degree programs in mental health
and human services in community colleges. From 1967 to 1973 some 7000 mental
health workers graduated from approximately 150 schools offering associate degrees in the United States, and another 10,000 were expected to graduate by 1977
(Young & True, 1973). These programs involve both specifically designed courses
and extensive field work.

There are more than 60 community or junior colleges that offer interpreting,
tutoring, counseling, and other support services for deaf students in architectural
drafting, photography, optics, and human service fields (Craig & Craig, 1980).
Mental health personnel with skills in working with deaf people should be encouraged to cooperate with administrators of community colleges and seek out
commitments from service agencies to hire deaf people with associate degrees in
mental health. As a good example, three deaf women recently completed their
associate degree studies in human services at the University of Minnesota and now
are working as human service generalists or human service technicians.

Deaf Professionals

In addition to training paraprofessionals, deaf mental health professionals
should be sought. Those professionals have a unique contribution to make to helping deaf individuals with emotional problems. Their fluency in manual communication and their deep knowledge of the deaf culture acquired through life-long

encounters with deafness make them, if trained as mental health specialists, invaluable. Sincere, well-adjusted, open, warm, and intelligent college graduates with good communication skills would make excellent mental health specialists to work with deaf people. The people sought should be willing, as I was, to undergo psychotherapy to overcome problems they have as a result of others' responses to their deafness. These people, who have knowledge of the deaf culture, would make excellent clinicians. I thus echo the call made by others to recruit deaf college graduates for advanced study in the many fields of mental health (Burke, 1969; Chough, 1973; Harris, 1976, 1980; Rainer & Altshuler, 1970, 1973). Yet despite the general recognition of the importance of recruiting deaf students for graduate study in mental health fields, little has been published on the special needs of deaf students in graduate programs in mental health (Harris, 1980).

SPECIAL CONSIDERATIONS IN RECRUITING AND
TRAINING DEAF GRADUATE STUDENTS

To begin with, deaf students are often denied admission to graduate school because of problems developing out of their deafness. For example, an adequate command of English is essential to success in graduate school. Yet deafness makes acquiring writing skills especially difficult. Directors of graduate programs should be made aware that deaf students can, with tutoring, learn to write adequately. If these directors were made aware that this problem could be overcome by determined students and if they knew also of the special potential some deaf students have as clinicians, they would, one hopes, accept deaf students into their programs and would understand that they were doing so without lowering academic standards.

Recruitment and admission of deaf students should not be an end in itself, however. Once admitted, the deaf student still requires special services if his or her full potential is to be realized. Deaf students need conscientious, professional supervision. Often, deaf graduate students are subject to inordinate pressures. Naive hearing professionals assume deaf graduate students are instant "experts" on all aspects of deafness. These professionals might assume, for example, that the deaf professional should counsel hearing parents of deaf children, ignoring the fact that the deaf student has never been a "hearing parent." Or the assumption is made, even by deaf students themselves, that they should be able to help every deaf patient, an assumption that fails to take into account those deaf patients who suffer severe, irreversible psychopathologic problems. Without adequate counseling and supervision, then, it is easy for deaf graduate students or interns to become frustrated—directing anger either at themselves, at hearing professionals, or at the parents of the deaf patients they are trying to help.

INTERPRETING SERVICES FOR DEAF
GRADUATE STUDENTS

In addition to counseling and supervision, a deaf student can gain considerable benefit from an interpreter. Thanks to the financial support of the Social and Rehabilitation Service, I was able to hire a full-time interpreter for 2 years of my doctoral internship at the University of Rochester Medical Center. As a result, I could participate in all the programs of a regular internship—including taking seminars in child therapy, psychodiagnostic testing, family therapy, group therapy, child and adolescent behavior, and behavior modification, attending grand rounds and various colloquia, and receiving supervised practice in individual and group therapy.

The interpreter also made it possible for me to benefit from the supervision of 12 mental health specialists, none of whom had experience in working with deaf students. Perhaps an example will shed light on the way a deaf graduate student aided by an interpreter and adequately supervised can perform in graduate or professional school. I began my internship by observing one of my supervisors interviewing a hearing patient through a one way mirror. The interpreter communicated to me the ongoing dialogue between my supervisor and his patient. After the interview, my supervisor explained the advantages and disadvantages of various interviewing techniques and discussed his responses to the interview. Later in my internship, I interviewed deaf students while my supervisor and the interpreter observed through the one way mirror. Still later, we again discussed the interview. Without an interpreter I would have been unable to take part in these training sessions—sessions through which I learned much about interviewing. For example, because of the presence of the interpreter, my supervisor was able to observe that I tended to ask close-ended questions. He suggested that I should ask open-ended questions so that I would obtain responses from the patient that would be more revealing and diagnostically meaningful.

Invaluable as an interpreter is, there are some limitations to what he or she can do. These limitations are especially apparent in group or family therapy sessions. For example, when a hearing therapist and I were co-leaders of a psychotherapy group for deaf teenagers, often more than one deaf student would speak at a time. The interpreter was able to read only the signs of one deaf student at a time, and as a result, much information was lost to the hearing therapist. Similarly, in a family session in which a hearing family therapist and I worked with one deaf patient and her family members, I had great difficulty trying to understand the myriad verbal and nonverbal interchanges between family members, particularly since I had to focus my attention on both the patient's sign language and the interpreter's.

Hearing Paraprofessionals

In addition to training deaf people in various ways to deliver mental health services to the deaf community, hearing people might serve in many other ways. Programs that might be undertaken include training interpreters to become acquainted with medical and mental problems in the deaf people they serve, training special education teachers to recognize and work with emotionally disturbed deaf children, enlisting hearing adults as big brothers and big sisters of hearing children of deaf parents, encouraging high school hearing students to learn sign language, and training hearing parents in both the communication modes and problems and the potential emotional problems of their deaf students.

CERTIFIED MEDICAL AND MENTAL
HEALTH INTERPRETERS

Interpreters interested in the medical and mental health of their deaf clients should be trained to increase their awareness of the health problems in deaf children and adults. It is presently possible for interpreters with comprehensive certificates to become certified legal interpreters by taking training sessions in the law (Reisman, Scanlan, & Kemp, 1977). A similar program providing training in medical and mental health might certify interpreters, who are highly skilled, interested, and sincere and respect deaf people and deaf culture, as official designated medical and mental health interpreters. Furthermore, Wolf (1976) proposed an orientation on deafness and interpreting as a model for nurses in medical and mental health settings. Through better understanding and communication between nurses and deaf clients and through the assistance of qualified medical/mental health interpreters, substantial progress could be accomplished in reducing the incidence on long-term and untreated medical complications. The value of interpreters has already been recognized. Four "counselor–interpreters" are part of the mental health program for the deaf at St. John Hospital and Health Center in Los Angeles (Kimberlin, 1977), while interpreters have been used at St. Paul–Ramsey Medical Center in programs treating drug- and alcohol-dependent patients (Reisman, Scanlan, & Kemp, 1977).

TRAINING TEACHERS IN THE MENTAL
HEALTH NEEDS OF DEAF STUDENTS

Increasing teachers' awareness of the mental health needs of deaf students would have many beneficial effects. It would, for example, enable teachers to help some deaf students who have minor adjustment problems. It would also provide teachers with the ability to assess realistically the potential for self-growth and academic learning of their deaf students and their own potential to help them. A teacher aware of the family problems and the medical, especially neurologic, dysfunctions many deaf students suffer from will be less frustrated, less disappointed with deaf students, and less impatient if deaf students fail to fulfill expectations. Studies indicating that teachers have the ability to recognize behavioral problems in hearing students (Bower, 1960; Cowen, et al., 1975) suggest that teachers of deaf students are capable of identifying students with emotional problems. Training could be a regular part of preparation programs for teachers of deaf students or it could be accomplished through a mental health consultation model, as was tried by Rothstein (1975) at the Lexington School for the Deaf.

BIG BROTHER AND BIG SISTER PROGRAMS

Hearing individuals could serve as big brothers and big sisters to the hearing children of deaf parents. These children frequently resent being cast as interpreters for deaf parents, who, often unintentionally, deprive their children from obtaining age-specific socialization experiences that are recommended for their personal growth. With this resentment often comes disobedience, passive–aggressive behavior, and a breakdown of respect and communication between child and parents.

Big brother and big sister programs might enlist hearing volunteers to help hearing children of deaf parents. In Minneapolis–St. Paul, Bunde (1976) and his assistant, a hearing woman of deaf parents, have led several groups of hearing children who have deaf parents.

HEARING HIGH SCHOOL STUDENTS AS
INTERPRETERS AND TUTORS

If sign language was taught and recognized as an alternative to the foreign language requirement in high schools, interested hearing students might become valuable helpers to deaf students, serving as interpreters, note-takers, or tutors. They could also serve as big brothers and sisters to deaf students, winning support in the hearing community for programs helping deaf children and adults. The hearing students would themselves benefit from their familiarity with a different culture, always a broadening experience.

PARENTS AS EDUCATORS–THERAPISTS
OF THEIR DEAF CHILDREN

Training hearing parents as ''home educators'' of their deaf children is another way of meeting the mental health needs of deaf children. This approach, which is called ''filial therapy'' has been successfully used for hearing parents who were trained to work as therapists with their hearing children who suffered emotional or behavioral problems (Fidler et al., 1969; Guerney, 1969; Stover & Guerney, 1967). Guerney and his colleagues trained parents by having them observe professional therapists in action. Other programs trained parents in behavior modification (Hawkins, Peterson, & Bijou, 1969; Shah, 1969). The parents of deaf children could benefit from similar programs, which would also include instruction in manual communication and an introduction to the learning problems of deaf children and the special resources—e.g., children's books written especially for deaf children—available to overcome them. Training parents has the special advantage of enabling children living far from organized programs for deaf children to receive the help they need.

A Cautionary Note

While I hope that specialists from many disciplines who are interested in the problems of deafness will find my suggestions for expanding the services to the deaf helpful and inspiring, I must add at this point that caution is called for. We should not allow our high hopes and willingness to work blind us to the real difficulties ahead. The following questions are raised to illustrate some of the potential difficulties surrounding but one of the suggested programs—the training of deaf and hearing paraprofessionals. Will these paraprofessionals be capable of overcoming personal limitations sufficiently to succeed as therapists? Such personal limitations—to name a few—include projecting their own problems on to others, panicking over their ignorance about mental health problems and/or inadequacy of skills in working with people, and dependency on other people for initiation and guidance. Will they all be able to keep clinical cases confidential? Will they be able to accept and assimilate their supervisor's suggestions? Will they be able to write adequate case reports? Will paraprofessionals be accepted and respected by professionals or will professionals view them as lesser qualified competitors who deprive them of clients? And will paraprofessional programs be funded adequately? Will career opportunities that take advantage of the paraprofessionals' training be available to the paraprofessional? One way of identifying and minimizing the effect of such difficulties is to implement each program on a pilot basis and to evaluate each program with reliable and valid instruments.

Despite the difficulties, we must move ahead with programs that will expand the helping services to deaf children and adults. The consequences of an imperfect program are not nearly so devastating as the consequences of doing less than we could because too few fully trained professionals are unavailable. The question should not be should we train paraprofessionals, but rather what roles should they play and how should they be trained. It is fitting to echo here the theme sounded by Cowen (1973) with its contrapuntal caution and hope:

A succinct, unequivocating, yet defensible summary for an area as complex and rapidly unfolding as this one is a sheer "pipe dream." It is not that such summaries haven't been ventured . . . rather they weigh much too heavily on soft data and glowing impressions from those who are actively caught up on the swirl of events. As such, the reports resemble the tidal wave of enthusiastic case testimonials in the early, golden days of psychotherapy. The fact of the matter, however, is that we are, as Sobey put it, in the middle of an nonprofessional "revolution." Events are moving with great speed, and for the moment our chips are placed on exploring an exciting, challenging, new world of usages rather than on hard-nosed evaluation. This balance will have to change before a trustworthy reckoning can be reached (Cowen, 1973).*

MENTAL HEALTH AND DEAF POLITICAL INVOLVEMENT

I believe that achieving the goal of improving mental health services for deaf children and adults—the creation of viable preventive programs and increasing quality and quantity of care—depends upon how much time and effort leaders of the deaf community are willing to devote to political action. Before effective political action can be taken, however, education must occur. The public must be made aware that the etiology of many of the mental health problems of deaf people are social. It is not only or especially hearing loss that causes emotional problems in deaf people but the reaction of others to deafness. Many of the mental health problems of deaf children and adults are the result of their alienation—in their families, in their neighborhoods, in the schools, and in society. In addition, other problems that partly contribute to the mental health problems deaf individuals suffer are as follows: the breakdown in communications between deaf children and their parents, siblings, teachers, neighbors; inadequate educational and socialization pro-

---

*Reprinted with permission from E.L. Cowen. Social and community interventions. *Annual Review of Psychology,* 1973, *24,* 448–449.

grams in schools; teachers untrained in the adjustment and emotional problems of deaf students; too few mental health personnel to work with deaf children and their parents; too little federal and state support for research into programs to help deaf citizens; too little legal help for deaf people to seek redress in the courts; too much job discrimination, especially in positions administrating programs for deaf people.

The solutions to these problems rest partly in political action. Deaf leaders and their hearing supporters must raise the political consciousness of deaf people. Workshops should be held for deaf consumers, parents of deaf children, representatives of public and private service delivery systems, government officials, and other concerned individuals or groups.

There are several political avenues that deaf leaders and those sympathetic to their cause can pursue. Pursuing them will help assure deaf people of their civil rights and increase the visibility of their cause.

Affirmative Action Policies

Two laws, recently enacted, offer opportunities for deaf adults to obtain decision-making positions or, at least, have the opportunity to contribute input to the decision-making process. These are the Rehabilitation Act Amendment of 1974 (Public Law 93–516) and the Education for the Handicapped Act (Public Law 94–142). Both laws require state and federal agencies to submit documents showing they have initiated affirmative action programs—that they are seriously committed to employing qualified handicapped people and that they have mechanisms that insure that handicapped people will be involved in the processes that shape decisions and policies affecting them.

Assuring that these laws are enforced takes time and effort. But if these laws can assure that qualified deaf people are placed in responsible, administrative positions, the time and effort are well-spent. Few deaf people are being placed in positions that give them authority over programs and policies that affect other deaf people. It is encouraging to note that lately a growing number of deaf persons have been hired as administrators in the field of education in deafness at Gallaudet College and a few other schools for the deaf. Unfortunately, it is only at a few schools, and few deaf persons with equal level of training are able to secure administrative positions in settings other than such schools. The effect of denying deaf people responsible, administrative positions is detrimental to all deaf people. Deaf persons in responsible positions make visible positive models to deaf children. Such models help deaf children accept their disability, increase their pride, and create the self-confidence that will make them aspire to become productive, successful citizens. When deaf applicants are denied positions as teachers because deaf children will not learn speech and lip reading from them, the deaf students are deprived of the models they need to become able to affirm their deafness. When no models are provided, self-denigration results. It is no wonder that many deaf people have low self-esteem and doubt their ability to pursue goals commensurate with those of their hearing counterparts.

National Center for Law and the Deaf

Established in 1975 through a federal grant from the Office of Education of the United State Department of Health, Education and Welfare, the National Center for Law and the Deaf is committed to assuring that deaf people's civil rights are protected. This organization can help deaf people seeking redress against discrimination in many ways. It can insure that local and state agencies adhere to affirmative action guidelines; assist deaf citizens in discrimination suits; set up workshops to educate deaf people on their rights under the law; pressure local and state advisory committees to appoint deaf people; and educate and encourage deaf students on the prospects of pursuing careers in law.

State Associations of the Deaf

The National Association of the Deaf could play a crucial role in helping the state associations of the deaf become effective political tools promoting a positive mental health climate for deaf children and adults. It is important to note that at the 1976 NAD convention in Houston a resolution that the NAD establish a Committee on Mental Health and Deafness was approved (Proceedings of the 33rd Biennial Convention of the NAD, 1976). The state associations can pressure state governments to be more responsive to the needs of deaf citizens. The following are the types of political goals they can pursue. For one, state associations can encourage state governments to create state commissions on deafness. Because of the low visibility of the problems of deafness, a commission coordinating the work of all programs, services, and agencies in a state is needed. The commission can also act as a safeguard to assure that there is deaf people's input in programs affecting deaf people. There is particular need for such coordination and safeguards in the area of education. The commission can demand specific assurance that the deaf community have input into decisions affecting the education of deaf children and that qualified deaf teachers and aides are hired whenever possible.

A second goal state associations can pursue is the creation by the state government of an agency for interpreting services. Such an agency will guarantee that no deaf person is deprived of services available to the hearing people because of the lack of an interpreter or the funds to hire one. This will insure that the state fulfills its responsibilities to all its citizens and will enable deaf people to avail themselves of services they have a right to obtain. If these services are more accessible, the medical and social problems that plague deaf people can be reduced. Mechanisms should insure that deaf people have the right to choose their own interpreters—perhaps by allowing the state to reimburse any qualified interpreter who works for a deaf person seeking use of local and/or state services. Instruction in the ways of selecting a good interpreter—what the requirements for certification are, what the interpreter's code of ethics is, etc.—should also be available.

Finally, in addition to pressuring state governments to be responsive to the needs of deaf citizens, state associations should develop their own plans and programs to actively meet personal, social, educational, vocational, and cultural needs of the deaf community.

Education

It is time that deaf people demand that the education of a deaf child be directed toward acquiring an *overall* sense of competence. We need to get away from the notion, perpetuated by well-intentioned teachers, audiologists, and administrators of special education, that intensive speech/speech-reading training is the primary goal of special education of a deaf child's needs. The exclusive emphasis on speech/ speech-reading training is a major cause of the failure of deaf people to realize their educational potential. We must look beyond a child's ability to acquire speech and speech-reading skills in deciding how a deaf child should be educated. We need to know how parents respond to their child's deafness—if they are willing to seek counseling, to learn sign language, to participate in the deaf community, and to change their life style and child-rearing practices to meet their deaf child's needs. We need to know whether and/or what community resources are available for the parents to obtain counseling and education regarding deafness. Are there sign-language classes, parent associations on deafness, opportunities to meet deaf adults at churches, clubs, organizations, and/or special events for the deaf community? This type of information is most relevant in assessing a deaf child's potential to develop into a confident, productive member of the community.

If speech/speech-reading training has been overemphasized, the acquisition of total communication skills cannot be. Although we do have excellent available measures to assess a deaf child's speech/speech-reading skills, we do need to be better able to measure progress in acquiring manual skills. I advocate the establishment of communication guidelines for deaf children's acquisition of sign language that parallel our measurement of hearing children's progress in acquiring speech. Just as we expect hearing infants to say a word by 1 year, to say "no" at about 18 months, and to be capable of 2-word sentences by 2 years, so also we should know what to expect of deaf babies—what gestures and signs they might be capable of at what age.

The goal of total competence that I propose as a model for the education of deaf students holds as the right of every deaf child the competence and confidence to communicate needs and aspirations to family, teachers, and to society. Deaf children should have the right to realize education goals and the right to a healthy social and emotional life.

CONCLUSION

In this paper, I have argued that new approaches are needed. The mental health problems deaf people suffer are the result of the isolation and alienation that results from the responses of others and of the deaf person to deafness. Remarkably few mental health personnel to work with deaf individuals, few decision-making opportunities for deaf consumers and professionals, and inadequate research and training funds in the area of mental health in deafness also contribute to the mental health problems in deaf children and adults. Thus we need not only to treat deaf people with mental health problems but also and especially to create positive mental health conditions for all deaf children and adults. Efforts should be directed toward modifying the educational environment and health services that reach the whole deaf community and toward strengthening the confidence and capabilities of every deaf individual.

To reach these ends, I propose a preventive mental health school program. This program includes a screening program for early detection and immediate amelioration of adjustment problems in deaf school children; the use of deaf mental health paraprofessionals to assure that sufficient, competent help is available to help all children who need it; deaf consumers' and parents' input into the governance of the programs; and the collaboration with a nearby mental health center to assure that the needed health expertise is available. In addition to the proposed preventive program, innovative methods are needed to create and tap new mental health manpower resources. These programs call for the training of deaf people as mental health paraprofessionals and specialists, programs that will not only expand mental health services to deaf children and adults but also increase new job opportunities. These programs also call for the use of hearing people in new ways—as certified medical and mental health interpreters, as big brothers and big sisters, and as home educators. Finally, it is time for deaf leaders and others to take political action. Affirmative action must be enforced. State associations, with the assistance from the National Association of the Deaf, must pressure the states to assure that deaf citizens' civil rights are protected, that they have access to all local and state services, and that their input is sought in creating and implementing programs that affect them.

But perhaps what the deaf community needs most is innovative, imaginative deaf people whom we might call futurists. A deaf futurist combines knowledge of what has worked in the past with an ability to anticipate the new and changing needs of the future and the courage to depart from traditional ways to meet those needs. The deaf futurist understands the importance of primary prevention to reduce the incidence of new cases of mental disorders in the deaf population. He or she realizes that to find the best solution to the mental health problems of deaf people one should focus on social trends, not create last-minute solutions to crisis situations.

Finally, while the deaf community must continue to welcome the cooperation and support of the hearing people, it must look to itself for leaders. The best response we can make to the patronizing and parental attitude many hearing people often take toward us is to point to our own leaders. And only by seeking out deaf leaders will we overcome the lack of confidence and lack of self-esteem that has so much impeded our progress. We must direct our own destiny if our success is to be real.

REFERENCES

Albee, G. The relation of conceptual models to manpower needs. In E. Cowen, E. Gardner, & M. Zax (Eds.), *Emergent approaches to mental health problems*, New York: Appleton-Century-Crofts, 1967.

Altshuler, K. Z. Personality traits and depressive symptoms in the deaf. In J. Wortis, (Ed.), *Recent advances in biological psychiatry,* (Vol. 6). New York: Plenum Press, 1964.

Altshuler, K. Z. Studies of the deaf: Relevance to Psychiatric theory. *American Journal of Psychiatry,* 1971, *127,* 1521–1526.

Altshuler, K. Z. The social and psychological development of the deaf child: Problems and treatment. In P. J. Fine, (Ed.), *Deafness in infancy and early childhood.* New York: Medcom Press, 1974.

Bower, E. *Early identification of emotionally handicapped children in school.* Springfield, Ill.: Charles C Thomas, 1960.

Brennan, E. C. College students and mental health programs for children. *American Journal of Public Health,* 1967, *57,* 1767–1771.

Bunde, L. T. *Deaf parents—hearing children: Toward a greater understanding of the unique aspects, needs, and problems relative to the communication factors caused by deafness.* Unpublished doctoral dissertation, Luther Theological Seminary, 1976.

Burke, D. Vocational rehabilitation and emerging mental health service needs of the deaf. In K. Z. Altshuler & J. D. Rainer (Eds.), *Mental health and the deaf: Approaches and prospects.* Washington, D.C.: U.S. Department of Health, Education and Welfare, 1969.

Cain, L. P., & Epstein, D. W. The utilization of housewives as volunteer case aides. *Social Casework,* 1967, *48,* 282–286.

Chough, S. K. Social services for deaf citizens: Some proposals for effectiveness. In A. G. Norris, (Ed.), *Deafness annual,* (Vol. 3). Silver Spring, Md.: Professional Rehabilitation Workers with the Adult Deaf, 1973.

Chough, S. K. The mental health needs of the deaf community: Implications for advocacy. *Mental Health in Deafness* 1977, *1:* 75–78. (DHEW Publication No. (ADM) 77-524).

Cowen, E. L. The effectiveness of secondary prevention programs using nonprofessionals in the school setting. *Proceedings of the 76th Annual Convention of American Psychological Association,* 1968, *2,* 705–706.

Cowen, E. L. Mothers in the classroom. *Psychology Today,* 1969, *2,* 36–39.

Cowen, E. L. Social and community interventions. *Annual Review of Psychology,* 1973, *24,* 423–472.

Cowen, E. L., Carlisle, R. L., & Kaufman, G. Evaluation of a college student volunteer program with primary graders experiencing school adjustment problems. *Psychology in the Schools,* 1969, *6,* 371–375.

Cowen, E. L., Chinsky, J. M., & Rappaport, J. An undergraduate practicum in community mental health. *Community Mental Health Journal,* 1970, *6,* 371–375.

Cowen, E. L., Dorr, D., Trost, M. A., et al. A follow-up study of maladapting school children seen by nonprofessionals. *Journal of Consulting and Clinical Psychology,* 1972, *36,* 235–238.

Cowen, E. L., Trost, M. A., Izzo, L. D., et al. *New ways in school mental health: Early detection and prevention of school maladaptation.* New York: Human Sciences Press, 1975.

Cowen, E. L., Zax, M., & Laird, J. D. A college student volunteer program in the elementary school setting. *Community Mental Health Journal,* 1966, *2,* 319–328.

Craig, W. N., & Craig, H. B. (Eds.). Programs and services for the deaf in the United States. *American Annals of the Deaf,* 1980, *125* (2): 200–204.

Davidson, G. C. The training of undergraduates as social reinforcers for autistic children. In L. P. Ullman & L. Krasner (Eds.), *Case studies in behavior modification*. New York: Holt, Rinehart & Winston, 1965.

Fidler, J. W., Guerney, B. G. Jr., Andronico, M. P., et al. Filial therapy as a logical extension of current trends in psychotherapy. In B. G. Guerney, Jr. (Ed.), *Psychotherapeutic agents: New roles for nonprofessionals, parents, and teachers*. New York: Holt, Rinehart & Winston, 1969.

Garmezy, N. Vulnerability research and the issue of primary prevention. *American Journal of Orthopsychiatry*, 1971, *41*, 101–116.

Garmezy, N. The experimental study of children vulnerable to psychopathology. In A. Davids, (Ed.), *Child personality and psychopathology, current topics*, (Vol. 2). New York: John Wiley & Sons, 1975.

Gentile, A., & McCarthy, B. *Additional handicapping conditions among hearing impaired students, United States: 1971–1972*. (Data from the annual survey of hearing impaired children and youth). Series D, No. 14. Washington, D. C.: Office of Demographic Studies, Gallaudet College, 1973.

Goldston, S. E. Mental health education in a community mental health center. *American Journal of Public Health*, 1968, *58*, 693–699.

Goldston, S. E. Primary prevention: A view from the federal view. In G. W. Albee & J. M. Joffe (eds.), *Primary prevention of psychopathology—Volume I: The Issues*. Hanover, N. H.: University Press of New England, 1977.

Goodman, G. An experiment with companionship therapy: College students and troubled boys—assumptions, selection, and design. *American Journal of Public Health*, 1967, *57*, 1772–1777.

Goodman, G. Systematic selection of therapeutic talent: The group assessment of interpersonal traits. In S. E. Golann & C. Eisdorfer (Eds.), *Handbook of community mental health*. New York: Appleton-Century-Crofts, 1972a.

Goodman, G. *Companionship therapy: Studies of structured intimacy*. San Francisco: Jossey-Bass, 1972b.

Gorlich, E. H. Volunteers in institutions for delinquents. *Children*, 1967, *14:* 147–150.

Goulder, T. J. & Trybus, R. J. *The classroom behavior of emotionally disturbed hearing-impaired children*. Series R, No. 3. Washington, D.C.: Office of Demographic Studies, Gallaudet College, 1977.

Grinker, R. R. (ed.). *Psychiatric diagnosis, therapy, and research on the psychotic deaf*. Washington, D. C.: Social Rehabilitation Service, Department of Health, Education and Welfare, 1969.

Guerney, B. G., Jr. (Ed.). *Psychotherapeutic agents—New roles for nonprofessionals, parents, and teachers*. New York: Holt, Rinehart & Winston, 1969.

Harris, R. I. Commentary: Dr. Denmark's paper: Deafness and mental illness: The rights of deaf mental patients. *Proceedings of the VIIth World Congress of the World Federation of the Deaf*. Silver Spring, Md.: National Association of the Deaf, 1976.

Harris, R. I. The relation of impulse control to parent hearing status, manual communication, and academic achievement in deaf children (Doctoral dissertation, New York University, 1976). *Dissertation Abstracts International*, 1977, *37*, 4682B. (University Microfilms No. 77-5410).

Harris, R. I. The relation of impulse control to parent hearing status, manual communication, and academic achievement in deaf children. *American Annals of the Deaf*, 1978, *123:* 52–67.

Harris, R. I. Education and training implications for professional psychologists who are deaf. *The Clinical Psychologist,* 1980, *33:* 7, 8, 10.

Harris, R. I. Primary and secondary prevention: A community-based mental health model for deaf children and adults. *Mental Health in Deafness* (an experimental publication of Saint Elizabeths Hospital, National Institute of Mental Health), in press.

Harris, R. I. Life events related to early childhood deafness as family stressors. In D. W. Holmes & E. H. Shroeyer (eds.), *Mental Health and Deafness.* Baltimore: University Park Press, in preparation.

Hawkins, R. P., Peterson, E. S., & Bijou, S. W. Behavior therapy in the home: Amelioration of problem parent-child relations with the parent in a therapeutic role. In B. G. Guerney (ed.), *Psychotherapeutic agents: New roles for nonprofessionals, parents and teachers.* New York: Holt, Rinehart & Winston, 1969.

Heilig, S. M., Farberow, N. L., Litman, R. E. et al. The role of nonprofessional volunteers in a suicide prevention center. *Community Mental Health Journal,* 1968, *4,* 287–295.

Hoffmeyer, B. E. In M. A. Locke (Ed.), *The Endeavor.* Silver Spring, Md.: International Association of Parents of the Deaf, 1976.

Jensema, C., & Trybus, R. J. *Reported emotional behavioral problems among hearing impaired children in special educational programs: United States, 1972–1973,* (Series R, No. 1). Washington, D.C.: Office of Demographic Studies, Gallaudet College, 1975.

Katkin, S., Ginsburg, M., Rifkin, M. J., et al. Effectiveness of female volunteers in the treatment of outpatients. *Journal of Consulting and Clinical Psychology,* 1971, *18,* 97–100.

Kimberlin, G. Personal communication, 1977.

Kreitzer, S. G. College students in a behavior therapy program with hospitalized emotionally disturbed children. In B. G. Guerney (Ed.), *Psychotherapeutic agents: New roles for nonprofessionals, parents, and teachers.* New York: Holt, Rinehart & Winston, 1969.

Linden, J. I., & Stollak, G. E. The training of undergraduates in play techniques. *Journal of Clinical Psychology,* 1969, *25,* 213–278.

Lowell, E. L. Higher education for the deaf. In D. Cutter, (Ed.), *Workshop for Baptists on deafness and rehabilitation.* Washington, D.C.: Vocational Rehabilitation Administration, Department of Health, Education and Welfare, 1965.

McWilliams, S. A., & Finkel, N. J. High school students as mental health aides in the elementary setting. *Journal of Consulting and Clinical Psychology,* 1973, *40,* 39–42.

Meadow, K. P. The development of an inventory for assessment of social and emotional behaviors in deaf children. *Directions* (an official publication of Gallaudet College), 1980, *1*(3): 11.

Meadow, K. P. & Trybus, R. J. Behavioral and emotional problems of deaf children: An overview. In L. J. Bradford & W. G. Hardy (eds.), *Hearing and Hearing Impairment.* New York: Grune & Stratton, 1979.

Mindel, E. D. Studies of the deaf child. In R. R. Grinker (Ed.), *Psychiatric diagnosis, therapy, and research on the psychotic deaf.* Washington, D. C.: Social Rehabilitation Service, Department of Health, Education and Welfare, 1969.

Mindel, E. D. & Vernon, M. *They grow in silence.* Silver Spring, Md.: National Association of the Deaf, 1971.

Mitchell, W. E. Amicatherapy: Theoretical perspectives and an example of practice: *Community Mental Health Journal,* 1966a, *2,* 307–314.

Mitchell, W. E. The use of college students in the outpatient treatment of troubled children.

In H. R. Huessy (Ed.), *Mental health with limited resources: Yankee ingenuity in low-cost programs,* New York: Grune & Stratton, 1966b.

Naiman, D. W. (Ed.). *Inservice training for afterclass staff in residential schools.* New York: Deafness Research and Training Center, New York University School of Education, 1972.

Naiman, D. W. A proposed model for preparation of personnel. In J. D. Schein, (Ed.), *Education and rehabilitation of deaf persons with other disabilities.* New York: Deafness Research and Training Center, New York University of School of Education, 1974.

Neale, D. C., & Mussell, B. Effects of big brother relationships on the school-related attitudes of disadvantaged children. *Journal of Special Education,* 1968, *2,* 397–404.

Newton, M. R., & Brown, R. D. A preventive approach to developmental problems in school children. In E. M. Bower & W. G. Hollister (Eds.), *Behavioral Science Frontiers in Education,* New York: John Wiley, 1967.

Perlmutter, F., & Durham, D. Using teenagers to supplement casework service. *Social Work,* 1965, *10,* 41–48.

Proceedings of the 33rd Biennial Convention of the National Association of the Deaf. *The Deaf American,* 1976, *29,* 37 (Bill 38), 52 (Resolution 36).

Rainer, J. D., & Altshuler, K. Z. *Comprehensive mental health services for the deaf.* New York: New York State Psychiatric Institute, 1966.

Rainer, J. D., & Altshuler, K. Z. *Expanded mental health care for the deaf: Rehabilitation and prevention.* New York: Research Foundation for Mental Hygiene, Rockland State Hospital, and New York State Psychiatric Institute, 1970.

Rainer, J. D. & Altshuler, K. Z. New directions in psychiatry for deaf people. In A. G. Norris (ed.), *Deafness annual* (vol. 3). Silver Spring, Md.: Professional Rehabilitation Workers With the Adult Deaf, 1973.

Rainer, J. D., Altshuler, K. Z., Kallmann, F. J., et al. (Eds.). *Family and mental health problems in a deaf population.* New York: New York State Psychiatric Institute, 1963.

Reinherz, H. College student volunteers as case-aides in a state hospital for children. *American Journal of Orthopsychiatry,* 1963, *33,* 544–546.

Reisman, G., Scanlan, J. M., & Kemp, K. Medical interpreting for hearing impaired patients. *Journal of the American Medical Association,* 1977, *237,* 2397–2398.

Rioch, M. J. Pilot projects in training mental health counselors. In E. L. Cowen, E. A. Gardner, & M. Zax (Eds.), *Emergent approaches to mental health problems.* New York: Appleton-Century-Crofts, 1967.

Rioch, M. J., Elkes, C., Flint, A. A., et al. National Institute of Mental Health pilot study in training of mental health counselors. *American Journal of Orthopsychiatry, 1963, 33,* 678–689.

Robinson, L. D. *Sound minds in a soundless world.* Washington, D. C.: Department of Health, Education and Welfare Publication No. (ADM) 77–560, 1978.

Rolf, J. F., & Harig, P. T. Etiological research in schizophrenic and rationale for primary prevention. *American Journal of Orthopsychiatry,* 1974, *44,* 538–554.

Rothstein, A. The preventive mental health program at the Lexington School for the Deaf. In D. W. Naiman, (Ed.), *Needs of emotionally disturbed hearing impaired children.* New York: Deafness Research and Training Center, New York University School of Education, 1975.

Sachs, B. B. The mental health needs of deaf Americans. *Task panel reports submitted to the president's commission on mental health.* (Vol. 3). Washington, D.C.: U.S. Government Printing Office, 1978.

Sameroff, A. J., & Chandler, M. J. Reproductive risk and the continuum of caretaking casualty. In F. D. Horowitz, M. Heterington, S. Scarr-Salapetek, et al. (Eds.), *Review of child development research* (Vol. 4). Chicago: University of Chicago Press, 1974.

Scheibe, K. E. College students spent eight weeks in mental hospital: A case report. *Psychotherapy: Theory, Research, and Practice* 1966, *2*, 117–120.

Schein, J. D. Deaf students with other disabilities. *American Annals of the Deaf,* 1975, *120*, 92–99.

Schlesinger, H. S., & Meadow, K. P. *Sound and sign: Childhood deafness and mental health.* Berkeley: University of California Press, 1972.

Shah, S. Training and utilizing a mother as the therapist for her child. In B. G. Guerney (Ed.), *Psychotherapeutic agents: New roles for nonprofessionals, parents, and teachers.* New York: Holt, Rinehart & Winston, 1969.

Shapiro, R. J., & Harris, R. I. Family therapy in treatment of the deaf. A case report. *Family Process,* 1976, *15*, 83–96.

Stover, L., & Guerney, B. G., Jr. The efficacy of training procedures for mothers in filial therapy. *Psychotherapy: Theory, Research, and Practice,* 1967, *4*, 110–115.

Tully, N. L., & Vernon, M. The impact of automation on the deaf worker. *American Federalist,* 1965, *72*, 20–23.

Umbarger, C. C., Dalsimer, J. S., Morrison, A. P., et al. *College students in mental hospitals.* New York: Grune & Stratton, 1962.

Vernon, M. The final report. In R. R. Grinker, (Ed.), *Psychiatric diagnosis, therapy, and research on the psychotic deaf.* Washington, D.C.: Social Rehabilitation Service, Department of Health, Education and Welfare, 1969.

Vernon, M., & Estes, C. C. Deaf leadership and political activism. *The Deaf American,* 1975, *28*, 3–6.

Vernon, M., Makowsky, B. Deafness and minority group dynamics. *Deaf American,* 1969, *21*, 3–6.

Walker, C. E., Wolpin, M., & Fellows, L. The use of high school students as therapists and researchers in a state mental hospital. *Psychotherapy: Theory, research, and practice,* 1967, *4*, 186–188.

Wolf, E. M. The deaf health care consumer in a hearing health care system. *Proceedings of the VIIth World Congress of the World Federation of the Deaf.* Silver Spring, Md.: National Association of the Deaf, 1976.

Young, E. C., & True, J. E. *The current status of the associate degree movement in mental health and the human services.* Paper presented at the 81th Annual Convention of the American Psychological Association, Montreal, Canada, 1973.

Zax, M., & Cowen, E. L. Early identification and prevention of emotional disturbance in a public school. In E. L. Cowen, E. A. Gardner, & M. Zax (Eds.), *Emergent approaches to mental health problems.* New York: Appleton-Century-Crofts, 1967.

Zax, M., & Cowen, E. L. *Abnormal psychology: Changing conceptions.* New York: Holt, Rinehart & Winston, 1972.

Zax, M., Cowen, E. L., Izzo, L. D., et al. A teacher-aide program for preventing emotional disturbance in primary grade school children. *Mental Hygiene,* 1966, *50*, 406–414.

Zax, M., Cowen, E. L., Rappaport, J. et al. Follow-up study of children identified early as emotionally disturbed. *Journal of Consulting and Clinical Psychology,* 1968, *32*, 369–374.

Zunker, V. G., & Brown, W. F. Comparative effectiveness of student and professional counselors. *Personnel Guidance Journal,* 1966, *44*, 738–743.

Index